Praise for *The Best Medicine*

"An ambitious, elegant meditation. . . . [Perri Klass] takes the most complex human patterns of all—history, medicine, politics, art—and knits them into something unique and beautiful."
—Christie Watson, *New York Times Book Review*

"Not too long ago, parents lived with the near certainty of losing a child or two; Perri Klass captures the drama of science and society's triumph over that abysmal reality. As we grapple with new and unimaginable scourges, the lessons in this gripping, personal, and beautifully researched chronicle could not be more relevant."
—Abraham Verghese, MD, author of *Cutting for Stone*

"With her broad pediatric knowledge and warm understanding of parental attachments, Perri Klass tells the dramatic story of how medical science transformed childhood in the twentieth century. . . . An important contribution to the history of childhood that can provide comfort and insight to all of us."
—Paula S. Fass, author of *The End of American Childhood*

"In today's world of pandemics and medical alarm, it is especially comforting to look to history for the paths that lay ahead. And there is no better place to begin than [*The Best Medicine*] by Perri Klass, the physician/writer known to millions of parents for her probing insights into the world of pediatric medicine. Starting at a time when Americans helplessly accepted the death of their children as a cruel fact of nature, Klass beautifully demonstrates how the fusion of medical science and public health led to the vaccines, antibiotics, safety measures, and self-help volumes that saved countless young lives while revolutionizing the ways in which we map our children's future. Elegantly written, filled with memorable characters and events, [*The Best Medicine*] is the perfect prescription for the uncertainties of our time."

—David Oshinsky, Pulitzer Prize–winning author of
Polio: An American Story

"In [*The Best Medicine*], the pediatrician Perri Klass describes how the world—and with it, parenting—has been transformed by declining infant and child mortality over the past century."

—Kate Julian, *Atlantic*

"A powerful story of the right of children to live and thrive from birth."
—*Kirkus Reviews*

"The result of Klass's erudition and nuance is a fascinating look at a seldom-sung but profound change in the human condition."

—*Publishers Weekly*

"Klass masterfully introduces readers to the people coming up with solutions for many of the dangers of childhood and shows how the pediatric specialty over time has worked to improve children's lives. Essential reading for parents."
—*Library Journal*

——

The
Best
Medicine

——//——

ALSO BY PERRI KLASS

Nonfiction

Treatment Kind and Fair: Letters to a Young Doctor

Baby Doctor: A Pediatrician's Training

A Not Entirely Benign Procedure: Four Years as a Medical Student

Quirky Kids: Understanding and Supporting Your Child With Developmental Differences, with Eileen Costello, MD

Every Mother Is a Daughter: The Never-Ending Quest for Success, Inner Peace, and a Really Clean Kitchen, with Sheila Solomon Klass

Two Sweaters for My Father: Writing About Knitting

The Real Life of a Pediatrician (editor)

Fiction

The Mercy Rule

The Mystery of Breathing

Love and Modern Medicine: Stories

Other Women's Children

I Am Having an Adventure: Stories

Recombinations

The
Best
Medicine

How Science and Public Health
Gave Children a Future

—————————— // ——————————

PERRI KLASS

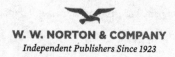

W. W. NORTON & COMPANY
Independent Publishers Since 1923

For information about permission to reproduce selections from this book,
write to Permissions, W. W. Norton & Company, Inc., 500 Fifth Avenue,
New York, NY 10110

For information about special discounts for bulk purchases, please contact
W. W. Norton Special Sales at specialsales@wwnorton.com or 800-233-4830

Manufacturing by LSC Communications, Harrisonburg
Book design by Lisa Buckley Design
Production manager: Beth Steidle

The Library of Congress has catalogued the hardcover edition of this book
as follows:

Names: Klass, Perri, 1958– author.
Title: A good time to be born : how science and public health gave children a
     future / Perri Klass.
Description: First edition. | New York, N.Y. : W. W. Norton & Company, [2020] |
     Includes bibliographical references and index.
Identifiers: LCCN 2020022472 | ISBN 9780393609998 (hardcover) |
     ISBN 9780393610000 (epub)
Subjects: MESH: Child Mortality—history | Infant Mortality—history |
     Child Health—history | Biomedical Research | Preventive Health Services—
     trends | United States
Classification: LCC HB1323.I4 | NLM WA 11 AA1 | DDC 304.6/4—dc23
LC record available at https://lccn.loc.gov/2020022472

ISBN 978-0-393-88238-4 pbk.

W. W. Norton & Company, Inc., 500 Fifth Avenue, New York, N.Y. 10110
www.wwnorton.com

W. W. Norton & Company Ltd., 15 Carlisle Street, London W1D 3BS

1 2 3 4 5 6 7 8 9 0

For Eileen Costello—
pediatric colleague and friend since our training days,
who understands how it all comes back to clinical medicine
and taking care of children—
and is always ready to hear or tell an interesting patient story

---

For the first time in my life I was really up against facts. No student, whether in law or medicine, is living a real life. . . . Here, in Boston, submerged in the hectic life of a big clinic, I was abruptly forced to translate what I had studied into actuality, to realize that the luridly colored pictures in ponderous medical texts meant actual fever and pain and delirium and mutilation, and that those crisp summaries of what to do about this or that physical ailment, which had sounded so reassuring on the printed page, were of distressingly little help to an inexperienced beginner.

—S. JOSEPHINE BAKER, *FIGHTING FOR LIFE*

Contents

The Waning of Child Mortality and the New Expectations of Parenthood

Our grandparents and great-grandparents and all the parents before, throughout history, expected that children would die. It was a known and predictable risk that went along with being a parent. Now we expect children *not* to die. We are the luckiest parents in history, we who are part of this wave, over the past seventy-five years or so, because we are the first parents ever who have been able to enter into parenthood in the hopeful expectation of seeing all our children survive and thrive. And we are also the luckiest children in history, born into an era when we could expect to grow up, along with all our sisters and brothers. Driving down child mortality in the late nineteenth and early twentieth centuries was in no way a single project, but it can be seen as a unified human accomplishment—maybe even our greatest human accomplishment, at least for pediatricians and parents. The entire world has relearned, with some shock and great sorrow, how vulnerable our precious human bodies are to the microorganisms that find ways to take advantage of how we live, what we eat, how we travel. Parents have taken some comfort in knowing that, for the most part, children have been less severely affected by Covid-19, but all through human history, babies and children have been a particularly vulnerable group, and parents have lived with the fear of contagion, infection, and death.

Children used to die, regularly and unsurprisingly. Babies died at birth or soon after, because they were premature or just "weak," because they were born with congenital anomalies, because they got infections. Older infants and one-year-olds died of summer diarrhea, often caused by microbes in the water or in the cow's milk they had started drinking after they had been weaned. Three-year-olds and four-year-olds (and five- and six- and seven- and eight-year-olds) died of scarlet fever and diphtheria and pneumonia and measles, of skin infections that turned into sepsis or influenza that turned into pneumonia. As recently as the late nineteenth and early twentieth centuries, almost every family in every ethnic group and every country, rich or poor, was touched in some way by the death of children. Childhood death was always there, in the shadows at the edge of the family landscape, in prayers and religious ceremonies, in the memorial portraits hanging on the wall, in popular sentimental poems and stories and dramas and paintings. Because they figured so consistently in childhood and family life, child deaths also figured in the art and literature and songs and stories of childhood and family life from a century ago, as they had all through human history.

"I am a lover of babies and yet I can't seems to have them," wrote Mrs. W.D. from Brooklyn in 1917. "I am married 11 yrs last July and would have six children and am about to become a mother again which I almost fear. I have now but 2 out of six, one boy 9 yrs and one 6 yrs." Two of them had apparently died some years ago—she didn't say how—but then within a year, she had two babies and ended up losing both of them: "I gave birth to a beautiful fat boy and it lived but 3 days." The doctor told her the baby had a "leaking heart." Three months later she was pregnant again; this son lived to be a year old, and then she awoke one morning "and found him dead along side of me." Now pregnant again, she worried constantly both about the "terrible long labor" she was likely to endure and about what would become of the baby: "I try and live a good honest life and my home is my heaven and babies are my idols. I love them but I am afraid something will happen to this one again."[1]

She was writing this letter to the United States government, to the Children's Bureau, established in 1912. This new federal office had published the pamphlets *Prenatal Care* (1913) and *Infant Care* (1914), which were immediately and enduringly popular; they were at first distributed free of charge and provided by politicians to their constituents, and were later available for purchase. By 1929, the government had estimated that these writings had touched the parents of half the babies born in the United States.[2] Mothers responded eagerly, sending more than 125,000 letters a year to the bureau, with their questions and their stories, including accounts of deaths. "You can think how I feel," Mrs. W.D. wrote to the author of the pamphlets. "I cry night and day for my big fat baby, [taken] from me like that."

Mrs. W.D. was not living in the Middle Ages, or even in the Victorian era. She was living in 1917, when my grandmother lived (and in New York City, where my grandmother lived), ten years before my own parents were born. In fact, Molly Ladd-Taylor, the historian who compiled the collection of mothers' letters to the Children's Bureau, was inspired by finding her own grandmother's letter in the files. Some of the letters came from women in rural areas, beyond easy reach of medical expertise during childbirth, but others, like Mrs. W.D., lived in big cities, where they were receiving full medical attention, and their letters are notable for a mix of tragic acceptance and hope for better answers, as they searched for government advice or medical wisdom that might change the story, going forward. And at that time, in 1917, when Mrs. W.D. wrote her letter, nearly a quarter of the children born alive in the United States died before their fifth birthdays.

"Just two years ago, after five years of married life, we became the proud parents of our first baby, a boy," wrote another mother, in 1918. "Four months later we buried our baby and it was then that I knew how helpless I was when it came to knowing what a mother should know. My baby was sacrificed thru mere ignorance. This happened in the capitol of Illinois and money or efforts were not spared to save him." She had been unable to nurse her son, she explained, and "he just faded away . . ."[3] Mothers told of deaths related to common everyday issues like nursing, weaning, and even constipation: "Our baby had not had an unaided movement of the bowels for more than a year when he died this June, at the age of two and a half years, [too] worn out to cut his last two baby teeth," wrote Mrs. F.W. from Michigan, also in 1918.[4]

They wrote, in those early decades of the twentieth century, with a certain hope for medical solutions, for advice that might protect the next baby, and even with a desire to extend that protection to all babies and children, to join in the larger project the Children's Bureau and its pamphlets represented. "I only wish I could take up the work of promoting baby welfare," wrote the woman who had lost her child in Illinois. Another mother, almost ten years later, in 1926, explaining that her daughter had died at twenty months of age, after an operation to correct injuries suffered at birth, pleaded, "So please try & help others through your department all you can & keep them from making the horrible mistake we made, & [from] the loss of the one whose place can never be filled."[5] And notably, the employees at the Children's Bureau, including Mary Mills West, the author of the *Infant Care* pamphlet, answered the letters individually and at some length. They attempted to provide specific information on topics from postnatal depression to breastfeeding and formula preparation; they sympathized with the grief of women who told of having lost children, and reassured them that they were not at fault. The mother whose child had died from birth injuries received an answer saying, "We are indeed sorry to hear of your great grief and sympathize with you most deeply," assuring her that "no matter what is done, whether a Caesarean section or an instrumental labor, there are always a certain number of babies who die from birth injuries."[6]

Some of the letters were from women who struggled with written language and spelling, others from the educated and the privileged. There was no segment of society in which children's lives were secure, nor had there ever been. Though the statistical evidence is incomplete, infant and child mortality in both Europe and America was extremely high through the seventeenth and early eighteenth centuries, with a third of all children—or in some cases even 40 percent or more—dying before they outgrew childhood. Child mortality rates—like adult mortality rates—fluctuated with food shortages and with epidemics. Mortality was often higher in cities, where crowded conditions made it easier for diseases to spread, but rural life could be deadly as well; in colonial New England in the early seventeenth century, one estimate has 60 out of every 100 children dying before the age of sixteen. "For the first three centuries of American history, infant death was the central reality of maternal experience," wrote historians Nancy Schrom Dye and Daniel Blake Smith, who examined the diaries and letters of American women from 1750 to 1920.[7]

"Infant mortality" means death before the first birthday, and "child mortality" usually means death before the fifth birthday (death from five to fourteen is a separate category). In the first decade of the twentieth century, when my grandmother was growing up, out of every 1,000 live births in the United States, more than 100 babies did not live to their first birthdays—and mortality rates were even higher among the rural poor, immigrants, and African Americans. By comparison, the infant mortality rate for the United States in 2017 was 5.8 deaths per 1,000 live births. The majority of these deaths before the first birthday actually occur in the first months of life, and most are due either to congenital anomalies—serious birth defects—or to prematurity. Now we are trying to get the infant mortality numbers down from 5.8 out of every 1,000 live births to between 2 and 3 out of every 1,000 live births, the best numbers achieved in some developed countries, such as Singapore, Finland, Japan, and Iceland (2 deaths per 1,000 live births in 2017). Compiling these statistics was a relatively new idea in the late nineteenth century, but infant mortality rates are now used as an indicator of the general health and the social welfare systems of a country, probably the most prominent public health score card we have.

The Best Medicine tells the story of one of our greatest human achievements, a remarkable fusion of science and public health and medicine that transformed our families, our emotional landscapes, and even our souls. All through human history, many babies died at birth, and many children died in infancy and childhood. This was true through the Middle Ages and the Renaissance, true in colonial America and in Victorian England, and it was still true in the early twentieth century. If you went around any table, pretty much everyone would have lost a sibling in childhood, lost a friend to death at a young age, lost a child. Infant and child mortality was a fact of life for almost every family, rich or poor (John D. Rockefeller, the richest man in the world, founded the Rockefeller Institute when his grandson died of scarlet fever), though mortality was higher among nineteenth-century disadvantaged populations, including enslaved children and the urban immigrant poor.

Poverty, privilege, and race affected—and continue to affect—childhood mortality in many ways. Richer children were in better shape nutritionally to begin with, and they were more likely to have access to better water and milk. Wealthy children—and white children—were more likely to get medical attention if they did get sick, but before antibiotics were available to fight infections, before effective rehydration techniques to counteract the deadly dehydration of diarrhea, there was only a limited amount that "medical attention"—however expert and expensive—could do. The children of physicians in the United States at the turn of the century had only marginally lower mortality rates than those of the population as a whole.[8] Throughout the eighteenth and nineteenth centuries and on into the twentieth, no wealthy family was untouched by childhood death. Tycoons and presidents called in the best doctors in the country, and their children still died. The nation is full of institutions founded by parents bereft of descendants to whom they could leave their fortunes, parents whose great wealth had not saved their sick children. Wellesley College was established in 1875 on five hundred acres outside Boston bought by Henry Fowle Durant, "originally intended as a country estate where Durant and his wife, Pauline, planned to build a pleasure palace for their gifted young son."[9] But the boy died of diphtheria at the age of eight, and so his pleasure palace became a college for women. Stanford University was founded by Leland and Jane Stanford in memory of their only child, Leland Jr., who died at fifteen of typhoid fever—in Florence, in 1884, on a luxurious Grand Tour.

By the time I was training in pediatrics, in the 1980s, there was no such thing as "routine" or "unavoidable" infant and child mortality; short of very rare and terrible diseases, almost every death was supposed to be preventable—and prevented. The vaccines of the 1950s and 1960s (polio, measles) were augmented with new vaccines to prevent diseases that were deadly but much rarer (such as the life-threatening infections caused by *Haemophilus influenzae* type b), and advances in neonatology had made it possible to save sick newborns who didn't breathe promptly in the delivery room and to keep tiny premature infants alive. We would go through our medical training without ever seeing a case of diphtheria or polio—those battles had been won. Instead, we would set our sights on eliminating SIDS, on making sure infants were properly strapped into car seats. Pediatric oncology offered a 90 percent cure rate even on the scariest ward; pediatric cardiology could save all but the most severe congenital heart defects. There were still battles to be won, but we had begun to see a world our grandmothers could not even have imagined, in which there was an implicit promise that if parents took the right precautions, every child could be expected to live to grow up. It was our obligation as pediatricians to help make the world even safer. Childhood deaths represented precautions not properly taken, treatments not properly applied, medical problems needing to be solved as quickly as possible.

This change in outlook represented a great tectonic shift in parenting, doctoring, and family life. Childhood death had always been part of the substance of loving children and living with children. The certainty that not all children would survive meant an imperative toward larger families and more frequent pregnancies for women, when childbirth carried risks of its own. We look back across a divide at a lost historical world in which great poets wrote of the sorrow of losing children—Longfellow, Emerson—and bad poets wrote sentimental "obituary verses" to order, to comfort grieving parents. Graveyards were full of tiny markers. Novelists from Charles Dickens to Mark Twain to Harriet Beecher Stowe used childhood deaths to wring their readers' hearts, and to make political and social arguments. But they also wrote those scenes because they had lived those scenes; they all lost children because almost everyone lost children. As Charles Dickens wrote to his wife, when their baby daughter died, "We never can expect to be exempt, as to our many children, from the afflictions of other parents."[10]

It was no single project that took us from a time when no parent could "expect to be exempt" to a time when all parents expect all children to grow up, when childhood death appears as the terrible exception. The 2003 Institute of Medicine manual *When Children Die* begins with the statement "Although dying is a part of life, a child's death, in a very real sense, is unnatural."[11] Childhood deaths seem unnatural today because they are rare and shocking events that we believe should be completely preventable. The manual goes on to say that "the death of a child is a special sorrow, a lifelong loss for surviving mothers, fathers, brothers, sisters, grandparents, and other family members."[12]

The conquest of infant and child mortality was a collective endeavor, pulling together public health and basic science: cities tackled sanitation and clean water, and bacteriology and virology

teased out the underlying mechanisms of the infections that killed
children. There was progress in nutrition and in pharmacology,
in medical care and technology. There were Nobel Prize–winning
feats of laboratory ingenuity. There were public health programs in
urban tenements, with visiting nurses going door to door. There were
"milk stations" to distribute clean milk to poor families, campaigns
to encourage breastfeeding, and coordinated efforts to educate mothers about how to keep their babies safe. And, of course, there were
parents, sometimes grieving parents, looking for answers, requesting
help, and demanding change.

Now, in response to the Covid-19 pandemic, we have witnessed
another collective scientific, medical, and social endeavor, moving
at a faster speed and using new and innovative ways of connecting,
from scientific researchers and doctors conducting accelerated clinical trials to frontline practitioners communicating on social media
hard-won advice gleaned from caring for patients sick with a new
disease. The times we have all been living through should help us
appreciate the last century's collective endeavor on behalf of children, as we think with new appreciation about the value of epidemiology, as we look with profound hope and gratitude to the scientific
and intellectual innovations of microbiology and pharmacology and
engineering, as we offer profound appreciation to frontline nurses,
physicians, and everyone else who assumes personal risk in caring
for the sick in a time of pandemic.

These were the disciplines that contributed to the work of reducing infant and child mortality, working and communicating more
slowly in the era before the Internet, but linked around the world
by the enterprise of keeping children alive. These were the people
who counted the number of babies born, recorded sickness and
death, figured out what caused mysterious symptoms, pushed for
practical hygienic measures in the home and education for parents,
and researched therapies to cure diseases and vaccines to prevent
them. Over time, these scientists, public health workers, doctors and

nurses, epidemiologists, and advocates collectively created a world in which parents could expect that their children would live to grow up.

The Best Medicine tells the story of this heroic collective endeavor, this combination of scientific discovery and public health mobilization that has made the world so much safer for our children. As a pediatrician, I feel a special sense of identification with some of the heroic early women doctors—Rebecca Crumpler, Mary Putnam Jacobi, Alice Hamilton, Josephine Baker—who brought new perspectives and energy to the project of taking care of women and children, and with the front-line public health nurses who carried the message that, even in the cruel summer in New York City tenements, mothers could take precautions and effectively protect their infants. The deadly "summer diarrhea" did not have to be accepted as inevitable, but could be prevented by breastfeeding and good hygiene; as Josephine Baker put it, "heat did not necessarily kill babies."

In previous centuries, no matter how rich and powerful parents were, no matter how many important doctors they could summon, they had a very limited ability to protect the children they loved. Today's routine immunizations mean that a sore throat cannot represent diphtheria (that's what killed Baby Ruth Cleveland, the twelve-year-old daughter of former president Grover Cleveland, in 1904). When today's children do get infections, they can be treated with antibiotics (there were no antibiotics to treat sixteen-year-old Calvin Coolidge Jr. in 1924 when he developed a blister on his toe after playing tennis on the White House lawn without wearing socks, and he died of a blood infection). There's a medical understanding now that makes it routine to provide lots of fluid to children with diarrhea, so that they don't die of dehydration (as perhaps did eleven-year-old Willie Lincoln after contracting typhoid from contaminated water in the White House). And we regularly mark our progress in neonatology by invoking a much more recent White House pediatric death: that of Patrick Bouvier Kennedy, the only child born in the twentieth century to a sitting president, who was born five and a half weeks premature in 1963 and died at the age of thirty-nine hours of premature lung disease, at Boston Children's Hospital, because there was no way to ventilate a premature infant.

The Best Medicine brings together this complex history, the stories of diseases that once terrified parents and terrorized families, the stories of parents, rich and poor, who did everything they could to keep their children alive, the stories of artists and writers who left records of children they had loved and lost. The book traces the discoveries of bacteriology and virology that elucidated the most terrifying diseases, and the scientific advances that made it possible to fight back, in powerful ways that had never before been remotely within reach. The perspectives of medical humanities, art, literature, and letters from the late nineteenth and early twentieth centuries are brought together with science and clinical medicine, to give a sense of how the reality of childhood mortality colored the world; how it figured in the lives of parents, doctors, politicians, artists, scientists, and activists; how parents at every level of every society grappled with the tragedy of losing children; and what it meant that this tragedy was both commonplace and inevitable. Even when these deaths were common, parents mourned and grieved with the same strong mix of emotions we feel today, and through history, many adult lives were shaped forever by that grief.

Parents today know, of course, that there are no guarantees, and we have all been most dramatically reminded of the power and reach of infectious disease by the 2019 coronavirus—as we were four decades ago by HIV, and by other infections such as Ebola, SARS, and H1N1. Still, we also know that the standard childhood infections, the ones everyone gets (or used to get), as well as the rarer but potentially deadly ones, can be either prevented or treated. Experts tell us how to keep our babies safe from day one: rear-facing baby car seats starting with the ride home from the hospital, sleeping position on the back to avoid SIDS, smoke detectors, carbon monoxide detectors, window guards to keep a small child from falling out. There are laws to regulate the sale of window blind cords so that children don't strangle, and to dictate how caps fit on medicine bottles so children don't poison themselves. These policy victories make it all the more striking that we have not succeeded in regulating guns or in applying technologies that might make them less accessible or less dangerous to the young, since guns remain a tragically significant cause of death in children, through accidents, suicides, and homicides. Racial disparities in maternal and infant mortality persist in the United States, with Black infants more than twice as likely to die in the first year of life than babies of other races (11.9 out of 1,000 live births versus 4.9) and Black mothers at least three times as likely to die from problems related to pregnancy. This disparity is not about poverty or education; highly educated Black women are more likely to lose their babies than are white women who didn't make it through eighth grade. These disparities are now being discussed in terms of the stresses of racism on women's bodies and women's lives and the effects of differential treatment by the health care system—as opposed to differential access, which is usually tied to poverty.[13] Studies show us over and over that minority children, like minority women, do not receive the same care that white children receive, and that racism continues to blight the health and growth of children in many different ways.[14] And, as always, infant mortality is also higher among the poor.

As a pediatrician, I have been aware all through my training and my clinical practice that I am living in a world where childhood death is rare, and I have wondered how my historical colleagues coped with the realities of taking care of so many children they could not save. Most of all, though, I have wondered, as a parent and as a pediatrician who often works with anxious parents, how mothers and fathers coped with the necessities of child-rearing in times of high infant and child mortality. How did parents—and doctors—handle the routine complaints that come into my exam room, and into every pediatric clinic and emergency room every day, the episodes of fever, diarrhea, rash, and stomach pain, when any one of those could have signaled the onset of something serious, untreatable, even fatal? For this reason, I focus in this book on the illnesses that worried all parents, including healthy parents of healthy children: the dangers of childbirth, the infections that carried off infants, the potentially deadly diseases that could strike down thriving children. Many other stories of progress and even triumph inform twentieth-century pediatrics, from the ability to repair congenital heart defects to the victories of pediatric oncology, to the advances in treating genetic conditions like cystic fibrosis and sickle-cell disease, and these, too, are part of creating a world where most children live to adulthood.

With the public health and sanitation and nutritional and medical victories that drove infant and child mortality down came a certain promise to parents: if everything is done right, it is possible to keep children safe. Buy the right car seat and use it according to instructions, feed the right healthy food, give the recommended immunizations on schedule; do all this and, barring rare and tragic events, your child will live to grow up—*should* live to grow up. The Institute of Medicine called it "unnatural" for a child to die because a child dying has come to seem like an outrage, a desperately unfair turn of events, and even, often, a tragedy that could have been averted if only the world had been made a little bit safer.[15]

This great good luck has brought with it a sense of responsibility that can leave parents feeling tremendously uneasy. It would not have occurred to my grandmother that it was up to her to keep her children absolutely safe, because she knew that this could not be done. She could no more have prevented accidents on the street than she could have kept the annual polio epidemics from sweeping through the city. The world, she knew, was dangerous for children, and not all of them made it to adulthood. But parents today have been promised safety, provided they make all the right decisions, buckling the newborn into a car seat for that first ride home from the hospital, putting the baby down in the proper safe sleeping position, and then moving on, as the child grows, to seat belts and bike helmets. All that advice is good and true and valid—I'm a pediatrician, and I reinforce it with my patients. Yet when a tragedy does take place, those unlucky parents can suffer a double burden of guilt and isolation, in a world where childhood death has become "unnatural." And all of us—the luckiest parents in history—may feel weighed down at least a little by the sense that so much is riding on our decisions, small and large.

We can look at parents from times past and feel that it must have been very difficult to relax and love your children in a world that was so full of dangers. Yet the possibility of watching our children grow up in a state of safety that my grandmother's generation could not have imagined carries its own anxieties and imperatives. And even while we worry over any remaining dangers, even as we keep a wary eye out for new problems and uncertainties, we should glory in the human endeavor that has brought us this far, and commit ourselves to extending the blessings of that safety more effectively and more equably to parents and children everywhere.

PART I

"The Desolation
of That
Empty Cradle"

CHAPTER 1

Postmortem Poetry and Comfort Books

Literary Echoes of Child Mortality

I n 1848, when Henry Wadsworth Longfellow's daughter Fanny died, he wrote a poem called "Resignation," acknowledging the universality of the loss:

> There is no flock, however watched and tended,
>> But one dead lamb is there!
> There is no fireside, howsoe'er defended,
>> But has one vacant chair![1]

In the nineteenth century, as in every century before it, childhood death was a part of the geography of the home and the geography of the heart. It is a lost world, a world that modern-day parents cannot imagine—one that we can evoke now only with the words and voices of the parents of that bygone era whose children could not be saved ("however watched and tended"). Recalling that era through the works of literature and art created to honor the many, many lost children by the grieving parents who mourned and remembered them individually helps us appreciate the glory of what we have accomplished in keeping children safe so that they live to grow up. The infant and child mortality numbers remind us how few are lost now, as compared to earlier eras, and offer us a sense of the scale of that accomplishment, but they cannot convey the emotional and mental triumph and joy of the modern era as vividly as the voices of the parents of the past can, or affect us as deeply as Longfellow's mourning for his daughter. He faced the loss with resignation, though in the second half of the nineteenth century, the idea of resignation itself began to change, as social reformers and scientists challenged the inevitability of the "vacant chair" that Longfellow took for granted would be found at every single fireside.

From the end of the nineteenth and the beginning of the twentieth centuries, many European countries, including England, France, Germany, and the Scandinavian nations, began calculating infant mortality in the way we do everywhere today: counting live births and determining a rate by tracking how many died out of every 1,000 of those live births. And they were counting those deaths and calculating those rates because, for the first time in human history, the death of the young was being treated not as a biological inevitability or a religious test of human faith but as an index of a society's welfare, its health and hygiene, and also its social progress.

In 1906, George Newman, a British physician who specialized in public health, published a historic work: *Infant Mortality: A Social Problem.* Newman was also the medical officer of a particular London borough, Finsbury, where for five years past, he had tracked both the health and the illnesses of the inhabitants. He began *Infant Mortality* by celebrating progress: the declining death rates for the general population, including adults and children, achieved over the previous half century, which he attributed to improvements in sanitation, medicine, and the general "standard of comfort of the people." But the death rate among babies, he said, was not declining, and he cited infant mortality rates from all over Europe, all between 100 and 300 babies dead before the first birthday out of every 1,000 live births. "Last year (1905) there was a loss to the nation," he wrote, "of 120,000 dead infants in England and Wales alone. . . . That is to say, that *one quarter* of the total deaths every year is of children under the age of twelve months"—"a vast army of small human beings that lived but a handful of days."[2] He was writing at a moment of great sentimental feeling, both about children and about the state of childhood: J. M. Barrie's play *Peter Pan*, with its "lost boys" and its children who never grow up, had been a tremendous success in 1904, two years before Newman's book, and was issued as a novel in 1911.

Newman was sounding the alarm about babies in part because older children were doing better; he was able to point to a declining mortality rate for those between one and five, which had, he said, dropped 14 to 16 percent in fifty years, and he celebrated even larger improvements in deaths among older children, which had fallen more than 50 percent. The improvements in public health and hygiene and in medical prevention and therapeutics over the second half of the nineteenth century had made a difference for children, as for adults. Still, despite all that progress, infants under the age of one continued to die at these disconcerting rates. In the preface to his book, on the very first page, he acknowledged that this "social problem" could never completely be solved because it reflected a profound biological vulnerability: "The young of all animals are more susceptible than the adult to the influence of environment and the approach of death. Hence, it is inevitable that, even under the most favourable circumstances, the deaths of infants will furnish a large contribution to the bills of mortality."[3] Positing as low, or even "ideal," an "infantile mortality rate" of perhaps 70 to 80 deaths for every 1,000 live births, he put forward the idea that this rate, and how close it came to that ideal, was an index to the health and the level of civilization of a given community—or nation.

Newman's book was a call to arms, and in it, he addressed issues from the exigencies of factory work, which separated poor women from their babies too early and prevented them from breastfeeding, to toxins in the environment, to the diarrhea epidemics that struck every summer

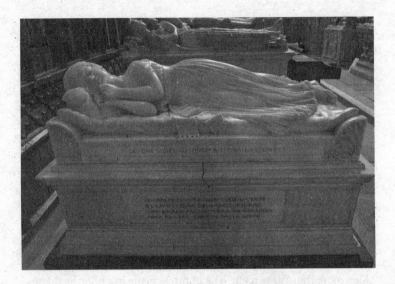

Parents memorialized their lost children according to their means and their artistic tastes. Penelope Boothby, the only child of a British baronet, died at the age of five in 1791. Her grieving father commissioned this monument, carved of Carrara marble by Thomas Banks, showing her lying on her side, head on a pillow, eyes closed, apparently asleep. *Alamy Images.*

and carried off many children under the age of two. He was also clear about the risk factor of poverty: "It is a well-known fact that communities in which there is a large measure of poverty have a higher mortality from all causes at all ages than communities better circumstanced."[4]

It's not hard to imagine reaching even across a century or so, to Newman's time or before, and identifying with a mother putting a baby to her breast or a father watching a toddler take a first few uncertain steps. But how was everyday life affected by the uncertainty that touched every family, sooner or later, and must have hovered somewhere in every parental consciousness? Biographers of eighteenth- and nineteenth- and even early-twentieth-century lives tend to compress the loss of a child into a paragraph or two and then it's over and done, while in more contemporary accounts of losing a child, such a death often becomes the central explanatory tragedy in

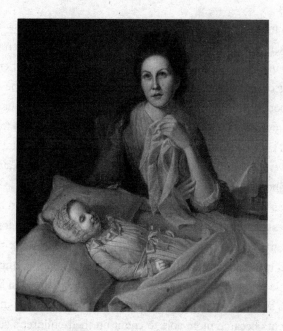

Margaret Peale, the daughter of the Philadelphia painter Charles Willson Peale, died in 1772 of smallpox. Her father originally painted this portrait of her, then later added in the image of his wife, Rachel. (The title, *Rachel Weeping*, evokes the biblical depiction of "Rachel weeping for her children" in Jeremiah 31.) Peale is said to have concealed the painting behind a curtain, with a warning: "Before you draw this curtain Consider whether you will afflict a Mother or Father who has lost a Child." *Philadelphia Museum of Art, Gift of the Barra Foundation, Inc., 1977-34-1.*

an adult's life. Newman was saying something relatively new when he suggested that many infant deaths could be prevented; the parents of the nineteenth century, rich and poor, had lived with the knowledge that nothing could reliably prevent infant death or reliably treat childhood illness, though, of course, religious belief and salvation offered a different kind of promise. Childhood death was always part of the landscape of family life, as perinatal death, for both infant and mother, was part of the landscape of birth.

In 1960, the historian Philippe Ariès put forward the idea that childhood had been in some sense "discovered" during the Renaissance. Earlier, during the Middle Ages, Ariès argued, children were dressed in miniature adult clothing and seen as small adults—that is, as workers who contributed to a family's economy. Children moved quickly into something very like adult life, rather than experiencing a prolonged period of education and further development. The state of childhood was not recognized as particularly distinct, although there was an awareness that children's hold on life was somewhat tenuous. Around the time of the Renaissance, the substance of parental feeling underwent a change as well, according to Ariès, with new attention to childhood as a distinct phase of life. And this newly "discovered" state was of interest to philosophers, who became intrigued by children's essential nature, children's brains, children's development, and to artists, who began to paint children's bodies more realistically, to represent their personalities more vividly. Declining infant and child mortality in the eighteenth century culminated in Edward Jenner's successful experiments with smallpox vaccination in 1796.[5] As parents became more able to count on their children's survival, Ariès argued, they allowed themselves to feel more interest and more affection. This thesis has provoked great debate over the past several decades, with extensive arguments among historians about how children and the state of childhood were viewed during the Middle Ages and the Renaissance in Europe, and with much debate about the connections between life expectancy and parental affection, as well as the larger understanding of the nature of childhood.[6]

During the nineteenth century, as the developed world built sewers, practiced better hygiene and better infant nutrition, and increasingly often vaccinated against smallpox, childhood mortality declined further. However, parents, rich and poor, continued to lose children. Perhaps influenced by Romantic sentiment, perhaps by somewhat improved survival odds, the combination of parental affection and regular parental loss gave rise to the Victorian era's flowering of intensely sentimental renditions of children so angelic that they were—inevitably—summoned up to heaven, dying in beautiful innocence, leaving behind a world that didn't deserve them.[7]

The Victorians were pious, and many of these death scenes were deeply religious, but childhood deaths were no longer seen to be sent directly from an all-powerful God, as they might once have been. Instead, they might reflect social evils and the cruelties of poverty and a callous world, or drive home the opposite social moral that even the wealthy and the powerful could not keep their children safe. In the work of Charles Dickens, a child might die in brutal poverty, reminding the reader that children lived in terrible and even murderous circumstances, or a child might die surrounded by useless wealth and helpless doctors. Either way, their deaths were meant to wring readers' hearts, and Dickens very much felt for his characters as he created them, while at the same time, he had a calculating eye for the marketability of child pathos. Dickens knew the ins and outs of childhood illnesses and parental worries; he and his wife had ten children of their own, some named after characters in his books. Of the ten, one died in infancy and one at the age of twenty-one (and a third at twenty-five), and there are persistent rumors that there was also a baby who died—and who was deliberately erased from history—born to Dickens and his mistress, the actress Ellen Ternan.

Children's deaths are central to every kind of writing before—and well into—the twentieth century: the private diaries and letters and personal narratives left by parents, the sermons and Puritan narratives written to frighten children into good behavior, the great novels of the Victorian era, and the worst, most sentimental potboilers. Bereavement poetry, often written by amateurs, commemorated individual lost children by name. The writers often had personal experience with childhood death—their own children, their siblings—and they could count on a readership full of people with such experience. Children's deathbeds and dying words, and their pieties and their miseries, recurred frequently both in factual accounts and in fiction, from the excruciatingly sentimental to the brilliantly and passionately original.

In 1630, during the reign of King Charles I (and fourteen years after the death of Shakespeare), a little book titled *A Handkercher for Parents Wet Eyes, Vpon the Death of Children* was published in London. Subtitled *A Consolatory Letter to a Friend,* the essay took the form of a letter from one father to another, discussing the death of a "beloved Sonne," who was no longer a newborn or a young child but a promising youth. It was, in fact, an early example of a "comfort book," a genre that would flourish particularly later on, in the Victorian era, with the popular obsession for romanticizing children's deaths. This early version, sterner and perhaps intended to be more masculine, still acknowledged the sorrow of losing a child. Grief was necessary, the author explained, and "must not be stopt too soone; for then the *Tears turn back to drowne the heart.*"[8] On the other hand, grief could be dangerous if too lengthily indulged: "you must not stay it too long; for then it playes the Tyrant." In the "consolatory letter," the author reminded the grieving father that he should not complain that his son might have been spared a little longer, since, after all, the boy could easily have died even younger. As further "consolation," he offered a catalog of early deaths: "Some are suffocated in the wombe; others crowz'd to death in the Birth. One is snacht away in the Cradle: Another mow'd off in his *May* of youth."[9] And finally, the writer tells his friend, the son had only been lent to him by God: "A great Duke or Prince lends you a dainty sweet Picture, of exquisite Worksmanship, to delight your Eyes withall; Will you powte . . . when after divers yeeres use, he re-demands it from you, to bee placed againe among the Ornaments of his Gallery?"[10] In fact, the father was advised to rejoice at his son's ascension: "He is not cleane gone, but onely gone before. His Mortality is ended, rather than his life. You have lost him for a *Time,* God hath found him for *Ever.*"[11]

The sense that God has deliberately called a child to heaven is mostly missing from public discourse in our era; it doesn't fit with our modern sense of medical causation or, for the most part, with the gentler religious teachings of our times. Families in different religious traditions may well believe in the power of God—and in the power of prayer—and they may take great comfort in the idea that a dead child is now with God or in heaven, without believing that the illness or the death has been deliberately sent and must therefore be accepted with gratitude.

It's not hard to imagine why people would have wanted to read narratives in which a child's death was, in fact, a happy ending—an early trip to heaven for a child who was being rewarded for living a life that had been perhaps so angelically good and holy that death represented an early promotion, rather than a punishment for a sinful parent. These stories must also have helped reinforce a sense of living in a just and ordered world, in which virtue and religious devotion would be rewarded. British historian Hannah Newton draws on a range of "biographies of pious children" from the seventeenth century in England that provide medical details of the children's illnesses but also offer the inevitably improving spectacle of their piety.[12] Stories of parental grief have been traced back further to medieval "miracle stories," in which the death of a child was followed by a divine miracle; the miracle offers comfort and meaning, but such stories also offer a description of the parent's grief and mourning.[13]

Such stories were not only aimed at parents; they were also meant to instruct and even prepare children for the potential trials of illness and early death. The earliest books for children in England were the guides to scare children into holy lives and holy deaths published in the 1670s. The most famous was Puritan minister James Janeway's collection *A Token for Children: Being an Exact Account of the Conversion, Holy and Exemplary Lives and Joyful Death of Several Young Children*, published in 1671, and its sequel, *The Second Part*, which came out in 1673, both reprinted many times over the course of the eighteenth century and on into the nineteenth. As one scholar put it: "Each exemplary child was divinely convicted of sin when very young—as young as two—and thereafter led a life of exemplary piety until his or her equally exemplary death, at which the young subject saw angels, uttered holy ejaculations, or offered other proof of his or her elect and blessed status."[14] These somewhat grisly tales—already in circulation orally when Janeway collected them—featured model children who were rewarded for their goodness with death. Janeway meant them to be read as facts, not fictions, and even cited witnesses in the second edition.

Over the course of the eighteenth and nineteenth centuries in England and America, that more severe and didactic religious narrative of the virtuous happy death of children, often wealthy privileged white children, evolved into something even more sentimental and etherealized. Instead of religion helping unfortunately—but realistically—stricken children face illness and death with courage and serenity, childhood death, especially in popular fiction, became an ennobling shaft of heavenly light, illuminating children who were by definition too good to remain on earth. These stories resolutely prettied up the difficult randomness of disease and death (suffocated in the womb, crushed in the cradle), and there is a continuum from those seventeenth-century stories, likely based on real individuals, of holy and beautiful childhood death to the later Victorian fictions in which an angelically good nature marks a child as too good to live.

Often saintly children who greet death with happy acceptance are subsidiary characters in nineteenth-century novels, tragic gravestones by the wayside as the narrative moves on. Think of Helen Burns in the novel *Jane Eyre*, who dies at the age of about fourteen at the cruel Lowood School, saying her good-bye to Jane:

> I am very happy, Jane; and when you hear that I am dead
> you must be sure and not grieve: there is nothing to grieve
> about. We all must die one day, and the illness which is
> removing me is not painful; it is gentle and gradual: my
> mind is at rest. I leave no one to regret me much: I have only
> a father; and he is lately married, and will not miss me. By
> dying young I shall escape great sufferings. I had not qual-

ities or talents to make my way very well in the world: I should have been continually at fault.[15]

Or think of Little Dick in *Oliver Twist,* a boy who is younger (and presumably smaller) than nine-year-old Oliver. Dick asks Mr. Bumble to send a message to his friend Oliver: "that I was glad to die when I was very young; for, perhaps, if I had lived to be a man, and had grown old, my little sister, who is in Heaven, might forget me, or be unlike me; and it would be so much happier if we were both children there together."[16]

While both of these children—tragic sidekicks to Jane and Oliver, two of the most famous eponymous children in literature—are deeply religious and look to their own deaths in religious terms, they are also aware that in very earthbound ways, they are extraneous and unwanted children. Helen was stowed at Lowood by her father, who will not miss her; he has a new family. Similarly, Dick is a workhouse child; the only loving family connection for him is a little sister, already dead, with whom he can be reunited in heaven. Their willingness to die can be seen as social criticism directed at the workhouse, the charity school.

"There is more child death in Dickens than in any other novelist," literary critic Laurence Lerner wrote in *Angels and Absences,* his book about the interplay between real child deaths and literary child deaths in the nineteenth century. "The Dickensian child leads a lively existence before dying, though that life is always touched (even enlivened) by the thought of death."[17] Dickens would create another pathetic child with a famously prolonged wasting away and death in thirteen-year-old Little Nell, no sidekick but instead the heroine of *The Old Curiosity Shop.* (Incidentally, "Little" as part of a fictional child's sobriquet is a poor prognostic sign in nineteenth-century fiction. Little Dick, Little Nell, and Little Eva, whom we will come to later—none of them get out alive.) So intense was her popularity, as the serialized novel appeared, with poor Nell's travails in the cold,

uncaring world making her a figure of such consuming interest, that
the story goes that crowds came down to the New York docks to meet
the ships bringing the magazines with the last installment, people
shouting to the sailors, demanding to know whether Little Nell had,
in fact, died.[18] This story—or perhaps this legend—is recounted in
many biographies of Dickens, and doubted in others, but there is no
question that the author himself, writing to his publisher, happily
counted up the letters he was receiving with every post, begging for
mercy for poor Nell.[19] And the great Irish parliamentarian Daniel
O'Connell read the death scene on a train, then threw the book out
the window, declaring, in tears, "He should not have killed her."

In *Dombey and Son,* Paul Dombey is the son of a very rich man,
his upbringing meant to be as luxurious as money can buy. The
bleakness of his life and the mixture of the deprivations and pressures that eventually lead to his death are a reminder that wealth can
be cruel in different ways than poverty, and that children need more
than money in order to thrive.[20] The description of Paul Dombey's
childhood is particularly interesting from a pediatric point of view,
because he is struck harshly by all the regular hazards of childhood.
You can certainly tell that Dickens had been around small children:

> Every tooth was a break-neck fence, and every pimple in
> the measles a stone wall to him. He was down in every fit
> of the hooping-cough, and rolled upon and crushed by a
> whole field of small diseases. . . . Some bird of prey got into
> his throat instead of the thrush; and the very chickens turn-
> ing ferocious—if they have anything to do with that infant
> malady to which they lend their name—worried him like
> tiger-cats.[21]

Dickens and his wife, who was born Catherine Hogarth, would
have ten children together, before their ugly divorce in which he
publicly repudiated her and criticized her as a mother. During their

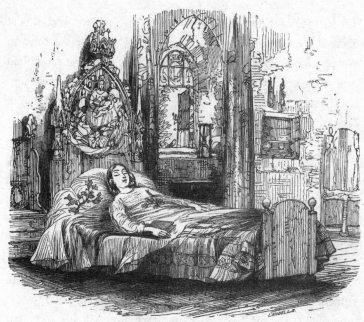

There, upon her little bed, she lay at rest.

Readers who had followed Little Nell's travails through the many episodes of the story finally said a sad goodbye to her in chapter 71: "There, upon her little bed, she lay at rest. . . . She was dead. Dear, gentle, patient, noble Nell was dead." Dickens's instructions to the illustrator, George Cattermole, for this scene expressed his own level of emotional involvement: "I want it to express the most beautiful repose and tranquility, and to have something of a happy look, if death can. . . . I am breaking my heart over this story and cannot bear to finish it." *Alamy Images.*

marriage, Hogarth also had two miscarriages and apparently suffered from severe postpartum depression. The first six of their children had been born by the time Dickens published the story of Paul Dombey, and it's hard to read that paragraph and not consider the multiple episodes of "small diseases," from thrush to whooping cough to measles to chicken pox, that must have swept through that home.

One of the Dickens daughters, Dora, died in infancy. (Dickens had a tendency to name his children after his characters, and Dora was named for the unfortunate "child wife" of *David Copperfield.*) Dora Annie Dickens, eight months old, went into convulsions one day in 1851 and died almost immediately. Neither parent was at home at the time; her mother was away at Malvern, a spa town in Worcestershire, famous for its mineral springs, and her father had gone to the London Tavern to speak at the annual dinner of the General Theatrical Fund. Dickens's best friend, the literary critic John Forster, informed him of Dora's death, and Dickens, that great author of serial fiction, chose to inform his wife of their child's death by authoring a kind of serial fiction: he wrote to Catherine the next day that "Little Dora, without being in the least pain, is suddenly stricken ill. . . . Mind! I will not deceive you. I think her *very* ill." He urged his wife to return home but enjoined her to come with "perfect composure," reminding her, "We never can expect to be exempt, as to our many children, from the afflictions of other parents."[22]

Dickens is celebrated as a creator of indelible fictional children, vulnerable outcasts in a dangerous and often uncaring world, tender innocents at the mercy of his many fascinating villains and charlatans, and serious literary protagonists like David Copperfield or Pip who can carry the weight of long and complex novels. He was interested in their adventures, and he was interested in their inner lives; he was interested in how they were shaped by the experiences he invented for them, and in what they would grow up to be. But the possibility of childhood death is a major preoccupation in his fiction. It hovers always over his work, as it hovered over that actual nursery, whether it is the social moral of the death that Oliver escapes and Little Dick does not, or how Paul Dombey, wealthy but not cherished tenderly, dies, while on the other hand, Tiny Tim famously does *not* die; the death forecast for him by the Ghost of Christmas Yet to Come is averted by the philanthropy of the reformed Ebenezer Scrooge. In Dickens's fiction, as in his own life, no child is safe; some die because their worlds are harsh and deprived, others because no one can "expect to be exempt."[23]

Samuel Clemens, writing as Mark Twain, was not in the business of creating saintly children. In fact, Tom Sawyer and Huck Finn, his most famous child creations, are invoked, nowadays, as boys who would no doubt run into serious trouble in the modern world. At best, they would be medicated for ADHD and oppositional behavior; at worst, they would be in juvenile custody for recurring attempts at running away or too much aggressive behavior.[24] There is a saintly deceased child in *Huckleberry Finn,* but Twain presents her satirically, offering a comment not just on the conventions of holy infancy but on the whole nineteenth-century high Victorian culture of memorials and sentimentality. Huck comes across her when he is invited in by the well-to-do Grangerford family, whose deceased fifteen-year-old daughter, Emmeline, drew sinister pictures of women in black, tombstones, weeping willows, and dead birds, giving her works appropriately doleful titles, including "Shall I Never See Thee More Alas" and "I Shall Never Hear Thy Sweet Chirrup More Alas." Huck finds these pictures quite depressing ("If ever I was down a little they always give me the fan-tods"), and although the family mourned the young artist's death, he comments shrewdly that "with her disposition, she was having a better time in the graveyard."[25] The dead girl's dark artwork also extends to poetry, including an ode composed to the deceased boy Stephen Dowling Bots:

> No whooping-cough did rack his frame,
> Nor measles drear with spots;
> Not these impaired the sacred name
> Of Stephen Dowling Bots.
> Despised love struck not with woe
> That head of curly knots,
> Nor stomach troubles laid him low,
> Young Stephen Dowling Bots.
> O no. Then list with tearful eye,
> Whilst I his fate do tell.
> His soul did from this cold world fly
> By falling down a well.

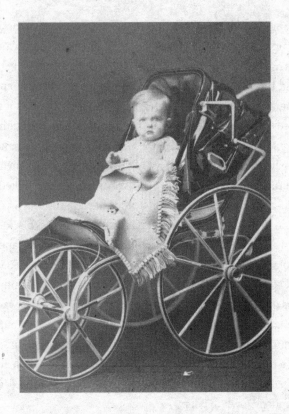

Langdon, shown here in his baby carriage, was the Clemens's only son. They had three daughters, only one of whom, Clara, survived her parents. Susy died of meningitis at twenty-four, and Jean, who suffered from epilepsy for many years, died at twenty-nine from the complications of a seizure. *The Mark Twain House & Museum, Hartford, Connecticut.*

. Huck, in his innocence, considers this "very good poetry," but it is most notable for its medical specificity, naming three plausible diseases that could have killed the boy yet didn't (measles, whooping cough, stomach troubles), then killing him off by accidental drowning. Twain, through Huck, makes great entertainment of satirizing the sentimental nineteenth-century cult of death and grieving.

For all his mockery, Mark Twain had suffered through the tragic loss of a child of his own, and he was tortured for years by the certainty that he was responsible. Langdon Clemens, the first child born to Samuel and Olivia Clemens, developed diphtheria, supposedly from a minor chill he contracted while out riding with his father, and died in June 1872 at the age of nineteen months—twelve years before the publication of *Huckleberry Finn*. His father was convinced that he was to blame for Langdon's illness and death. The child had a cough but seemed to be recovering, and his father took him out in the carriage. During the long drive in an open carriage, Twain fell into "a reverie," he said many years later, and let the fur blankets slip off Langdon, and by the time the coachman noticed this, "the child was almost frozen." When they reached home, the boy was sick again. In 1906, a full thirty-four years later, Twain was still penitent: "I have always felt shame for that treacherous morning's work and have not allowed myself to think of it when I could help it."[26]

Two years before the death of his own son, Twain wrote a scathing essay titled "Postmortem Poetry," in which he mocked the terrible verse published in children's obituaries, offering real samples of memorial poetry, changing only the last names. Of a poem about four children who burned to death in a house fire after their parents had left them on their own, Twain remarked, "There is something so innocent, so guileless, so complacent, so unearthly serene and self-satisfied about this peerless 'hog-wash,' that the man must be made of stone who can read it without a dulcet ecstasy creeping along his backbone and quivering in his marrow."[27] This quote very explicitly evokes the famous Oscar Wilde aphorism that "one must have a heart of stone to read the death of little Nell without laughing." In that lost world in which dead children and mourning parents were routine and regular parts of life, morbid humor clearly had its place.

His own experience with childhood death did not blunt Twain's satirical rejection of the comforts of sentimental poetry. Emmeline

Grangerford is sometimes identified by critics with Julia Ann Moore (1847–1920), the "Sweet Singer of Michigan," who, starting as a teenager, wrote dependably clunky and tragic verse for mournful occasions. Her career was marked by that same strange juxtaposition of truly tragic stories and intense mockery brought on by sentimental cliché and terrible writing. Moore bore ten children of her own, six of whom survived to adulthood. Her profoundly sentimental verse was published in the 1876 volume *The Sweet Singer of Michigan Salutes the Public,* by a publisher who treated it as a joke; it was reviewed in such terms as "Shakespeare, could he read it, would be glad that he was dead."[28] However, the book sold well, and it may not have been read ironically by most of its purchasers; "obituary poetry," usually published in newspapers along with death notices, was generally popular in America in the 1870s. The bad verse that Twain wrote for Emmeline Grangerford certainly bears a strong resemblance to Moore's, and to the contemporary ear, these poems also evoke Edward Gorey's more macabre humor—but Moore was certainly not joking. Here is Moore's "tribute" to "Little Andrew":

> Andrew was a little infant,
> And his life was two years old;
> He was his parents' eldest boy,
> And he was drowned, I was told. . . .
> This little child knew no danger—
> Its little soul was free from sin—
> He was looking in the water,
> When, alas, this child fell in.[29]

And consider the death of "Little Libbie" (the real thing, not a parody):

> One morning in April, a short time ago,
> Libbie was active and gay;

Her Saviour called her, she had to go,
E're the close of that pleasant day.

While eating dinner, this dear little child
Was choked on a piece of beef.
Doctors came, tried their skill awhile,
But none could give relief.

She was ten years of age, I am told,
And in school stood very high.
Her little form the earth enfolds,
In her embrace it must ever lie.[30]

Twain may have been thinking of Moore, who was widely read, but there was another model for the "Sweet Singer" even closer to home. Right in Hartford, where the Clemens family lived, Lydia Howard Huntley Sigourney (1791–1865) was a hugely successful poet and journalist, and a specialist in sentimental elegies. She was a best-selling author, famous enough that a town in Iowa was named after her and important enough that, like Harriet Beecher Stowe, she met Queen Victoria. She was also an influential educator, concerned with the education of deaf children, among other issues, and deeply engaged with questions of slavery and the treatment of the Indians. But it was for her writings on domestic life and families that she was loved by her wider reading public, mostly women, to whom she addressed herself both in poetry and in a series of books: *Letters to Young Ladies*, *Letters to My Pupils*, and *Letters to Mothers*.[31]

In *Letters to Mothers*, perhaps her most successful book, published in 1838 and still in print today with a religious Christian publisher, the Sweet Singer of Hartford offered this most graphic, ghoulish, and yet sentimental of stories:

I once saw a sight, mournful, yet beautiful. Twin infants,
in the same coffin. . . . Death united them. . . . Bright rose-
buds in their little hands, as they slumbered side by side.
Together they had entered the gate of life, and at the gate of
death were scarcely divided. When after the silent lapse of
time, the mother was able to speak of her bereavement with
composure, she said, that from among the sources whence
she had derived comfort, was the thought that they would
be *always together*.[32]

This story, to our ears, suggests unspeakable tragedy; think of
that poor mother who had given birth to twin babies and then seen
them die, one after the other. In Sigourney's telling, the twins' mother
was able to find comfort in the idea of a Christian afterlife, but she
struggled before she could speak about it with proper pious acceptance. Although the comfort was real enough, so was the struggle;
the attainment of composure required, at the very least, "the silent
lapse of time."

In the overlays of sentiment and sentimentalism, of mourning
and grieving and narrating loss, the figure of the "poetess" occupies
a peculiar place. Julia Ann Moore, like Lydia Huntley Sigourney,
had buried several of her own children. The comfort they reached
for, like the comfort they provided—through the mix of obituary
memories, devotions, and tributes—was grounded in the harsh daily
reality of infant and child mortality. The lost world of parents in the
past, remembering their children, is reflected by the great writers
of the age, but also by the lesser and by the amateurs, all of them
touched themselves by the common everyday tragedy of losing children.[33] The hunger for a kind of rhyming folk narrative, complete
with promises of beautiful memories that would not fade and joyful celestial reunions, was as real and sincere as the countervailing
urge to mock the awkwardness and the schmaltz. As Dickens, who

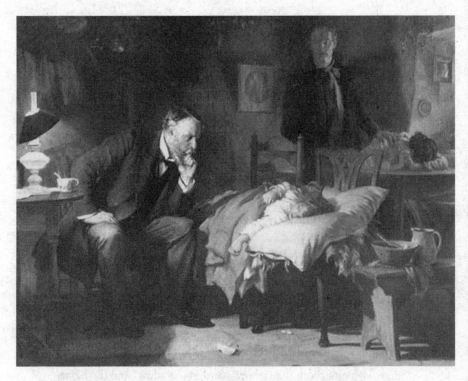

In this 1891 painting, Luke Fildes, a Victorian artist, recalled the death of his own son, Philip, at one year of age, and the doctor who had cared for the child with dedication but had not been able to save him. The painter suggested that unlike his own son, this child might recover, with dawn bringing "the first glimmerings of the joy which is to follow." *David Croat Thomson,* The Life and Work of Luke Fildes, R.A. *(London: J. S. Virtue and Company, 1895), 13; Alamy Images.*

shamelessly marketed dying fictional children, reminded his wife when their daughter died, no parent could expect to be exempt. The sentiment was real, and so was the sentimentality. The grief was real, and so was the guilt. Mark Twain never forgave himself for letting his son catch cold.

CHAPTER 2

"Ma'am, Have You Ever Lost a Child?"

Child Death in Civil War America

"American Mothers! Can you doubt that the slave feels as tenderly for her offspring as you do for yours? . . . Will you not raise your voices, and plead for her emancipation—her immediate emancipation?" The call came in an 1832 essay in the influential anti-slavery newspaper *The Liberator,* under the pen name "Zillah," which is both the Hebrew word for "shadow" and the name of a woman in Genesis, married to a descendant of Cain. Zillah was Sarah Mapps Douglass, an African American woman in her twenties who had grown up in Philadelphia, the daughter of parents who were themselves very involved in the anti-slavery movement. She taught in New York City before opening a school for African American girls back in her hometown. Zillah's essay was published as harsh legislation was enacted in many states, making it harder for free African Americans to move across state borders and easier for southern slaveholders to pursue escaped and fugitive slaves.

"Does thy heart swell with anguish, when thy helpless infant is torn from thy arms, and carried thou knowest not whither?" Zillah asked, and went on to answer: "Yes, I know thou dost feel all this."[1] But the question was only rhetorically addressed to enslaved women; instead, the author was invoking the sense of losing a child in a delib-

LADIES' DEPARTMENT.

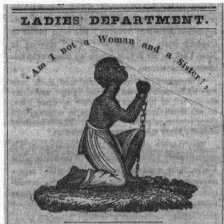

"Am I not a Woman and a Sister?"

☞ Our word for it, there are few young white ladies who can prepare an essay for the press with more accuracy in regard to orthography and punctuation, or written in a more beautiful hand, than the following, by a young colored lady. We beg for other favors.

For the Liberator.

UNNATURAL DISTINCTION.

I have often thought of the distinction made in places of *Public Worship* between white and colored persons, and have wondered that the latter should humble themselves so much as to occupy one of those seats provided for them.

A reverend gentleman who addressed the audi-other feeling, and she again tied her child, and returned to the labors of the field.

American Mothers! can you doubt that the slave feels as tenderly for her offspring as you do for yours? Do your hearts feel no throb of pity for her woes? Will you not raise your voices, and plead for her emancipation—her immediate emancipation?

At another time, when assisting her mistress to get dinner, she dropped the skin of a potato into what she was preparing. The angry woman snatched the knife from her hand, and struck her with it upon the bosom! My countenance expressed so much horror at this account, that I believe the poor woman thought I doubted her veracity. Baring her aged bosom, 'Look,' said she, 'my child, here is the scar'—and I looked and wept that woman should have so far forgot her gentle nature. Soon after this, she was sold to another person, and at his death freed. She then went to reside in a neighboring city. Her old mistress, after a series of misfortunes, was reduced almost to beggary, and bent her weary footsteps to the same city; and would you believe it, reader? She sent for the woman she had so cruelly wronged, to come and assist her. Her friends persuaded her not to go; but she, noble creature! woman-like, weeping that a lady should be so reduced, obeyed the call, and waited upon her as faithfully as if she had been her dearest friend.

Calumniators of my despised race, read this and blush.   ZILLAH.

Philadelphia, July 8th, 1832.

Sarah Mapps Douglass, writing in the Ladies' Department of *The Liberator*, made the case that white American mothers should identify with the affection that enslaved women felt for their offspring and end the system which ripped families apart. *The Library Company of Philadelphia.*

erate attempt to galvanize white women and compel them past political sympathy to identification and a sense of urgent action. In an era in which all women, at every social level, knew very well the fear of being permanently parted from a child, abolitionists consistently and successfully called on those maternal emotions, purposefully connecting the fear of losing a much-loved child with the forced family separations produced by the slave system.

Abolitionists cited infant and child mortality among the enslaved to show the cruelty of the system, while slaveholders, aware that they were being judged for childhood deaths, used those same figures to blame mothers for being inadequate caretakers, thereby justifying extending and intensifying control over the daily lives of enslaved families. They might attribute infant death, for example, to "overlaying" by mothers at night, so that they inadvertently suffocated their babies while sleeping with them. Narratives written by those who had escaped slavery emphasized and illuminated the agonies of separated families, and *Uncle Tom's Cabin,* the most famous abolitionist text of them all, returned again and again to the theme of family separation and childhood death, to the power of maternal love and maternal grief. The national discourse on slavery regularly cited the very real children living harsh and often shortened lives under an evil system that viewed them as figures on a balance sheet.

Because these humans were viewed as property, the births and deaths of slaves represented profit and loss, and so records were kept. The economist Richard Steckel was the first to pull together a great deal of this data, in "A Dreadful Childhood: The Excess Mortality of American Slaves," originally published in 1986. Of every 1,000 live births, as many as 350 infants died, thus duplicating the mortality rates from previous centuries in Europe. When stillbirths were included, the total rate of loss by the age of one was almost 50 percent of pregnancies. Another 201 children in every thousand died by the age of five. These mortality rates, he calculated, were roughly double those of the entire U.S. population at the time. Every stage carried excess risk for enslaved children, from the pregnancies, which were shadowed by brutally hard work and inadequate nutrition, to the conditions of birth and medical care available to the mothers and infants to the vulnerable early weeks of life. Steckel argued that much of the excess mortality occurred in the first month of life, and that a great deal of it was due to low birth weights, which he attributed to maternal and fetal infections, to the forced hard work done during the pregnancies, and to the malnutrition of the mothers—both a general impoverished diet and specific vitamin deficiencies.[2] He was also able to show that infant mortality was higher on larger plantations, perhaps because in those settings, infants were likely to be grouped together, away from their mothers, and less likely to be breastfed. In every population, rich or poor, maternal breastfeeding reduced infant mortality, and any other kind of nutrition for babies increased it.

The historian Daina Ramey Berry assembled a large database tracing these lives; she wrote in 2017: "After analyzing 15,256 appraisal and sale values for male and female children between the ages of zero and ten, I found that the commodification of black bodies evolved as enslaved children aged. We know that when they were young, their monetary values were low, for several reasons. First, there was a high incidence of infant mortality as enslaved children had a low survival rate in the first few years of life."[3] Successful pregnancies increased the slaveholder's human "property," but conditions favoring successful pregnancies might decrease the profits to be extracted from the labor of the enslaved mothers. Some slaveholders allowed pregnant women a little bit of ease, while others held firm to racist assumptions about the toughness of Africans and their descendants and their ability to tolerate extreme conditions. Many individual records tell stories of women who worked up until labor began: "The slave Betty worked in the Alabama cotton fields during the spring months of 1845 almost to the day she bore her child, which may explain why her baby died within the week. In the fall of 1844, Charity's owner did not excuse her from cotton picking until the day of her baby's birth."[4]

Some doctors in the South marketed their services to slaveholders, both in determining whether enslaved women were actually pregnant (if they were suspected of trying to avoid work) and in attending them at delivery. Still, it was more common to follow the less expensive practice of having those births attended by enslaved midwives, possibly in tandem with the slaveholder's wife, if she had any experience. Some doctors used enslaved women for surgical experiments—that is, for practicing and perfecting new surgical procedures, including cesarean sections and the repair of vesicovaginal fistulas.[5] Childbirth was dangerous for all women during this period, of course, and medical attention did not necessarily make it less dangerous. Women who are malnourished or sick with other chronic diseases, from intestinal worms to tuberculosis, have always been at greater risk in the physiologically demanding circumstances of pregnancy. That the living conditions of slavery were particularly hazardous to women and, most especially, to children was borne out by the extraordinarily high rates (possibly even higher in the Caribbean than in the American South) of pregnancy loss, maternal mortality, infant mortality, and childhood death among those who were enslaved. This registered both with abolitionists and with those who drew their profit from enslaved labor.

Thomas Affleck, who owned a Mississippi plantation and later one in Texas, published the *Southern Rural Almanac and Garden Calendar*. He observed that "the mortality of negro children is as two to one when compared with the whites."[6] Babies were born into conditions of high risk, including neonatal tetanus, often spread when dirt from farm animals comes into contact with the newly severed umbilical cord and its large blood vessels serve as gateways for infection to enter the baby's body. Perhaps as many as 5 to 10 percent of infants born to enslaved mothers died of this devastating infection, which was not widely understood by either midwives or doctors.[7] J. Marion Sims, the doctor who is now notorious for his repeated gynecological experiments on enslaved women, had his own theory about what caused tetanus, and carried out a horrendous series of "treatments"—or experiments—with enslaved newborns that involved puncturing their skulls.[8] Affleck blamed the enslaved midwives for neonatal tetanus: "A vast proportion die under nine or ten days, from the most unskillful management of negro midwives, who do not know how to take care of the navel, and doses the infant with nasty nostrums from the moment of its birth;" while older children, he claimed, might die

This 1860 list of prices for enslaved people, described by gender, age, and height, who were sold at auction, serves as a vivid reminder of the harsh realities of the slave system—boys about four feet tall, their names not noted, became anonymous property to be bought and sold. Records like this one, with the carefully measured heights of the children being sold, have allowed scholars to trace the physical realities of the brutalized childhoods experienced by enslaved children. *David M. Rubenstein Rare Book & Manuscript Library, Duke University.*

"from having access to green fruit, eating acorns, etc., and from dirt eating."[9] As a plantation owner, he did not blame the slave system. Nowadays, in pediatrics, we might look at the tendency to eat dirt, a form of what we call pica (eating non-nutritive substances), as possible evidence of iron-deficiency anemia or other vitamin or mineral deficiencies in a nutritionally deprived child.

Slaveholders were aware that the high rates of infant and child death did not make them—or their systems—look good and that these rates were cited by critics of slavery as evidence that the system was cruel and immoral. And so, in response, plantation owners tried hard to blame those mortality rates on the mothers. There were accusations of "overlaying," or smothering infants in their sleep: "Last week," wrote Robert Hubard to his brother Edmund, "Tilla overlaid / when asleep / and killed her youngest child—a boy 6 or 7 months old. This was no doubt caused by her own want of care and attention."[10] Affleck, another plantation owner, at least conceded that those mothers might be exhausted: "Not a few are over-laid by the wearied mother, who sleeps so dead a sleep as not to be aware of the injury to her infant." Some have interpreted this phenomenon, historically, as including examples of infanticide, perhaps acts of resistance by parents who were unwilling to bring their children up into slavery. More recent scholars have argued that these were examples of what we now call sudden infant death syndrome, with the deprivations of slavery increasing the risk factors, including malnourished infants and exhausted parents.[11]

Accusations of maternal neglect and incompetence served the same overarching economic agenda for slaveholders, providing a pretext to keep the babies together in a nursery, thus making it possible for the mothers to put in a full day's work. But the supervision in such nurseries was very scanty, with adults often made to do other work in addition to caring for the group of infants and young children, or with children told to watch over those only a few years younger than themselves. As Schwartz described it: "Children as young as two or three rocked babies or protected them from wandering off or getting too near the fire."[12] Similarly, in an effort to reduce that high mortality rate in coastal rice-growing areas, which were swampy parts of the country where malaria was extremely dangerous to babies, planters created "pineland camps" and dispatched enslaved children there for long periods, ostensibly to keep them safer from infection but also to separate them from their parents, who could then be made to work without interruptions for child-care responsibilities, in those same dangerous swampy malarial zones.

Steckel, working from slave manifests, was able to show that younger enslaved children were extremely small for their ages, stunted in their growth even in comparison to children in the twenty-first century growing up in the most extreme slums of the poorest countries.[13] Poorly nourished, harshly treated, cared for by parents who were themselves maltreated and exploited, and sometimes sold away from their parents, they died of infections, complicated by malnutrition, of accidents and wounds, and of abuse and maltreatment. Sojourner Truth, in her autobiography, said that her father repeatedly told "a thrilling story of a little slave-child, which, because it annoyed the family with its cries, was caught up by a white man, who dashed its brains out against the wall. An Indian (for Indians were plenty in that region then) passed along as the bereaved mother washed the bloody corpse of her murdered child, and learning the cause of its death, said, with characteristic vehemence, 'If I had been here, I would have put my tomahawk in his head!' meaning the murderer's." Truth went on to offer another instance of brutality, in which a developmentally delayed child, a five-year-old who could neither walk nor talk, was kicked and tormented to death by a cruel slaveholder who found the child's moaning annoying.[14]

Many narratives and personal histories testify to the strong bonds between the children experiencing this "dreadful childhood" and the parents whose attempts to care for them and nurture them were so hampered and twisted by the exigencies and cruelties of the slave system. In 1834, the twenty-year-old William Wells Brown escaped slavery in Kentucky and traveled north, but it meant parting from his mother, who was being sent "to New Orleans, to die on a cotton,

sugar, or rice plantation!" He blamed himself—she had been captured after trying to escape with him—but she assured him that he
had only done his duty, and urged him toward liberty.

He wrote, "As I thought of my mother, I could but feel that I
had lost

'—the glory of my life,
My blessing and my pride!
I half forgot the name of slave,
When she was by my side.'"[15]

Sojourner Truth spoke caustically of how she "found herself the
mother of five children, and she rejoiced in being permitted to be
the instrument of increasing the property of her oppressors! Think,
dear reader, without a blush, if you can, for one moment, of a *mother*
thus willingly, and with *pride,* laying her own children, the 'flesh of
her flesh,' on the altar of slavery—a sacrifice to the bloody Moloch!
But we must remember that beings capable of such sacrifices are
not mothers; they are only 'things,' 'chattels,' 'property.'"[16] The 1854
book *The Experience of Thomas Jones, Who Was a Slave for Forty-Three
Years* began with an account of two generations of parental love, and
parental agony: "My dear parents were conscious of the desperate
and incurable woe of their position and destiny; and of the lot of
inevitable suffering in store for their beloved children. They talked
about our coming misery, and they lifted up their voices and wept
aloud. . . . I am a father, and I have had the same feelings of unspeakable anguish, as I have looked upon my precious babes, and have
thought of the ignorance, degradation and woe which they must
endure as slaves."[17]

The greatest fear that Jones remembered his parents having was
their terror that their children would be sold, separated from the
family and sent away forever. Similarly, the 1849 book *The Life of*

Josiah Henson, Formerly a Slave, Now an Inhabitant of Canada, Narrated by Himself, began with a searing memory of Henson watching his mother as, one by one, her six children were sold, until it was his turn as the youngest and she tried appealing to the man who had already bought her: "She fell at his feet, and clung to his knees, entreating him in tones that a mother only could command, to buy her baby as well as herself, and spare to her one of her little ones at least. Will it, can it be believed that this man, thus appealed to, was capable not merely of turning a deaf ear to her supplication, but of disengaging himself from her with such violent blows and kicks, as to reduce her to the necessity of creeping out of his reach, and mingling the groan of bodily suffering with the sob of a breaking heart?"[18] Henson was bought by another man, but when he fell ill, he was subsequently reunited with his mother; his book was a source of inspiration and material for Harriet Beecher Stowe, and a scene very much like the one described here takes place in *Uncle Tom's Cabin.*

The slave system, which regularly and systematically separated parents and children, almost by definition discounted the significance of their affection, both in legal rulings and in general attitudes: "Although the system discouraged parents from forming strong bonds, the slave mother was nevertheless constantly accused of neglecting her children, and the father of brutality. Indeed, slaves were cursed as both immoral and incompetent parents."[19] Sojourner Truth also opened her autobiography with an account of her parents' grief, countering "all who would fain believe that slave parents have not natural affection for their offspring" with recollections of how her parents "would sit for hours, recalling and recounting every endearing, as well as harrowing circumstance that taxed memory could supply, from the histories of those dear departed ones, of whom they had been robbed, and for whom their hearts still bled."[20]

In *Uncle Tom's Cabin*, the hugely influential abolitionist novel aimed squarely at a white readership, Harriet Beecher Stowe returned to the subject of losing children again and again, deliberately juxtaposing the inevitable sorrows of infant mortality with the horrors of a system that deliberately and cruelly snatched children away and left their mothers to grieve. Parental grief is one of the main narrative engines of this most notorious of American novels, which did so much to shape the public vision of the slave system.

"All good causes owe their success to the push of women," wrote Mary V. Cook in 1887.[21] Although she was one of the founders of the National Association of Colored Women, abolition and racial equality were not the "good causes" that she referenced specifically; by 1887, at least, she was more intent on the temperance movement and on missionary work. But the good cause of anti-slavery activism in the United States in the decades before the Civil War did indeed owe much of its success to "the push of women," and the call of mutual motherhood aimed to extend empathy across the barriers of race and social class. The grief that a mother, Black or white, might feel at the loss of a child was a rhetorical rallying cry in a mixture of political activism, sentimentality, fact, and fiction.

The shadow of being separated from a child turns up early in *Uncle Tom's Cabin*, in one of the most famous scenes in American literature. In the chapter titled "The Mother's Struggle," Eliza runs away with her son because he has been sold and is about to be taken from her, in that most common and terrible fear of enslaved parents, the same fear Zillah had referenced at the beginning of her essay. Eliza and Harry make it all the way to the Kentucky side of the Ohio River, where she sees the "great cakes of floating ice" and learns that the ferry is not running, only to spy her pursuers arriving. And then come the two paragraphs that have been so often illustrated, so regularly enacted on the stage: Eliza grabs up her son, and before the astonished eyes of her pursuers, "nerved with strength such as God gives only to the desperate, with one wild cry and flying leap, she vaulted sheer over the turbid current by the shore, on to the raft of ice beyond." Her pursuers cry out in astonishment, but on she goes: "With wild cries and desperate energy she leaped to another and still another cake;—stumbling—leaping—slipping—springing upwards again! Her shoes are gone—her stockings cut from her feet—while blood marked every step; but she saw nothing, felt nothing, till dimly, as in a dream, she saw the Ohio side, and a man helping her up the bank."[22]

The kindly man who helps her up the bank directs her to a house where she will find aid; that home belongs to the Birds, a couple who have, in a pointed nineteenth-century novelistic coincidence, just been arguing about the fugitive slave laws. The man of the house is in fact a statesman, Senator Bird, who has voted for legislation making it illegal to help or abet runaway slaves, and his wife is angry about it and has just announced to the senator, "It's a shameful, wicked, abominable law, and I'll break it, for one, the first time I get a chance; and I hope I *shall* have a chance, I do!"[23] And she *shall* have that chance; it is soon after that dramatically opportune moment that Mrs. Bird is called into the kitchen and finds her own servants tending to the swooning Eliza.

Harriet Beecher Stowe continues Eliza's story with a chapter that takes the moral questions of slavery and the fugitive slave law to a whole new level, "In Which It Appears That a Senator Is but a Man," which Henry Louis Gates and Hollis Robbins describe in *The Annotated Uncle Tom's Cabin* as "Stowe's most powerful and political chapter title."[24] *Uncle Tom's Cabin* was written very specifically in response to the Fugitive Slave Act of 1850; it was after reading a letter from her sister-in-law detailing the horrors of the act and the new vulnerability of those who had escaped slavery but could now be hunted down even in the city of Boston that Stowe declared, "I will write something. I will if I live."[25]

This is Eliza's chance to make the case against the hated legislation—and, by extension, against the evils of slavery. You can almost feel Stowe hitching up her skirts, relatively early in the book, in the ninth of forty-five chapters, seizing her pulpit. Her characters are on the other side of a dramatic, even climactic scene of physical peril and maternal heroism, panting on the shore in relative safety—but the danger is still near. She has proven herself, as a writer, a master of plot, drama, and danger, and created an escape scene so strong that it is still instantly recognizable more than 150 years later—and this is her moment to claim her audience for the novel's cause.

Eliza looks at Mrs. Bird with a "keen, scrutinizing glance" and notes that she is dressed in mourning.

"'Ma'am,' she said, suddenly, 'have you ever lost a child?'"[26]

And indeed they have—a month before, the Bird family had buried their darling little Henry. And it is on this connection—from the departed and deeply mourned Henry to the threatened Harry, for whose sake Eliza is fleeing—that Stowe is building an identification that will reach across the racial divide and stir the mothers of America. When Mrs. Bird, crying, acknowledges her recent loss, Eliza says, "Then you will feel for me. I have lost two, one after another,—left 'em buried there when I came away; and I had only this one left . . . and, ma'am, they were going to take him away from me,—to *sell* him,—sell him down south, ma'am, to go all alone,—a baby that had never been away from his mother in his life!"[27]

And at that point, Eliza's case is made. Mrs. Bird is weeping, as are her two surviving sons and her servants, while the senator himself is blowing his nose and wiping his glasses. Even as the senator goes off to ready his carriage to carry Eliza to safety himself, he suggests to his wife that there is children's clothing to be found in "that drawer full of things—of—of—poor little Henry's."[28] The senator's two sons follow their mother as she unlocks the drawer. And Stowe then dispenses with the intervening characters and seizes the

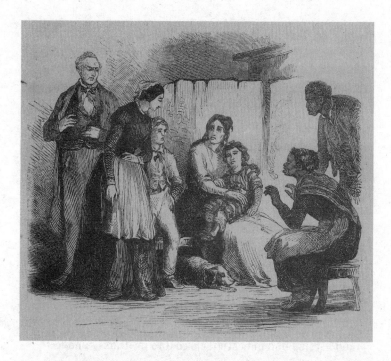

In this illustration by Hammatt Billings for the 1853 illustrated edition of *Uncle Tom's Cabin*, Senator Bird stands to the left, behind his wife and son, listening to Eliza tell her story as she holds her son, Harry (remember that Eliza in the book is fair enough to pass for white as she makes her escape), while the two family servants, Cudjoe ("the black man-of-all-work") and Dinah ("their only colored domestic, old Aunt Dinah"), listen on the right. *From* Uncle Tom's Cabin; or, Life Among the Lowly. *PS2954 .U5 1853. Clifton Waller Barrett Library of American Literature, Special Collections, University of Virginia, Charlottesville.*

nineteenth-century novelist's prerogative of directly apostrophizing her readers:

> And oh! mother that reads this, has there never been in your
> house a drawer, or a closet, the opening of which has been
> to you like the opening again of a little grave? Ah! happy
> mother that you are, if it has not been so.[29]

Stowe was drawing on a reality with which her readership—middle-class, educated women, domestic and dutiful—would be profoundly familiar. They would also have their secret drawers full of lovingly folded child-sized clothing, their mourning outfits, and their tiny graves. Stowe herself certainly did, as she wrote to a friend in the summer of 1849, after her son Charley died in a cholera epidemic in Cincinnati:

> No one knows fully what it is to live till they have stood
> helpless by, to see the death struggle of what was dearest to
> them— Poor Charley's dying cries and sufferings rent my
> heart— even so let it be— for thro the baptism of sorrow we
> come to a full knowledge of the sufferings of God— who has
> borne for us all that we bear— Those dying agonies were to
> him only the birth pangs of a joyful and glorious existence
> and now he remembereth no more the anguish for joy—
> and I seeing him in heaven rejoice thro my tears— and feel
> myself the mother of an angel—

But after these exalted sentiments, she then returned to the crushing sorrow of having lost the real earthly child she loved:

> Yet when I read your letter it brought my lost darling so plain
> before me— as he used to look when tired and sleepy and
> going to you for his welcome pillow— it affected me just as
> the sight of his little brown hat or his little coat or shoes—
> all treasured away with care just as he wore them last.[30]

Indeed she knew that drawer, that closet, that she would invoke in *Uncle Tom's Cabin*, the opening of which would be like the opening of a small grave, and understood that this grief would resonate with mothers—and fathers—everywhere.

Uncle Tom's Cabin was published as a serial in the *National Era* in

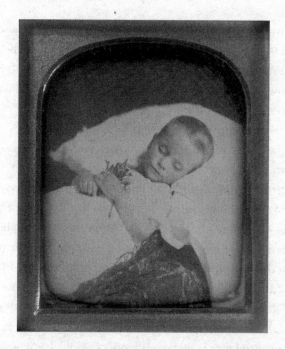

Harriet Beecher Stowe wrote to her husband when their son Charley died that "he has been my pride and joy. . . . Yet I have just seen him in his death agony, looked on his imploring face when I could not help nor soothe nor do one thing, not one, to mitigate his cruel suffering, do nothing but pray in my anguish that he might die soon." It was a Victorian custom, both in the United States and England, to take a photo of someone who had recently died. In this photograph, Samuel Charles Stowe is posed as a sleeping angel, perhaps allowing his family an alternative image to the memories of his suffering and death. *Schlesinger Library, Radcliffe Institute, Harvard University.*

1851–52, starting two years after Charley's death; it was an immediate sensation, selling three hundred thousand copies in the United States in its first year and a million in England, where Stowe traveled as a visiting celebrity, meeting Queen Victoria and carrying home volumes of signatures to anti-slavery petitions. A year after the novel was published, in response to an inquiry from London asking for an account of the circumstances of how *Uncle Tom's Cabin* had been written, she responded:

I have been the mother of seven children, the most beautiful
and the most loved of whom lies buried near my Cincinnati residence. It was at his dying bed and at his grave that I
learned what a poor slave mother may feel when her child is
torn away from her.[31]

In the course of writing the book she claimed had its origins in
her own grief for her "beautiful, loving, gladsome" child,[32] Stowe
also created the most saintly and most celebrated childhood death
scene of the entire nineteenth century, the death of Little Eva from
childhood tuberculosis, an infection that proves fatal in spite of the
best medical care that a great deal of the slaveholder's money can
buy, for that disease could neither be prevented nor cured. Eva is not
a particularly realistic child, but she dies of a real disease: an infection of slow-growing bacteria, now called *Mycobacterium tuberculosis*,
in her lungs. It's the same disease that killed off Helen Burns in *Jane
Eyre*, and also four of Charlotte Brontë's sisters, two of them when
they were only ten and eleven, and another two by the age of thirty.

Tuberculosis is a waxing and waning disease, a slow dying. At
one point in *Uncle Tom's Cabin*, Eva seems better, but it is only "one of
those deceitful lulls, by which her inexorable disease so often beguiles
the anxious heart, even on the verge of the grave." Eva herself knows
the truth, and there is nothing that her father's wealth and luxury
can do to alter that truth, just as there is nothing the most expensive
physician in the city can offer. Eva is dying, "though nursed so tenderly, and though life was unfolding before her with every brightness
that love and wealth could give."[33] Cousin Ophelia, nursing the child,
speaks to Eva's father, Augustine St. Clare, in the language of religious
acceptance: "Has not God a right to do what he will with his own?"
And St. Clare answers with words that must surely have resonated
with many nineteenth-century parents, possibly including the author:
"Perhaps so; but that doesn't make it any easier to bear."[34]

Stowe's Charley had died from cholera, a disease that kills by intractable diarrhea, which washes the necessary salts and sugars out of a small child's body and leaves it dehydrated and unable to function. Eva's death—she wastes slowly away, pale and lovely, with full religious acceptance, in a flower-filled room in a lavish lake house— is more beautiful in every way.[35]

In working with her private grief and generalizing it to be somehow reflective of the grief of enslaved mothers all over the South whose children had been taken from them, Stowe also found a target for anger. She found a way to frame the loss of children as a wrong that could be corrected, a battle that could be fought and won. She was in a kind of dilemma, as are all those who must reconcile a belief in a personal and omnipotent deity with the shock and misery that come from some of that deity's actions, and what she found was a way to make parental bereavement into a righteous cause.

Lydia Huntley Sigourney had struck the same note in her 1838 *Letters to Mothers,* arguing that any mother who mourned a young child must be "moved to deeper sympathy with all who mourn . . . more strongly incited to every deed of mercy. . . . When she sees a little coffin pass, no matter whether the mother who mourns, be a stranger, or a mendicant, or burnt dark beneath an African sun, is she not to her, in the pitying thrill of that moment, as a sister?[36]

In chapter 45 of *Uncle Tom's Cabin,* Stowe launches full bore into her sermon: "And you, mothers, of America," she writes, "you who have learned by the cradles of your own children, to love and feel for all mankind." She reminds them of all the emotional bonds between mother and child—the love, the joy, the worry over education—and she begs them, accordingly, to pity enslaved mothers with all those same "affections" and yet "not one legal right to protect, guide, or educate" their children. Then she appeals to those who could not fight back and defend their own children from illness to fight now against something that can actually be defeated, and end the parallel agonies of slavery and the loss of children:

By the sick hour of your child; by those dying eyes, which
you can never forget; by those last cries, that wrung your
heart when you could neither help nor save; by the desolation of that empty cradle, that silent nursery,—I beseech
you, pity those mothers that are constantly made childless
by the American slave-trade![37]

————————//————————

"Mid-nineteenth-century Americans endured a high rate of infant
mortality but expected that most individuals who reached young
adulthood would survive at least into middle age," writes Drew
Gilpin Faust in *This Republic of Suffering: Death and the American
Civil War*. The Civil War destroyed that expectation and touched
so many people with death and loss that it "transformed the American nation," she argues, and established sacrifice, mourning, and
memorials as the ground for ultimate reconciliation, the common
experience binding the nation back together.[38] Many of those who
fell as soldiers were boys of eighteen and nineteen, even sixteen
and seventeen. Some 204,000 soldiers died on the battlefields—but
twice as many, another 419,000, died of disease, in training camps,
in military hospitals, and in crowded prisoner-of-war camps on
both sides.[39]

And though soldiers who died during their army service were
hardly part of the common picture of childhood death, Civil War
culture repeatedly invoked the image of the grieving parent, especially the tragic mother, recalling the dead soldier as all too recently
a promising child, mourning the loss of a sturdy toddler or a happy
schoolboy now having perished in harsh and brutal conditions. On
both sides of the conflict, songs emphasized the emotional anguish
that war brought to the mothers left behind, like "Dear Mother, I've
Come Home to Die" and "I'm Glad to Be the Mother of a Soldier
Boy."[40] Eleanor Cecilia Donnelly, a Philadelphia poet whose Civil War
poems were widely reprinted, invoked a biblical trope, Rachel weep-

ing for her children and refusing to be comforted, in the prophecy of Jeremiah, in her poem "Rachel in the North:"

> My boy—my pride—my strong-limbed Absalom!
> Dead! dead? Who dared to whisper *"dead"* of thee?
> Dead on the field,—thy bright locks stained with loam.

Here the death of a young man on the battlefield does not evoke images of young manhood or battle glory; instead Rachel recalls:

> My only son,—the nursling of my breast,—
> The blue-eyed boy who sat upon my knee,
> And in my mother-arms took cradled rest.[41]

The two first ladies of the Civil War, Mary Todd Lincoln in the Union White House and Varina Howell Davis in the Confederate White House, were, in some ways, parallel figures. Both were in fact deeply unpopular, and both were suspected of divided loyalties during a war that literally divided a nation and split many families. Both were extremely well educated for women of their time, and both were mocked as unattractive. But the most remarkable parallel between the two privileged and powerful women may be their devastating maternal trajectories: each woman outlived almost all her children. Mary Lincoln was survived by only one of her four sons; Varina Davis, by one daughter out of her six children. They were emblems of tragic maternity and loss in a country—across the North and the South—that was full of bereaved parents. Their stories offer a perspective on grief and grieving at a moment when on top of the usual dangers to children, war was consuming teenaged boys in great numbers. The great and powerful, both military and political leaders, made their decisions and speeches and fought their battles while worrying about sick children and mourning dead children. Neither the wartime White House nor the war's most iconic moments—such as the Gettysburg Address—can be fully understood without taking into account the constant shadow of childhood death.

Mary and Abraham Lincoln had four sons in all; the oldest was Robert, born in 1843, when the Lincolns were living in Springfield, Illinois. Their second son was Edward, born while the family was still in Springfield; he came down with what was initially diagnosed as diphtheria in the winter when he was three, suffered for fifty-two days, and died in February 1850, before he reached his fourth birthday.[42]

Both parents grieved when Edward died, but Mary's grief was so uncontrolled, her fits of weeping so extreme, that her husband reached out to a minister for help in consoling her. The neighbors remembered, years later, that she had been deeply distressed, "how she lay prostrated, stunned, turning away from food, completely unable to meet this disaster. Her haggard husband, himself sunk in the deep melancholia which death always produced in him, bent over her, pleading, 'Eat, Mary, for we must live.'" The minister's counsel proved helpful, and she later joined his church; she also wrote a memorial poem for Eddie, which was printed in the *Springfield Journal*:

Angel boy—fare thee well, farewell
Sweet Eddie, We bid thee adieu! . . .
Bright is the home to him now given
For of such is the Kingdom of Heaven.[43]

In an era in which grief and mourning for the death of a child were common experiences, Mary Lincoln's behavior was seen as extreme. In the drama of her grieving, in her refusal to follow the religious imperatives of acceptance, and in her lack of balance, she was somehow deeply disturbing to those around her. Abraham Lincoln's "deep melancholia," by contrast, is presented as ennobling and, at the very least, not insane. It may be that one factor in Mary's emotional state after the death of her younger child was that she was almost immediately pregnant again, with her third son, William Wallace, who was born in 1850, the same year his brother died. In the nineteenth century, losing children and bearing children were commonly closely linked in time, so that women bore grief and pregnancy simultaneously.

When Abraham Lincoln was elected president, the oldest Lincoln son was away at Harvard, and the second was dead and buried in Hutchinson's Cemetery in Springfield, Illinois. The Lincolns brought with them to Washington two boys, Willie and Tad, ages ten and seven, whose doings were chronicled by an avid press, which then, as now, found White House children a ready source of human interest. In early 1862, a year into the Civil War, the Lincoln boys both fell ill in February—probably with typhoid caused by salmonella bacteria, which may have come to them via contaminated water drawn from the Potomac River. The sanitation systems of Washington, D.C., were overtaxed by the exigencies of a wartime population boom and encamped soldiers with very cursory sewage arrangements (a formal sewer system would not be built until twenty years later). The story of the sick boys was followed closely by the press and played out in a city full of sick and dying soldiers, politicians, and military leaders directing a war that now seemed likely to go on and on.

Tad recovered eventually, though it took a while, but Willie deteriorated. He was attended by Dr. Stone, the Lincoln family doctor, who treated him with Peruvian bark, also called cinchona and Jesuit's bark, a natural source of quinine that was a celebrated South American remedy for malaria. Willie also was given calomel, a mercury powder, which was a popular purgative and would have served only to dehydrate him further, and perhaps, if he had survived, to leave him with mercury poisoning. (This is what some biographers have thought happened to Louisa May Alcott, author of *Little Women*. As a Civil War nurse, she was treated for typhoid with mercury, which she believed destroyed her health.) And finally, he was given jalap, another purgative drug, this one derived from the roots of a Mexican plant. He was also offered beef tea and blackberry cordial.

Medical knowledge at the time of the Civil War was still without a theory of bacteriology; infectious diseases were still thought to be "miasmic," caused by bad air or bad odors, and sanitary precautions to prevent diarrheal disease were unknown. (And, for that matter, sanitary precautions around surgery and childbirth were not yet practiced.) Only eight years earlier, in 1854, Dr. John Snow in London had identified a particular pump as the source of infection in a cholera epidemic. In a story famous in epidemiology and infectious diseases, he took the pump handle off and stopped the spread of cholera—though there was not at that point any understanding of bacteriology to support his observations. The bacterium that causes typhoid would not be identified until 1880, and the antibiotics to treat it would not be discovered until decades after that, though decent sewer systems and an understanding of the process of sterilizing water would help a good deal to lower the risks. The idea that a child who was suffering from diarrhea was actually at risk of fatal dehydration had not yet entered medical thought and, in fact, would not until the very end of the century. Instead, diarrhea might well be treated with emetics and purgatives to clear the disease out of the system, which would have the result of increasing the dangerous loss of fluids and electrolytes. Willie Lincoln's death was very much a nineteenth-century death, from an era not just before antibiotic medicine but before there was a clear understanding of the infectious risks of contaminated water—even the knowledge that it could be rendered safe by boiling—and before any awareness of the medical imperative to keep a sick child hydrated.

Willie's death was miserable, with diarrhea and painful abdominal spasms, and probably much like Charley Stowe's death thirteen years earlier. "His mother, frantic with anxiety, hung over him with loving care, oblivious of every other thing in the world. If she could only save the life of her little blue-eyed boy, nothing else mattered." This is how the story was narrated in the very first biography of

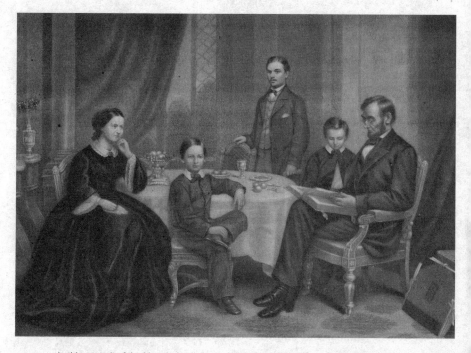

In this portrait of the Lincoln family in the White House in 1861, we see the president looking at a book with one child while the First Lady gazes fondly at another. Their oldest son, Robert (the only child who would survive his parents), stands behind the table. *Alamy Images.*

Mary Lincoln, *The True Story of Mary, Wife of Lincoln,* published in 1928 by her niece, who may have been responding, in part, to criticisms that Mary had allowed an elaborate White House ball to take place two weeks earlier, while her son was sick.[44] The biography goes on to quote a Washington news clipping: "Mrs. Lincoln has not left his bedside since Wednesday night, and fears are entertained for her health. This evening the fever has abated and hopes are entertained for the recovery of the little sufferer." But he did not recover; Willie Lincoln died on February 20, 1862, and "the grief of his parents was too deep for them ever to allude to this sorrow."[45] Tributes poured forth, eulogizing the manly and charming qualities of the child who had died.

Mary grieved, but she ignored many of the conventions of grief: she gave his relics away, she never again entered the rooms at the White House where he had died and been embalmed, and she refused to have Bud and Holly Taft, the brothers who had been the regular playmates of both her sons, invited to the White House again, lest they remind her of the son who had died. Mary Lincoln was very far indeed from one of Harriet Beecher Stowe's bereaved matrons, cherishing a tragic "drawer, or a closet, the opening of which has been to you like the opening again of a little grave," clinging to the sacred relics of the beloved departed child but also bravely carrying on in her womanly duties as center and heart of the family.

The most famous—and perhaps prophetic—story told of Mary Lincoln's mourning was recounted by Elizabeth Keckley, who described herself on the title title page of her 1868 memoir, *Behind the Scenes in the Lincoln White House: Memoirs of an African-American Seamstress*, as "formerly a slave, but more recently modiste and friend to Mrs. Abraham Lincoln." She described Abraham Lincoln leading his grief-stricken wife to the window and pointing out a lunatic asylum: "Mother, do you see that large white building on the hill yonder? Try and control your grief, or it will drive you mad, and we may have to send you there."[46]

Abraham Lincoln's grief for his son, on the other hand, has evoked sympathy and admiration. Lincoln scholar Harold Holzer has claimed that out of that paternal grief emerged a new and more martial Abraham Lincoln, determined to win the war for all the grieving patriotic fathers who had given their sons: "Thousands of fathers had lost sons without losing their love of country or dedication to its preservation. A tougher-than-ever Lincoln now identified with such fathers, emerging from his testing loss a warrior. Willie's death might have been, in its way, the turning point of the Civil War."[47]

Before the country split in two, Jefferson Davis served as secretary of war to President Franklin Pierce. Varina Davis had befriended the first lady (back when there was only one White House with one first lady in it), the tragic Jane Appleton Pierce, a reclusive and diminu-tive woman from New Hampshire who had not wanted her husband to go into politics, let alone run for president. The Pierces had three sons; the first died at the age of three days, the second when he was four years old. The third, Benjamin, was twelve when his father was elected. Two months after the election, the family was on a train near Andover, Massachusetts, on the Boston & Maine line, when one of the train's axles broke and the car derailed. There was only a single fatal injury, as the newspaper report put it: "The little boy's brains were dashed out" before his parents' eyes. The newspaper correspon-dent went on to express concern that "considerable apprehension is felt here lest this melancholy casualty may prove serious in its con-sequences to Mrs. Pierce. She has been for several years in delicate health caused partly by the loss of her first child. The boy killed to-day was almost idolized by his mother and father."

However, a dispatch the following day reported that "the lady of Gen. Pierce is much more resigned to the sad calamity, and the fears which existed that she might not be able to bear up under it are now removed."[48] But, in fact, Jane Pierce did not bear up under the loss of her last son; she did not attend the inauguration, and thus she did not hear her husband begin his inaugural address with the words "It is a relief to feel that no heart but my own can know the personal regret and bitter sorrow over which I have been borne to a position so suitable for others rather than desirable for myself."[49] Though she did eventually move into the White House, she avoided all hostess duties for two years, and she struggled with severe depression for the rest of her life. She blamed her husband and his political career for Benny's death, and she wrote long letters to her dead son and held séances in the White House, hoping to reach him.

Franklin Pierce was also severely affected by the accident, which left husband and wife estranged and unable to comfort each other. Like Lincoln, he is often said to have suffered from melancholia, or depression, and his tenure in the White House was marked by solitary alcoholism, leading to his death from cirrhosis of the liver. Did the violent death of his only living child have something to do with transforming him from a successful military leader turned promising politician into someone now generally listed as one of the worst presidents in our history? Certainly, it tipped his wife over from an already "delicate" state into profound depression and deep hostility toward his political career.

Before the war, Jane had "borrowed" her friend Varina Davis's first child, Samuel, now and then, for the pleasure of holding a baby. But Samuel died of measles in 1854, shortly before his second birthday, leaving Varina deeply depressed and Jefferson Davis so sad that he "could hardly bear the sound of a child's voice."[50] Yet Varina was also pregnant, and she gave birth to a daughter, Maggie, in February 1855. Jefferson Jr. was born in 1857, after which Varina developed puerperal fever, a dangerous infection of the uterus following childbirth, and came very close to dying herself. But she survived and went on to bear three more children over the next seven years, as the nation moved into the Civil War.

At the former White House of the Confederacy, part of the American Civil War Museum in Richmond, there is a group portrait of the Davis children in the former nursery. The one who died in that very room, during the Civil War, was a little boy named Joseph Evan Davis, the fourth child, born in 1859 and said to be his father's favorite. On April 30, 1864, at the age of five—while the Civil War was being fought—he fell off the porch, dropping about fifteen feet to the pavement, and broke his neck—or, in some accounts, fractured his skull—and was carried back into the nursery. Word was sent to his parents, who were both out of the house, at Davis's office in the Custom House, and they arrived while their son was still breathing; he died about forty-five minutes later. "Varina gave way to a 'passionate' outburst of grief while Jefferson began pacing the floor and praying aloud," says her biographer.[51] There was a public funeral, at Hollywood Cemetery in Richmond, where a large crowd watched the

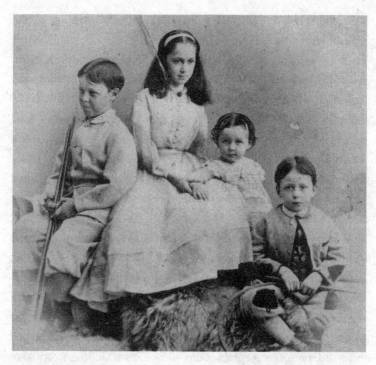

This ghostly portrait of four of the Davis children was taken after the Civil War, and therefore does not include Samuel, who died at a year of age, or Joseph, who fell to his death from a window of the White House of the Confederacy. From left, Jefferson Jr., who died at twenty-one of yellow fever; Margaret, the only child to outlive her parents; Varina, who died in her thirties; and William, who died at ten of diphtheria. *Alamy Images.*

burial; the children of Richmond took up a collection and raised forty dollars for a special memorial stone. A week later, Varina wrote to her mother that she was struggling to accept what had happened; later that spring she was described as depressed and very doubtful about the progress of the war and the future of the slaveholding, white-supremacist Confederacy. She was also pregnant with her last child, a daughter, Winnie, born eight weeks after her brother's accident.

Joey Davis's death, unlike Willie Lincoln's, was not particularly a nineteenth-century child's death; yet it was one that, today, we consider preventable (thanks to window guards, protective fencing, and close supervision). Billy Davis died of diphtheria at the age of ten, several years after the war. The last remaining son, Jefferson Davis Jr., died at twenty-one, on the anniversary of his brother Billy's death, in a terrible 1878 yellow fever epidemic in Memphis. His mother, who had chosen to stay with her husband rather than go to her son, could not forgive herself for that, "and she missed her 'manly witty good son,' the last of the 'four bright strong sons,' the one she expected to rely on in her old age," reports Varina's biographer.

In May 1871, Mary Lincoln and Tad returned to the United States from Germany, where they had been living, to visit her oldest son, Robert, now married and living in Chicago. But Tad, who had just turned eighteen, caught a cold on board the ship, and by early June he was lying "very dangerously ill" in a hotel room in Chicago, attended by several different physicians, "listening with their stethoscopes to Tad's heart and lungs, tapping his pleural spaces to see if there was liquid, encouraging his mother to use hot poultices on his chest, and, to relieve the painful stitch that occurred when the boy breathed, prescribing opium compounds such as Godfrey's cordial or Dover's powders."[52] Whether it was tuberculosis or pneumonia—or, most probably, the one complicated by the other—Tad grew sicker and sicker, and he died miserably of respiratory failure on July 15, in a scene as tragic and melodramatic as any sympathetic biographer could describe: "There were several hours of agonizing distress; then Mary saw her youngest son fall forward in his chair, and the light went out of the dear eyes that had looked at her with Lincoln's own understanding love. . . . For the fourth time in her life Mary lay utterly prostrated with the grief of an irreparable loss. . . . 'I feel that there is no life to me, without my idolized Taddie,' she wrote."[53] Her only remaining son was her oldest, Robert, who had long had doubts about her stability, and who would have her tried for insanity and briefly institutionalized four years later.

Plagued by a variety of medical ailments, Mary survived Tad by only eleven years, dying at the age of sixty-three in one of those melancholy—and melodramatic—coincidences beloved by nineteenth-century authors, the day after the anniversary of his death, July 16, 1882. Or perhaps it was not a coincidence: she experienced great grief and stress on the death anniversaries, and there had come to be so many of them. Perhaps the sorrow and weight of that particular anniversary contributed to her collapse the day before her death, and to the stroke that killed her.

Those two most high-profile children's deaths during the Civil War—Abraham Lincoln's favorite child in the White House and Jefferson Davis's favorite child in the White House of the Confederacy—were small-boy variants of the challenges to nineteenth-century medicine that loomed so large during the Civil War: infection and injury. After the war, slavery would be abolished, but those who had been enslaved would continue to face poverty, racism, and disproportionately high infant and child mortality, though not the horrifyingly high death rates and the systematic death and disease that the slave system had produced. By the 1880s, around one in four African American children died by the age of five, while for white children the number was perhaps closer to one in five, though there was great variation in both rates by region and family circumstance.[54] But for infants and children who got sick, white and Black, there was often relatively little that could be done. Infant and child mortality was in no way an "equalizer," but the ways that abolitionists had used it so effectively to conjure the horrors of slavery perhaps pointed to a certain sad commonality, a knowledge that no children were truly safe. There would continue to be tragic secret drawers, like little graves, in the homes of the rich and powerful, as well as the homes of the poor. Children died and parents treasured their relics, remembered their sad anniversaries, mourned sometimes for the rest of their lives. But the deaths were not preventable, and the illnesses, for the most part, could not be treated—even with ample funds and the finest nineteenth-century medical expertise.

PART II

"The Birth
of a
Great and New Idea"

CHAPTER 3

"We Might Rather Wonder That Any Survive"

Mortality, Miasmas, and Mother's Milk

As a young woman from a good upper-middle-class family in Poughkeepsie, New York, in the late nineteenth century, Sara Josephine Baker had not planned on having a career. But when her father died and she needed to support herself and her mother and sister, she went to medical school. After she graduated, in 1898, she started working as a young novice doctor in poor Boston neighborhoods. One day she was summoned to help a woman who had gone into labor in a top-floor room. "I thought I already knew something about how filthy a tenement room could be," she wrote in her autobiography, *Fighting for Life,* published in 1939. "But this was something special, particularly in the amount of insect life." In one corner was the patient, on a heap of straw, in another, "four stunted children, too frightened to make any noise." Dr. Baker went to examine the woman and discovered that "her back was one raw, festering sore."[1] The woman said her husband had burned her by throwing a kettle of scalding water on her, and at that point the husband himself, who had been lying drunk on the floor, rose to his feet in anger and began to threaten both women, his pregnant wife and the young doctor.

Baker ran out into the hallway, and the husband followed, waving his fist and cursing. "But then," she wrote, "as he lurched after me, he crossed the stair-head and, with instinctive reaction, I doubled my fist and hit him. It was beautifully timed. I weighed hardly half as much as he, but he was practically incapable of standing up, and this frantic tap of mine was strategically placed. He toppled backward, struck about a third of the way down the rather long stair and slid to the bottom with a hideous crash. Then there was absolute silence. I had taken my opportunity and the result was evident. I went back into the room, pushed a piece of furniture against the closed door and delivered the baby undisturbed."[2]

Later on, she wrote, she became somewhat anxious that she might perhaps have committed murder, but "only when the delivery was finished, the room partly cleaned up, the children cared for and the patient made relatively comfortable."[3] When Baker did think about the husband she had so efficiently disposed of, she was too exhausted to be anxious. "It had been sheer reflex instinct; he was in the way and not fit to live anyhow and I had taken the first handy means of getting rid of him. I was not sorry; I was not glad either—it had just been part of the exigencies of this particular job. Well, I thought, as calmly as I could, there is the end of your medical career and probably jail to follow."[4] To her great relief, however, the man was alive and cursing at her as she descended the stairs.

The young Josephine Baker didn't know it yet, when she attended that Boston delivery, but her cause was to be saving babies, in great numbers, and with the maximum possible efficiency. She was training and beginning her career as medical science was fully waking up to the idea that infant death was not an unalterable, unpreventable event—and that awakening may have happened in part because of the growing presence in medicine of women like Baker and her teachers.

As she was beginning her medical practice in the early twentieth century, on average 10 percent of infants in the United States died before their first birthday.[5] In some cities, 30 percent of the babies died in that first year, and those high numbers were of great concern to the progressive reformers focused on urban poverty, including Jane Addams, who in 1889 founded Hull House, a pioneering settlement house in Chicago to serve poor families, and Jacob Riis, who chronicled the conditions in New York City tenements in his 1890 book, *How the Other Half Lives*. Urban infant mortality among the poor was a source of shame, and a problem to be tackled and solved. To give a sense of how much tragedy has in fact been averted by the work done to bring down infant mortality rates, the CDC in 1997 calculated that if those turn-of-the-century mortality rates had prevailed in 1997, 500,000 babies born that year would have died, rather than the 28,045 who did die (note that every death is now registered and counted).[6] Numbers like that are hard to grasp—the reverberating tragedy of half a million families each grieving the loss of a child is impossible to imagine, just as you can't actually rejoice at the idea of only 28,045 of them.

Sara Josephine Baker was born in 1873—thirty-three years before that other, more famous Josephine Baker, the celebrated dancer, whose career she followed with interest and delight, as she pursued her own life of public health work and her healthy babies crusade. *Fighting for Life* is at once idiosyncratic, humorous, and remarkably plainspoken; a physician reviewing the reissued volume in the *New York Times* in 2013 cites Baker's "startlingly modern voice."[7] Baker's story about taking on the drunk husband defines her approach: pick the imperatives, then do what it takes. This meant whatever the "exigencies of this particular job" required: clean up, take care of the children, and so on. To read her book is to hear the direct and humorous voice of a genuinely heroic physician, driven in her life's work by a strong sense of mission allied to what I can only call a strong sense of medical fascination, which drew her into the profession and kept her focused on the dilemmas of health and disease.

Before the Civil War, the American Medical Association noted "the fearful *increase* of infant mortality in New York," and asked the question, "Why should infant mortality in American cities be greater than even in Paris! 8 per cent. above Glasgow, 10 per cent. above Liverpool, and nearly 13 per cent. greater than in London?"[8] The 1857 AMA *Report on Infant Mortality in Large Cities, the Sources of Its Increase, and Means for Its Diminution* placed much of the blame on poverty, hereditary disease, and "abortionism." With increasing urgency as the century drew to an end, such questions were asked as around the world cities and nations began to quantify infant mortality. Early death rates became a matter of national (or urban) pride or shame. Cities were particularly dangerous places for children: industrialization and immigration had moved many poor people into the urban centers of Europe and America, severely stressing their housing, water supplies, and sanitary facilities. In New York, Boston, and Chicago, immigrants were packed into tenements, along with migrants from rural areas, drawn by industrialization and the possibility of factory jobs. Even if children outside cities were dying of the same diseases (and in many cases they were, though much less attention was being paid to rural infant and child mortality at the time), the urban setting meant that many children died in close proximity, giving rise to horrible scenes that seemed out of place in these cities, which also prided themselves on leading the civilized world in fashion, art, and education. Sociologist Viviana Zelizer, in *Pricing the Priceless Child,* places perspectives on child mortality in the context of a "profound transformation in the economic and sentimental value of children" during the late nineteenth and early twentieth centuries: "While Victorian sentimentalists eulogized children, turn-of-the-century American activists were determined to avoid their death. . . . The romantic cult of the dead child was therefore transformed into a public campaign for the preservation of child life."[9]

Richard Meckel's book *Save the Babies: American Public Health Reform and the Prevention of Infant Mortality, 1850–1929* traces the phases of the American response to infant mortality. The first involved recognizing the important role of urban poverty and realizing that government intervention was necessary to prevent diseases that were fostered by filth and sanitary overload; people could not stay clean and healthy simply through individual effort. The British sanitarian movement (what we would now understand as public health, with an emphasis on sanitation and hygiene) took place for the most part within government agencies; the sanitarian reformers in the United States modeled themselves to some extent on the British, but the Americans, at least at the beginning, were doctors and reformers working outside government institutions.[10] The American sanitarians were also, in many cases, training their reformist zeal on immigrant populations, and there was a certain xenophobic tendency to blame "unsanitary" foreign habits for some of the problems that led to the high mortality rates in the cities.

Smallpox drew strength from crowded conditions; cholera rode on the contamination of drinking water with sewage. When the sanitarian movement began, early in the nineteenth century, no one yet understood that disease was caused by microbes; the discoveries of bacteriology and germ theory would come closer to the end of the nineteenth century and the beginning of the twentieth. Yet the sanitarians believed that by cleaning up the environment, they could prevent the spread of many diseases, from cholera to diphtheria to scarlet fever to measles, which were regarded as "miasmatic" diseases, caused by bad odors, bad air, bad vapors, and sewer gas. In fact, the English sanitarians were particularly focused on miasmas, which were understood to concentrate, rather than dissipate, in crowded urban areas. Edwin Chadwick, the author of the very influential 1842 British Poor Law Commissioners' *Report on the Sanitary Conditions of the Labouring Population of Great Britain* liked to say, "All smell is disease."[11]

The miasma theory did include a certain element of contagion. This was the state-of-the-art science in the middle of the nineteenth century, at the moment that Dickens was writing his novels, in a London quite literally plagued by infectious diseases. A further elaboration, the zymotic theory of disease, developed by William Farr, a British sanitarian, argued that fermentation processes within the body of a sick person produced poisonous miasmas that could be breathed in by others. Those same fermentation processes could take place wherever filthy conditions existed, and again, the danger was greatest in cities, where people and waste were concentrated. For all these reasons, the primary focus of these early reform efforts was on garbage and sewage removal, clean drinking water, and home ventilation. The sanitarians believed that these measures would bring about major improvements in infant mortality more quickly and effectively than trying to change parental practices, and in some cases they were correct. In particular, they were concerned about impure air. The 1857 AMA report that noted the high mortality in cities, claimed that many infants in urban slums "perish in a few weeks or months for lack of pure air; and instead of marvelling at the extent and increase of fatality among such, we might rather wonder that any survive."[12]

Recognizing, counting, and combating infant mortality among the urban poor was not a straightforward task—but Baker and her colleagues four decades later were part of a systematic public health attack on childhood death. This campaign would stumble at times but would eventually change the statistics for rural babies as well as urban, and for the children of the wealthy as well as the children of the poor. In an early chapter of her book, Baker tells the story of a reporter who was determined to find an explanation for her unwomanly desire to become a doctor; he decided that it could all be traced to a knee injury she suffered as a young girl, which kept her on crutches and under the care of doctors for some time. "If little Josephine Baker had not hurt her knee, 90,000 babies now alive would have died," she quotes the sappy news story saying, and goes on to argue the point about the knee—but not about the 90,000 babies.[13]

No, she didn't think her knee injury had anything to do with her choice of a medical career. Her life course had been set not by an isolated accident but by a deadly encounter with an infectious disease; such illnesses were by no means confined to the poor, or to

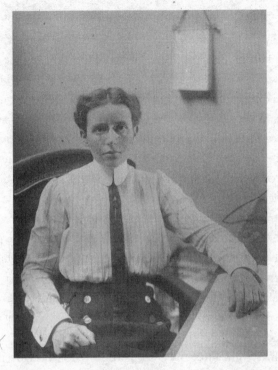

"If I was to be the only woman executive in the New York City Department of Health," Josephine Baker wrote, "I badly needed protective coloring. . . . My man-tailored suits and shirtwaists and stiff collars and four-in-hand ties were a trifle expensive, but they more than paid their way as buffers." *Jessie Tarbox Beals Photograph Collection, The New-York Historical Society.*

the cities. Her prosperous lawyer father died in a typhoid epidemic, his will to live already destroyed, Josephine thought, by the death of her thirteen-year-old brother a few months before. (Despite her medical training, she says only that her brother died "suddenly," and she doesn't seem particularly surprised that such things happened, just as she matter-of-factly mentions that one of her sisters died in infancy.) Faced with the need to support herself, her mother, and an invalid sister, Josephine Baker decided on medicine, and found her way to the New York Infirmary for Women and Children. That institution was headed by Dr. Emily Blackwell, who pioneered medical education and medical practice for women together with her sister Dr. Elizabeth Blackwell, the first woman to attend an American medical school and become a doctor (in 1849). The New York Infirmary was one of quite a number of women's medical schools in late-nineteenth-century America. By the time Baker graduated, in 1898, there were nineteen such institutions, and more than seven thousand female doctors had graduated from them—a dramatic increase in the half century since Elizabeth Blackwell had qualified. By 1868, twenty years after Blackwell, five hundred women had followed her into medicine, and then in the next thirty years, another sixty-five hundred were trained.[14] Baker's training and her career suggest that these first pioneering generations of women doctors brought a new perspective to the practice of medicine, especially to the medical care of women and children.

Baker worked hard at her studies, and she failed only one course. It was called "The Normal Child," taught by Dr. Anne Sturges Daniel, and was the sort of course that was not offered at any other medical school, because no one spent time in medical school studying the normal. Anne Sturges Daniel, born in 1858, was herself a pioneering woman doctor, committed to educating the tenement populations and to helping women in prison; among other things, she persuaded the authorities to hire female wardens for women prisoners. Dr. Daniel was also convinced that doctors needed to understand child health and development. But healthy children did not appear in medical textbooks or medical conversations, and Baker, as an arrogant medical student, scorned the class, did no work, and, accordingly, flunked.

"That was my first, and only, failure," she wrote. "It not only gave a severe jolt to my pride but roused in me a fierce anger at having to take the course over again the following year. I made up my mind that, stupid as it might seem, I intended to learn all there was to know about the normal child." What she learned in that class in 1895 included all kinds of truths and essentials of preventive health and hygiene—the basic elements of keeping children well, rather than caring for them when they got sick—and these principles were still true and essential in 1939 when she sat down to write her life story. "The lectures, I discovered, once I started listening to them, were very fine; the bits of sought-out information most intriguing. As a result, that little pest, the normal child, made such a dent on my consciousness that it was he, rather than my lame knee, who is undoubtedly responsible for the survival of those 90,000 babies the reporter mentioned."[15] The class Baker had failed would be the foundation of her career, and Dr. Daniel's insight that doctors would not understand how to handle sickness in children unless they understood normal health and development was far ahead of her time. "Neither she nor I had any idea that she was preparing me for thirty years of child welfare crusading," Baker wrote. "But, when the opportunity came, I was ready and eager for it, and I, as well as the babies, owe a debt of gratitude to Dr. Daniel which I can never repay."[16]

What was killing off those normal children in their infancy? Diarrheal diseases were a major scourge among infants, with particularly high death rates in hot weather. "More than a quarter of the children born in the civilized world of the second half of the nineteenth century died before their fifth birthday, and nearly one-half of these deaths were caused by the summer diarrheas," Thomas Cone wrote in his *History of American Pediatrics*.[17] The seasonal nature of the "summer diarrhea" led people to see it as a looming epidemic, a menace to be feared, as it came back every year with the hot weather. Newspapers wrote of "the annual epidemic slaughter of innocent babes."[18] The medical name for the sickness was *cholera infantum*, not to be confused with the disease called cholera, the one that caused the epidemic in Cincinnati and killed little Charley Stowe. That cholera, justifiably dreaded throughout the nineteenth century, was a very specific bacterial infection that came out of India in the early 1800s to cause huge epidemics in many Asian, European, and American cities, wiping out children and adults alike with a characteristic copious watery diarrhea that could severely dehydrate·an adult in a matter of hours. *Cholera infantum*, on the other hand, was just another name for diarrhea and vomiting; it described a baby sick with what we would now call a GI (or gastro-intestinal) bug, caused by any of the many viral or bacterial patho-gens that result in those symptoms. Diarrheal disease is still a killer in the developing world; we now vaccinate against rotavirus, which is particularly likely to cause diarrhea in the young and, before the vaccine, as recently as 2003, was still causing over a hundred mil-lion cases of gastroenteritis a year worldwide, and close to half a million deaths in children under five.[19] (Rotavirus was not neces-sarily a major cause of historical "summer diarrhea"—in the United States now, it is largely a winter disease, though it is less seasonal in other countries.)

It was not a new idea in the late nineteenth century that stomach illnesses could be dangerous to babies and small children. Doctors had been worrying over *cholera infantum* for a long time. Many doctors thought it might be connected to teething, which was generally—all the way back to Hippocrates—considered to be a dangerous process, fraught with serious complications, ranging from infections to con-vulsions.[20] Benjamin Rush, a colonial doctor in Philadelphia who was a friend of Benjamin Franklin's, named the disease; one year after he signed the Declaration of Independence, he wrote an article about it, "An Inquiry into the Cause and Cure of the Cholera Infantum."[21] The illness was directly related to the hot weather, he said. "It affects children from the first or second week after their birth, till they are two years old. It sometimes begins with a diarrhoea, which continues for several days without any other symptom of indisposition; but it more frequently comes on with a violent vomiting and purging, and a high fever." His suggestions for how to treat the illness included exacerbating it—giving medications that would make children vomit more (for example, ipecacuanha, derived from a South American root, a powerful emetic, which up until the 1990s we used to give to children who had ingested poisons) or increase their diarrhea (castor oil, for example), so as to get the dangerous "bile" out of their gastro-intestinal tracts.

This was the kind of treatment Willie Lincoln got, as he lay dying of typhoid in the White House. But when sick babies seemed to have naturally purged themselves, Rush advised doctors to soothe them with opiates—which slow down the GI tract, as anyone who has ever been constipated by the painkillers prescribed after surgery would know. Rush suggested a range of other therapies that might alleviate stomach pain and soothe the babies but concluded, "After all that has been said in favor of the remedies that have been mentioned, I am sorry to add, that I have often seen them all administered with-out effect." The best remedy, he thought, was often country air; even before the sanitarian reform movement, there was a sense that clean air might help children stay healthy.

By the time Josephine Baker was training, in the late nineteenth century, reformers looked at *cholera infantum* as an epidemic disease of the tenements, but "summer diarrhea" struck middle-class chil-dren as well, particularly those who were bottle-fed or weaned, since they would have been exposed to potentially contaminated cow's milk or water. Diarrheal disease was responsible for 20 percent of the deaths in children under two across the United States, according to an 1880 count.[22] And depending on who was affected, the disease might be attributed to different causes.

Dr. Rebecca Crumpler, the first African American woman to earn a medical degree in the United States, and a physician who had prac-ticed extensively among the Black population, both in the North and the South, noted in her 1883 *Book of Medical Discourses*: "It has been argued, authoritatively, no doubt, that the causes of cholera infantum are, poor milk, bad air arising from old water-soaked cellars, of tene-ment houses, or when it affects those of all conditions in life, the rich, the poor, the Black and the white,—its cause is said to be in some atmospherical phenomena."[23] So when poor children died of diarrhea, it was thought to be bad air in poor housing (and immigrant parents

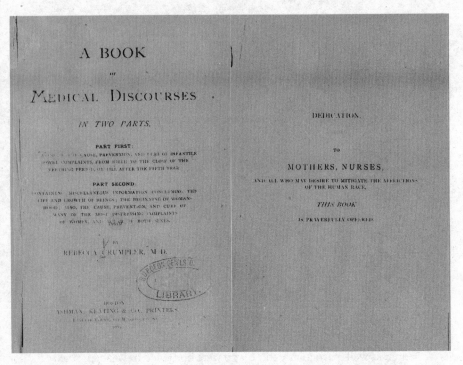

Rebecca Crumpler, the first Black woman to earn a medical degree in the United States, graduated from the New England Female Medical College. She published her *Book of Medical Discourses* in 1883, dedicating it to mothers and nurses (as well as "all who may desire to mitigate the affliction of the human race"). In the introduction, she wrote, "There is no doubt that thousands of little ones annually die at our very doors, from diseases which could have been prevented, or cut short by timely aid." *Courtesy of US National Library of Medicine.*

who kept windows shut against drafts); when wealthy children died, Crumpler remarked ironically, the whole atmosphere was at fault.

Whether children were rich or poor, Black or white, the connection to bottle-feeding was clear; breastfed babies were at much lower risk. In fact, the "second summer" was particularly dangerous for children, because they were more likely to be weaned by then, and drinking cow's milk. Similarly, the long-standing association between teething and diarrhea may have arisen because children got weaned as their teeth came in; they stopped drinking breast milk, with its helpful bacteria and protective maternal antibodies, and started getting cow's milk—which had spent varying amounts of time sitting around, back before refrigeration.

My pediatric training instilled in me a healthy fear of dehydration in small children, and even today part of every physical exam on a sick baby or toddler involves assessing the child for hydration status. We ask how many wet diapers today and how wet were they; we look for abrupt weight loss, especially in young babies, who are regularly weighed at the doctor's office, and who, if they've dropped a pound or two, may have lost a significant percentage of their total body weight. We pinch the skin, checking whether the "skin turgor" is normally elastic; as children get dehydrated, their skin becomes less springy, less able to rebound immediately when pinched. We notice if a baby's anterior fontanel—the soft spot on the top of the head—is slightly depressed, rather than flat, if the mouth is dry or tacky to the touch, if the eyes are sunken. We get a quick index of blood volume by pressing on the skin, squeezing out the blood in the capillaries that supply the skin and then observing how quickly it comes back. And we note all this in the kind of medical language that becomes second nature: anterior fontanel open and flat, mucous membranes moist, eyes not sunken, skin turgor normal, capillary refill good. (Well, what this actually looks like in the physician's note is "AFOF MMM . . .")

All diseases that result in fluid loss are more dangerous to children than to adults, and more dangerous to babies than to children. Babies live on a narrower margin physiologically; they have less fluid in them, and relatively small losses from diarrhea and vomiting can dehydrate them much more quickly. And they have disproportionately large skin surfaces for their weight. That means that anything that is lost across the barrier of the skin is lost disproportionately faster by smaller bodies; it's why babies can get dangerously cold very fast, and even die after delivery if they aren't well wrapped or held against the mother's body. It's also why fluid evaporates quickly out of their bodies across their skin, especially if they're feverish.

When babies show evidence of dehydration, we treat it as a medical emergency; we hydrate them aggressively, often admitting them to the hospital for D&D—diarrhea and dehydration—which we remedy with IV fluids and electrolytes. We know that otherwise their cells will shrivel, and in their blood vessels the thick blood will turn to sludge; they'll also suffer from the accompanying disturbances in body chemistry brought on by dehydration: the imbalances in sodium, potassium, chloride, and other electrolytes, severely disturbing a whole range of body functions. When I was a resident, most of those babies had rotavirus; nowadays they are specifically protected by the vaccine, and there are many fewer such hospitalizations, but babies still get other viral and bacterial infections. And so when we talk about childhood illnesses with parents, we emphasize over and over again that the diarrhea itself is not dangerous to the baby, but the dehydration is.

In modern terms, almost all those hundreds and thousands of *cholera infantum* deaths were probably dehydration deaths, babies drying up and expiring under the eyes of their parents—and their doctors—because they had infectious diarrhea, and because their fluids were not replenished. The nineteenth-century medical writers who described the disease noted the frequent and watery stools, the persistent vomiting, the loss of urine output. They never used the term "dehydration," but they described all the same consequences of fluid loss that I learned to check for a hundred years later: sunken eyes, dry skin, change in skin tone, and a look of emaciation, with the skin in folds. *Cholera infantum* must have been a terrifying disease for parents to witness.

Although fluid and electrolyte theory was still a long way off, Josephine Baker's medical training at the end of the nineteenth century could take advantage of important advances in hygiene, antisepsis, and, finally, germ theory, with the gradual acceptance of microbes, rather than poisonous vapors or miasmas, as the causative agents in many diseases, from cholera to diphtheria to tuberculosis.

In 1856, the French scientist Louis Pasteur, trying to help the French wine industry, found that he could keep wine from spoiling by heating it, thereby inventing the process we call pasteurization. His family's business was tanning leather, and they lived in a wine-making region. Both processes harness microbes, though that was not understood at the time, and much of Pasteur's early research involved unraveling the complexities of fermentation and showing that it could take place only with the help of microscopic organisms. He disproved the idea of spontaneous generation, in which microbes supposedly appeared from nowhere, by showing that if flasks containing meat broth were boiled and then covered, no microbes would appear, while if they were left uncovered, they would become contaminated and microorganisms would grow.

At around the same time, in Germany, Robert Koch was studying anthrax, a deadly disease that attacks cows, sheep, and goats and can be very dangerous to humans as well. Like Pasteur, Koch was focused on threats to important elements of the economy; Pasteur was looking at winemaking and dairies—and also silkworms—while Koch was concerned with farms and livestock. We tend to think of anthrax now in the context of terrorism, but it was another agricultural hazard in the nineteenth century, striking people who worked with domestic animals. Koch purified out the infectious element from animals with anthrax, managed to culture it in the eye fluid of an ox, and injected what he had cultured into healthy animals, showing that they would then develop the disease. He was also able to demonstrate that the anthrax bacteria could form spores, which could survive for a long time in the soil, then start to grow and multiply when they were inside an animal.[24] Pasteur and Koch disliked each other (and played out the national enmity between France and Germany); they are the two great rival fathers of microbiology, for whom the great European institutes of biomedical research are named, and their research established that bacteria could cause spoilage, disease, and death.

In 1866, Pasteur published, in his *Studies on Wine,* a method he had found for destroying organisms that would spoil wine—or milk. He was able to kill these organisms by heating the wine to a temperature just below boiling. His work in bacteriology, however, was not immediately useful in his own family: only two of his five children survived to adulthood; the other three died of typhoid, one of the quintessential diseases of contaminated food and water.

The early version of pasteurization was initially used by milk producers more to slow down spoilage of the milk than to prevent infections, though by the mid-1890s, it was understood to have that effect as well.[25] By 1897, the pediatric textbook authored by Dr. Luther Emmett Holt, the superintendent of New York City's Babies Hospital, had assigned blame for summer diarrhea where it actually belonged, to bacteria, and in 1902, Dr. Henry Koplik said in *The Diseases of Infancy and Early Childhood:* "No matter how carefully it is handled before it reaches the infant, milk passes through many channels, and in each of these it is exposed to infection. The intense heat of summer also favors the increase of infective agents."[26] Infant feeding and pure milk were critical, but for the first time the role of the milk was clear: spoiling in the summer heat, it was serving as a breeding ground for pathological microorganisms.

These American pediatric textbooks, with their careful attention to infant feeding, reflected the growth of a new medical specialty. Doctors in every era and in every culture had always cared for sick children, and some had written about children's diseases, as far back as ancient times. Chinese pediatric specialists in the Sung dynasty (960–1279), and brilliant Persian doctors like al-Razi and Ibn Sina (sometimes called Avicenna) left clear descriptions of the child's body and childhood diseases in the 900s, during the golden age of Islamic medicine. According to British historian Hannah Newton, parents and the medical practitioners in early modern England had a clear sense that children were biologically different from adults:

the doctors of the time argued that children's bodies and brains were dominated by "moist" humors.[27]

Even so, in the western medical tradition, pediatrics as a separate medical specialty, with distinct training and dedicated scientific research, was a relatively new field in the nineteenth century. The great children's hospitals had been established in Europe in the nineteenth century, and American cities had followed suit (in Philadelphia in 1855, in Boston in 1869). Abraham Jacobi, the revolution-minded German immigrant who is usually credited with being the true father of American pediatrics, introduced the term "pediatrics" in the States, and helped to found it as a field that was linked, from the beginning, to advocacy for children. He was much preoccupied with the question of how to feed infants safely and would write extensively on the subject throughout his career.

Jacobi was from a poor Jewish family in Westphalia; he got his MD at Bonn in 1851, but, after being arrested for his revolutionary activities, fled Germany and went to England. He upset Friedrich Engels by appearing at his house in Manchester in the middle of the night, asking to join the revolution. Engels suggested that the "wild Westphalian" might do better in New York, as indeed he did; he arrived in New York City in 1853, and in 1860 he was appointed a clinical professor of the diseases of children at New York Medical College, the first such medical school appointment in the world.[28] Jacobi would later teach pediatrics at Columbia, and his contemporary Job Lewis Smith would have a professorship at Bellevue Medical School.

Jacobi and Smith were, respectively, the first and second president of the first U.S. professional pediatric organization, the American Pediatric Society, founded in 1887.[29] As a professional model, the group tended to envision the new specialty as a smaller and more exclusive group of hospital-based specialists, caring for the sickest children. In contrast, many of the women physicians drawn to working with children were focused on public health and prevention.

Abraham Jacobi fought hard for many years to see pasteurization implemented, bringing over a new German apparatus in 1889; it was welcomed among doctors who worked with poor urban populations, but elsewhere there was a lot of resistance, with even pediatricians objecting to it. As the pasteurization process was refined and improved, the milk came to taste better, and the process gained acceptance. But even in 1912, more than half of the members of the American Pediatric Society believed that babies could get digestive disorders from drinking pasteurized milk.[30]

The discoveries of germ theory were not universally accepted even, among doctors, and the "miasmatic" ideas about disease would still have influence well into the new century. Still, many doctors were now practicing and teaching with a fuller awareness of the infectious origins of much of the disease and death they saw. The new information did not help doctors treat children sick with diarrhea, but it did prompt them to think about preventing infection. And if the problem was that infectious agents were present in the milk babies were drinking, then the milk would have to be purified.

In Europe, the French had taken the lead in the effort to address the problem of infant mortality. The death rate among babies in France was high, as was typical across Europe in the late nineteenth century, and the birth rate was low compared to the rates in Germany and England. The population was not increasing from immigration, either, unlike that of the United States. It became a matter of public and political pride in France to see that as many babies as possible should live to grow up, to work and fight for their country. In earlier eras, medical experts had felt that the only possible (albeit less preferable) substitute for a mother's breast was the breast of a wet nurse and had offered advice on how to choose the right nurse, bearing in mind the general conviction that moral character could be imbibed with breast milk. Although artificial feeding—via bottles of cow's milk or infant formula—was becoming popular in the nineteenth century, the French medical establishment made a better bet than the American milk reformers, who sought to sanitize commercially available cow's milk. The French, instead, put their national money on breastfeeding, right from the beginning, perhaps in part thanks to the legacy of Jean-Jacques Rousseau, whose 1762 book *Émile* had proposed that maternal breastfeeding might lead to a total moral and social transformation of society: "Let mothers deign to nurse their children, morals will reform themselves, nature's sentiments will be awakened in every heart, the State will be repeopled."[31]

Marie Antoinette, as queen of France, tried hard yet failed to nurse her first child in 1778. She went on to subsidize ordinary mothers in France with monthly stipends, which were higher if the mother nursed her own child than if she employed a wet nurse. This movement was not about science; breastfeeding was a spiritual and moral imperative. The goal was to bind families—and, therefore, societies—closer together. But the effect was to establish a French custom of breastfeeding, even by those wealthy enough to employ substitutes, while celebrating the virtue of the nursing mother.

The eighteenth-century breastfeeding movement spread through Europe and crossed to America. Women were assured, often by men, that nursing was easy, beautiful, natural, and sacred. From other women came a more realistic acknowledgment that nursing a baby was not always either simple or beautiful, and that many women, then as now, struggled to succeed at it and were sometimes desperate for alternatives. In Great Britain, in 1798, as part of the breastfeeding cultural moment, William Roscoe, a poet, scholar, abolitionist, and botanist in Liverpool, published an extremely successful breastfeeding tract in verse, a translation of a poem written more than two hundred years earlier by an Italian poet, Luigi Tansillo. The English edition was dedicated to Roscoe's wife, who had nursed their own ten children, and it went through several editions. It urged women, however wealthy or poor they might be, to nurse their children:

Let the sweet office be your constant care;
With peace and health in humblest station blest,
Give to the smiling babe the fostering breast.[32]

Those lines reached the United States, where they were quoted in the first chapter of *The Maternal Physician*, published in 1811 by "An American Matron," who built on the health and well-being of her own eight thriving children to advise mothers that they could be their own children's doctors.

The author, Mary Palmer Tyler, felt that any woman could breast-feed successfully, but Tyler also clearly felt that she would need to argue some women into it, and to that end, she recounted a some-what harrowing story of her own persistence: "My first child had the thrush when about a fortnight old." Thrush, a fungal infection that can thrive in young infants' mouths, is still one of the most common problems a pediatrician sees—and the worry is always that it will pass back and forth between the baby's mouth and the mother's breast, where it can cause severe irritation. "Now I took the humour from his mouth, and for two months he seldome sucked without throwing up fresh blood afterwards, which he had swal-lowed with the milk. The torture I endured can better be conceived than described." Her friends urged her to wean the child, but "my own mother, who watched over me and my babe with more than maternal tenderness, and who, I am convinced, felt all I suffered with redoubled anguish, constantly exhorted me to persevere with fortitude, nor let any thing I endured tempt me to tear my babe from the breast, and by improper food occasion ill health, if not endanger his life; for amidst all my distress I had the inexpressible delight of seeing him thrive surprisingly." She listened to her mother and was richly rewarded for doing so, "for the days of affliction passed away as a dream, and left the sweet consciousness of having done my duty as a recompense for suffering; a recompense, how right, how lasting, how consoling!" And so the American Matron urged her readers to do likewise: "I entreat every mother to undergo every thing short of death or lasting disease, rather than refuse to suckle her child."[33]

Dr. Rebecca Crumpler, in her 1883 *Book of Medical Discourses,* echoed the American Matron in encouraging all women to breast-feed, but also in acknowledging that many of her readers might struggle, especially in the first month of an infant's life: "It is well to bear in mind that a scarcity of milk during the month should never be taken as an excuse for refusing to nurse the child; for if it can get but a spoonful a day, it greatly encourages the chance for increasing it." She did not hesitate to stress the essential value of nursing: "The mother's milk is the fountain of life to the babe, and therefore seldom dries up unless there be some unnatural obstruction." Furthermore, and perhaps alone among the medical authorities writing on the topic (maybe because she had practiced among a recently enslaved population), she gave a thought to the wet nurse's own child and pointed a rather severe moral about selfishness at those who expected others to nurse their children: "A lady of wealth may get discouraged and give her babe to the care of another, whose baby may in consequence have to be put in some charity-house or otherwise to board. Her baby may thrive and live; while that of her wet-nurse may soon pine away and die. No one can avoid distressing others unless he strives, to the best of his ability, to bear his own burdens."[34]

The health benefits of breastfeeding went well beyond protection against impure milk. Pasteurization could make cow's milk safe, but it could not replace other essential ingredients in breast milk. In an era in which infectious diseases were major causes of mortality, breastfeeding meant that when babies were youngest and most vulnerable, they were receiving maternal antibodies against many common infections, though that immunity was not understood at the time. Since a mother was almost certain to have had measles, the baby would get antibodies against measles. Babies were less likely to get scarlet fever than older children, because their mothers passed along antibodies. These maternal antibodies, manufactured by the mother's immune system against the various infections to which she has been exposed, everything from measles and diphtheria and whooping cough to chicken pox and cholera, cross the placenta to the fetus and are also passed in the breast milk. The process, which we call passive transfer, does not provide lasting immunity to the baby, because the antibodies last only while they are circulating in the baby's blood, and the baby's immune system will not take over and produce more until there is an actual infectious exposure (unless the baby is vaccinated, but more about that later on). The late-nineteenth-century reformers who urged mothers to nurse were telling them that they had the ability to care for their babies in ways that would significantly change the odds of surviving beyond the age of one, and that the way to do this involved close skin-to-skin contact between mother and baby. Thus, they were indeed changing family life, promoting the most basic biologic bonding.

Meanwhile, most American pediatricians and public health reformers in the late nineteenth century focused less on encouraging breastfeeding and more on making the non-human milk supply safe, as well as figuring out the correct scientific way to mix it into baby formula. Prophetically, the author of The Maternal Physician had complained, back at the beginning of the century, that not all doctors were sufficiently supportive of nursing by well-to-do women: "I have often been vexed with physicians who, while they exhort us to follow nature, from a misplaced indulgence to the prevailing fastidiousness of the age, adopt the absurd notion that a mother cannot endure the fatigue of suckling her own child."[35]

Josephine Baker wrote that "the pasteurizing process was already known, but the great bulk of milk consumed by the poorer people was 'grocery' or 'loose' milk, unpasteurized, originating from all sorts and conditions of dairies, sold in dubious containers, and undoubtedly one of the most prolific sources of babies' and children's diseases." Milk came into New York from many different states, all with different rules and standards, and it sat without refrigeration in stores and in

homes. "Under those circumstances," Baker pointed out, "telling a tenement mother to give her child so much milk a day was like telling her
to give him a diluted germ-culture daily."[36] The effort to improve the
milk supply and, especially, to make it safe for young children, would
represent the next major phase of the American battle to prevent diarrhea and bring down the number of summer deaths.

As far back as 1842, Robert Hartley had published "An Essay on
Milk," describing the filthy—and unregulated—conditions prevailing
in the dairies that supplied New York City's milk; a particular object of
reform was "swill milk," distributed by dairies adjacent to distilleries,
where cows were fed on distillery waste.[37] This diet, essentially boiled
grain with very limited nutritional value, was particularly unhealthy
for the cows. They would initially refuse to eat it, and when they were
finally driven to it by hunger, they lived very short and unhealthy
lives, during which they produced a thin bluish milk; this was then
adulterated with chalk and other additives to make it look better and
was widely sold. There were public health and temperance campaigns
against these dairies for decades, and eventually better train service
throughout the Northeast meant that milk could be brought in from
the country and sold relatively cheaply in the city. But that unadulterated milk was not necessarily safe, either. Rural cows could have
tuberculosis, and rural dairies were not necessarily sanitary. Every
stage of getting the milk from the cow to the child was fraught with
opportunities to introduce germs and impurities: the milk was often
diluted by the sellers or doctored with various substances to hide
signs that it had spoiled; the containers were not necessarily clean or
covered; homes had no means of refrigeration; and cups and bottles
might be washed with contaminated water.

The American Public Health Association was founded in 1872,
seven years after the end of the Civil War. The organization grew in
part out of the older "sanitarian" movement, which had held a series of
National Quarantine and Sanitary Conventions, trying to set standards
for reducing the spread of infections. In its early years, the new public

health organization focused especially on the control of tuberculosis, even before the infectious nature of the disease was clearly understood; it also took on other major epidemic diseases, such as yellow fever.

By the turn of the century, the public health movement was looking at milk and its dangers, as well. Between 1880 and 1895, in response to the public outcry against swill milk, many cities passed ordinances designed to regulate the sale of milk and to prevent adulteration. Inspection and enforcement were difficult, especially given the complex chain from dairy to middleman to seller. In 1905 the American Public Health Association published *Standard Methods for the Examination of Milk*. The problem was not only that milk might be deliberately diluted; there was increasing evidence that even unadulterated milk could cause infectious disease, from typhoid to tuberculosis. Milk came to the cities by complicated paths, and there were so many points at which it could be contaminated with bacteria and viruses.

By then, most states had boards of health, applying the new science to check the chemical composition of milk, but the real responsibility—and expense—in this field fell at the municipal level, where issues like water supply and sewer systems were understood to be essential for the health of all. Germ theory—the understanding that microbes caused human disease—meant that even the wealthy had to worry about what might be lurking in the water or the milk, and had to understand that the well-being of others in the city who perhaps handled their food or cared for their children might have a direct bearing on their own health.[38]

Pasteurization was first made compulsory in Chicago in 1908. Mandatory purification came to New York City in 1912; a year earlier, only 15 percent of the milk supply in New York had been pasteurized.[39] The New York City Department of Health initially ruled that two kinds of milk were acceptable, pasteurized milk or milk from "certified" carefully inspected dairies with high standards of hygiene. But after some cows with tuberculosis were found even in the model dairies, certified milk had to be pasteurized as well.

In the United States, many leaders in the new pediatric profession placed great emphasis on the proper feeding of infants. Unfortunately, this often meant denigrating the expertise—and experience—of mothers and nursemaids, who did not have the benefit of full medical training and a pediatric specialization. In the name of medical science, some practitioners managed to create such scientific "mystery" around the feeding of babies that bitter controversies about how to get it precisely correct raged even among medical professionals. Meanwhile, the advice given to those actually caring for and feeding the babies was sometimes too complex for anyone to follow without a laboratory and laboratory assistants.

Two of the most important figures in the founding of American pediatrics, Thomas Morgan Rotch and Abraham Jacobi, speaking from Boston and from New York, respectively, ran up against each other in a long-lasting debate about how formula should be prepared and what mothers could be asked to do. Dr. Rotch, the first professor of pediatrics at Harvard Medical School, developed a system of preparing food for infants that was called "percentage feeding" or the "American method." He believed that formula had to be individualized for infants, that "what is one infant's food may be another's poison."[40] The milk proteins, fats, and sugars had to be carefully regulated or indigestion would result, and the proportions had to be changed as the child grew—thus the term "percentage feeding." This method was widely adopted by American pediatricians during the 1890s, though it never gained much support abroad. This medicalization of infant feeding was part of how pediatrics established itself, for if scientific measurement was necessary for safe infant nutrition, then highly educated men in white coats were essential intermediaries. Rotch's formulas were so complex that, complained one pediatrician, they "required almost the equivalent of an advanced degree in higher mathematics, employing algebraic equations to compute the food mixture for a baby."[41] The Walker-Gordon company, working together with Dr. Rotch, established laboratories in many cities—twenty by 1907—and began producing "laboratory milk" for the doctors to use.[42]

Dr. Abraham Jacobi, Rotch's New York colleague, had no patience for percentage feeding; his comment on the method, famously, was "You cannot feed babies with mathematics, you must feed them with brains."[43] In his 1885 work *Infant Diet,* he argued for a simple mixture of boiled cow's milk and cane sugar, diluted with barley water or oatmeal water; the degree of dilution could vary according to the infant's age and weight. Unlike many doctors, Jacobi was notable for his early and consistent advocacy of boiling the milk: "It destroys the germs of typhoid fever, Asiatic cholera, diphtheria and tuberculosis, also the many bacteria which cause the change of milk-sugar into lactic acid and the rapid acidulation of milk with its bad effects on the secretion of the intestinal tract."[44]

Rotch and Jacobi disagreed on how to mix formula, but they both believed it was important to get the recipe right, because so many women were not able to breastfeed adequately. Jacobi, who would later reverse his position on this and come back to breastfeeding, wrote that "a woman with a markedly nervous temperament is generally unsuitable for the office of nursing, since her milk is liable to become deficient in quantity or perverted in quality." Rotch, the high priest of precision formulas, worried that human milk production was highly complex, and "when from any cause this sensitive machinery is thrown out of equilibrium its product is at once

Opposite, top: As part of the movement to make purified milk available to the poor, the philanthropist Nathan Straus established milk dispensaries in New York City; here, a young girl picks up milk at one such dispensary. (The sign to the left of the door reads "Pasteurized Milk Depot Open.") *Library of Congress, Prints and Photographs Division, LC-B2-4374.*

Opposite, middle: Nurses working in a milk laboratory at the Infants' Hospital in Boston around 1915. *Boston Children's Hospital Archives, Boston, Massachusetts.*

Opposite, bottom: At the Pure Milk Depot at the Morningside Presbyterian Church in New York City, milk was provided to mothers and young children. *Courtesy of the New York Academy of Medicine Library.*

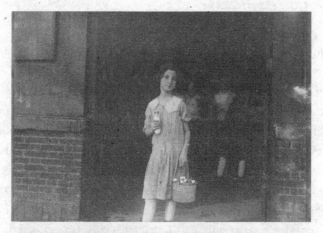

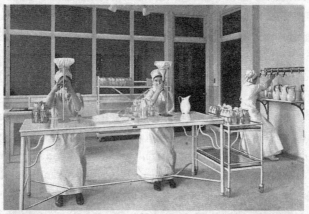

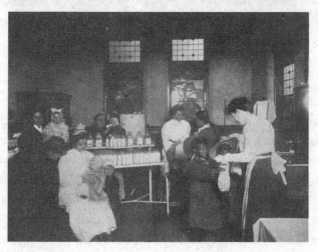

changed, sometimes but slightly, but again to such an extent that the most disastrous consequences may follow when it is imbibed."[45] And in his popular 1894 book, *The Care and Feeding of Children,* presented in question-and-answer form, Luther Emmett Holt, speaking from Columbia University, wrote directly to mothers: "Worry, anxiety, fatigue, loss of sleep, household cares, social dissipation, etc., have more than anything else to do with the failure of the modern mother as a nurse. Uncontrolled emotions, grief, excitement, fright, passion, may cause milk to disagree with the child."[46] This is a long way from the confidence of the author of *The Maternal Physician,* advised by her own mother, valiantly nursing her way through pain and blood, to a confident happy outcome.

Abraham Jacobi also urged setting up places "where the poor could buy clean milk at a fair price," and in response, Nathan Straus, a department store owner and philanthropist, established pure milk depots and pasteurization plants in New York City. There was certainly demand; the dispensaries were established in 1893, and by the summer of 1895, they were selling more than six hundred thousand bottles a summer, each for the price of one cent (infant formula) or one and a half cents (regular milk). Within fifteen years, they were up to four million. The milk was packaged in specially designed bottles with round bottoms, so they could not be left standing unstoppered, which was supposed to prevent later contamination.

———————— // ————————

In the United States, the census of 1900 asked women how many children they had borne and how many of those were still alive. The numbers brought home the fact that infant mortality was still high throughout the country. Though the highest infant mortality rates, up to 30 percent of live births, were in cities, it was a rural problem, too. Those numbers for the United States represented more complete data than had ever been available before. In their 1991 monograph, *Fatal Years: Child Mortality in Late Nineteenth-Century America,* Samuel

H. Preston and Michael R. Haines carried out a sophisticated demographic and statistical analysis of that census and were able to show high mortality figures toward the end of the nineteenth century among the wealthy and privileged as well as among the poor. The Bureau of the Census, established by Congress in 1902, began to publish regular—and standardized—reports of deaths by age and by cause in what was called the Death Registration Area (comprising ten states, the District of Columbia, and more than 150 individual cities). Most of the infant deaths were attributed to three causes: diseases of the digestive system, which would have included all forms of diarrhea; diseases of the respiratory system, which covered everything from influenza to pneumonia to TB; and congenital problems, which included prematurity, congenital malformations, and "congenital debility" or weakness.[47]

Josephine Baker had opened her private practice in New York City in 1899, but soon after, needing extra income, she responded to a notice in the newspaper and took a test for a civil service job, to be a medical inspector for the department of health, because it paid thirty dollars a month. She found the job dispiriting: she was supposed to go to schools and check children for infectious illnesses, but she was expected to visit three or four schools in an hour, and the medical attention was perfunctory at best. Many inspectors, she thought, didn't even bother to go to the schools and look at the children. The department of health, she wrote, was ineffectual and full of political hangers-on; the place "reeked of negligence and stale tobacco smoke and slacking."[48]

But the following year, 1902, saw changes, with a new mayor and a new commissioner of health. She was offered a position for the summer in tracking down and caring for sick babies, and she accepted. "It was an appalling summer too," she wrote, "with an average of fifteen hundred babies dying each week in the city; lean, miserable, wailing little souls carried off wholesale by dysentery." She worked in Hell's Kitchen, mostly among Irish immigrants, though the northern part of the district also had a Black population. Everyone was desperately poor. "I climbed stair after stair, knocked on door after door, met drunk after drunk, filthy mother after filthy mother and dying baby after dying baby. It was the hardest physical labor I ever did in my life: just backache and perspiration and disgust and discouragement and aching feet day in and day out." She was never mealymouthed, never out to make herself seem selfless or saintly. She said things about her patients that would certainly not pass today as sufficiently sensitive but that clearly reflected her own willingness to knock on those doors and to come to grips with the conditions in which people were actually living: "The babies' mothers could not afford doctors and seemed too lackadaisical to carry their babies to the nearby clinics and too lazy or too indifferent to carry out the instructions you might give them."

But she felt for the mothers, and she could see that "lazy" or "indifferent" did not imply uncaring. "I do not mean," she explained, "that they were callous when their babies died. Then they cried like mothers, for a change. They were just horribly fatalistic about it while it was going on. Babies always died in summer and there was no point in trying to do anything about it. It depressed me so that I branched out and went looking for healthy babies too and tried to tell their mothers how to care for them. But they were not interested. I might as well have been trying to tell them how to keep it from raining."[49]

The new chief of the health department, Dr. Walter Bensel, started looking into situations where no sick babies were being reported in certain poor districts and found that many doctors were not actually keeping track. A major shakeup occurred, with dozens of inspectors losing their jobs and Josephine Baker herself promoted to Dr. Bensel's assistant, in a position to think about addressing the problems of infant mortality on a much larger scale: "The more I thought of it," she remarked, "the more I could see that this was a matter between me and the babies."[50]

In the first decade of the twentieth century in the United States, babies were still dying in large numbers of summer diarrhea. "Even New York's worst slums have now forgotten what dysentery epidemics were like," Josephine Baker wrote in 1939. "But we knew thirty years ago."[51] By 1913, there were 297 stations providing milk to the poor in 38 cities, most run by charities, some by municipal health departments, but they did not end the summer diarrheal deaths.[52] For all the large numbers of milk bottles given away and sold, the total added up to only a small portion of the milk being consumed by poor urban children.[53] Most poor mothers could not come every day to pick up their supplies, and so the result was that instead of being used to prevent disease, as the only pure food given to a child after weaning, the clean milk was sometimes used when children got sick and their parents became worried.

The milk stations would eventually use the milk as a kind of lure: mothers would come because they could buy safe milk, but they would also be educated, taught how to mix that milk into formula for their infants, which some doctors felt was a complex process beyond the reach of the ordinary mother.

As pasteurized milk became the rule in American cities, in the second and third decades of the twentieth century, summer diarrhea mortality did indeed go down, and it dropped most quickly in the cities that were earliest in requiring pasteurization, such as New York.[54] "Like everyone else in the medical profession of the day," Baker wrote, "I had been trained in the then unimpeachable Rotch school of milk-modification, which was based on consideration of the baby's age, health, complexion, nationality, color of eyes and numerological and astrological data—or at least so it seemed when you started working with it." She directed the stations to use—and teach—a much simpler formula, based on Abraham Jacobi's directions, which simply called for mixing milk, lime water (a solution of calcium hydroxide), and sugar, according to the baby's weight—but the pediatricians who supported her efforts requested anonymity, expecting a furor. "Once again high and mighty medical associations called me a murderer," she wrote. "And once again I was able to demonstrate with figures that the babies I was murdering were much livelier little ghosts than the city had ever known before."[55]

CHAPTER 4

"Each Has a Right to Live"

Educating Mothers and Keeping Babies Alive

I n the summer of 1908, New York City was anticipating the deaths of fifteen hundred babies a week, based on what had happened in earlier summers. The milk stations were operating, but it was not clear that they were preventing the summer diarrhea deaths, and pasteurization was not yet the law. Josephine Baker was allowed to try an experiment, employing the thirty nurses used for school inspections, who were free for the summer. She selected "a complicated, filthy, sunless and stifling nest of tenements" on the Lower East Side of Manhattan, inhabited mostly by newly arrived Italians—she referred to the generic "Mrs. Capozzi." She hoped that these mothers might be receptive to "learning the American way of caring for babies," for as each new birth was registered, a nurse would be sent out to visit the home, ideally within hours.[1]

What did the nurses teach? "Nothing revolutionary; just insistence on breast-feeding, efficient ventilation, frequent bathing, the right kind of thin summer clothes, out-of-door airing in the little strip of park around the corner—all of it commonplace enough for the modern baby, but all of it completely new to Mrs. Capozzi and all of it new in public health." In fact, she wrote, the mothers did not object to having perfect strangers show up, but tended to regard the visits as part of the strangeness of a new country. "Many of these mothers were a little flattered to have an American lady take all that trouble about little Giovanni, and were likely to go out of their way to learn and to cooperate." In Baker's voice, it is possible to hear the persistent condescending attitudes about immigrants and poverty that often accompanied public health interventions, though she also makes it clear that babies were dying as well in the supposedly hygienic nurseries of the well-to-do.

There were tensions and disagreements between the nurses and doctors and the mothers, and certainly the mothers were selective about which pieces of advice they chose to follow. And there was teaching and learning in both directions. Dr. Alice Hamilton, a pioneer in the field of occupational health, worked as a physician at Hull House in Chicago at the turn of the century, that early and exemplary settlement house that provided social and educational opportunities to a working class and largely immigrant population. She wrote in her autobiography that with the immigrant mothers, "I gave what I had been taught was the best advice about feeding babies—nothing but milk till their teeth came. When I see the varied diet modern mothers give their babies, anything apparently from bacon to bananas, I realize that those Italian women knew what a baby needed far more than my Ann Arbor professor did. I cannot feel I did any harm, however, for my teachings had no effect."[2] (She went on to say that seeing a baby chewing on salami had come to suggest to her that the baby was getting the benefit of garlic, "full of most valuable vitamins.")

But much of the advice on preventing infections was new and useful (as it would be useful to mothers all over the country when the Children's Bureau published its pamphlets), and mothers in the tenements were aware of the dangers threatening their infants and willing to try new strategies to protect them. The practice of sending what we would now call "home visitors" to help at-risk families with newborns has become one of the most reliable ways of helping babies and mothers stay healthy. New mothers who were far from their own families may well have been happy to have female "experts" come to the home to offer help and advice, as Baker wrote: "As soon as they saw that their babies were flourishing, despite the cruelly hot weather, they became our most efficient aides."

Baker herself had the sense that the nurses were making a difference, but she was surprised by how great a difference. Although the death rate in the rest of the city was as high as ever, there were twelve hundred fewer deaths in her chosen district than there had been the summer before. "We had saved more babies than there were men in a regiment of soldiers and I had learned one certain thing: heat did not necessarily kill babies." Late that same summer, she was made chief of the new Bureau of Child Hygiene within the New York City Department of Health, the first such bureau in the world, she wrote. They had figured out how to save babies in large numbers, and she had found her true mission: preventive public health and the education of mothers. "There," she wrote, "if we have to be dramatic about it, was the actual beginning of my life work."[3]

Milk activists had been working for decades to make the milk supply safe, sanitarians had fought to clean up the cities, but the new century was underway and babies were still vulnerable. Josephine Baker, working with a group of statisticians, had learned that a third of the deaths in New York City were those of children under five, and a fifth involved babies under a year. Now, armed with this information, in 1908, her first year as head of the new Bureau of Child Hygiene, she remembered back to her days of going from house to house, several years before: "Interesting figures beyond any doubt; perhaps they impressed me so particularly because they were not just cold statistics to me at all. I had served my time in that long, hot summer in Hell's Kitchen when I walked up and down tenement stairs to find in every house a wailing skeleton of a baby, doomed by ignorance and neglect to die needlessly." And thus Dr. Baker realized that she was approaching a "startling idea," one that would shape the rest of her life: "The way to keep people from dying from disease, it struck me suddenly, was to keep them from falling ill."[4]

The visiting nurses could also check on pregnant women, though Baker would later regret that prenatal care had not been more heavily emphasized. The milk stations and dispensaries that had been opened in poor urban neighborhoods could become places where babies received not only milk but also medical care. Richard Meckel cites a New York health report from 1909 in which a visiting nurse recorded a mother bringing her sick infant to the Bellevue Hospital dispensary on July 15: "The doctor says child has not been getting enough nourishment." This was followed by two visits by the nurse to the home: "I ordered milk and showed mother how to prepare it." The baby came back to the dispensary: "Doctor told mother to alternate breast feeding with a prescription of milk. Nurse showed mother how to make prescription." There were more visits to the home, more trips in to the dispensary, and by August 8, still in those dangerous summer months, the nurse recorded: "Called. Mother and baby are looking better. Baby is doing very well. House was in better condition than nurse has ever seen it before. Baby is now getting along upon its mother's milk. . . . I shall keep the family under observation until the mother and baby are both perfectly well."[5]

Josephine Baker and her New York City Department of Health colleagues were part of a burgeoning international movement. The network of milk dispensaries had brought together a new array of philanthropists and activists, committed to the idea of bringing down infant mortality, and they would continue to play an important role in the child welfare movement.[6] The problem of infant mortality and the challenge of bringing it down had become a much more widely discussed, more urgent public concern, throughout both Europe and the United States. "The first two decades of the twentieth century witnessed a virtual explosion of public concern over infant mortality and the consequent emergence of an international infant welfare movement of truly immense dimensions," Meckel wrote.[7]

This public concern, this new sense that infant deaths could and should be prevented, had grown in part out of the nationalist feeling that the fate of a country's babies was more than a domestic family-by-family issue; there was a sense of civic and political ownership, as in those patriotic French attempts to bring down infant mortality for the sake of increasing the population of future citizens, workers, and soldiers. The deaths of children were no longer considered just intimate—and inevitable—domestic tragedies, private family matters occasioning personal sadness, and reflections of the will of God. If population increase was a national goal, then infant mortality truly was a "social problem" and could be mitigated by social improvements. The popular images of child death would no longer center on the "neat little white funeral" that Baker described encountering again and again in the poorest streets of Hell's Kitchen, or on the sentimental verses that a bereaved mother might write—or read—for her own comfort, or memorial photographs or a keepsake drawer full of abandoned tiny clothes. Instead, there was a growing idea that child deaths were in fact, in many cases, preventable and that it was not just a parental obligation to prevent them but a social responsibility. Over the course of the twentieth century, infant mortality would become (and remains) an index to how a country is doing, a kind of global scorecard, a gauge of progress and of commitment to the well-being of the most vulnerable members of the population.

During the first several decades of the new century, infant mortality rates would come down dramatically. The many people in many disciplines who took on the problem and the organizations that worked to bring about decreasing rates thus deserve huge credit for saving lives and, in fact, for bringing about a major change in the collective experience of family life. But there were also more problematic elements that informed this new discussion on how to save babies, ranging from the rhetoric of blaming poor families for their poverty, to the patronizing—and sometimes frankly racist—ideas about immigrants, to the troubling conversations about racial purity and eugenics.

In 1906, George Newman published *Infant Mortality: A Social Problem*. Newman was trained in both medicine and public health, and he was a Quaker with a strong social conscience. His book claimed that infant mortality had not really been lowered by the many attempted sanitary and public health reforms of the second half of the nineteenth century and argued that neither cleaning up the milk supply nor any other single answer could solve what was, as the title suggested, a social problem. He argued that while infant mortality was often higher in poor communities, there were also many exceptions: geographical or ethnic subgroups where the poor did not lose disproportionate numbers of children in infancy. "Under some of the worst external conditions in the world the evil is absent," he observed. "It is difficult to escape the conclusion that this loss of infant life is in some way intimately related to the social life of the people."[8] So the social problem was not just poverty. It was more specific to the way people lived. If babies did not have to die, then along with an increased sense of social responsibility came an increased sense of parental responsibility.

Thus, Newman's tremendously influential book helped draw attention to the ongoing issue of infant mortality but also helped reformulate it as a problem of maternal education. "The social life of the people" would come to mean the domestic, hygienic, and maternal skills of the mother, above all, and the way to save the babies would become, increasingly, to teach mothers how to do their job properly. Reformers would continue to argue that the mother's job also required social supports—prenatal and pediatric medical care, maternity leave after giving birth so that breastfeeding was possible, clean water supplies and decent housing—but in many cases, those reforms, which continued to loom as complicated, expensive, and politically difficult, took a back seat to the idea of maternal responsibility and the imperative to educate women.[9] If infant deaths were unavoidable in the warm weather, then a fatalistic acceptance was the only possible rational attitude on parents' part, together with the insurance payments that would cover that sad little funeral. (Baker notes that even the poorest families, perhaps knowing how common it was for babies to die, always insured their infants.)[10] But if proper hygiene and good parenting practices could keep more babies alive, then it became the responsibility of the parents to learn those practices, and the responsibility of society to teach them, and perhaps even enforce them.

There is a long and not terribly honorable tradition in medicine, including in my own field of pediatrics, of blaming mothers. Most dramatically, this happened with the disgraceful attempt to claim that cold, rejecting "refrigerator mothers" caused their children to develop autism, a classic case of doctors and researchers who hadn't found an explanation deciding that it must be the mothers' fault. Recently I was talking to a pediatrician who studies childhood obesity in the twenty-first century, one of the biggest health problems with which pediatricians in the United States are currently grappling, and not very successfully. "When medicine does not understand a problem, we blame it on personal responsibility," she said. "We blame it on bad parenting." So let's be clear: housing conditions and poverty can in fact pose serious dangers to the health and growth of children, at the beginning of the twenty-first century just as at the beginning of the twentieth. While it is always a good thing to provide parents with education and support, it is completely false to suggest that scrupulous attention to the rules of good parenting and hygiene can offset the depredations and dangers of poverty and racism.

But in the first decade of the twentieth century, it was maternal education that became the major rallying cry of the new international alliances that were emerging to save babies. One after another, European countries responded to the problem: the Ligue contre la mortalité infantile was founded in France in 1902; the Dutch National

League (Nederlandsche Bond tot Bescherming van Zuigelingen) in 1908, and the German Union for the Protection of Infants (Deutsche Vereinigung für Säuglingsschutz) in 1909. There were national conferences and international conferences, and in 1907, the formation of the International Union for the Protection of Infant Life. What is perhaps most striking about this is that none of these organizations had existed before, in countries with long traditions of organized medicine. Infant mortality was not only being discovered—or rediscovered—but it was being formulated as a problem to be solved, nationally or internationally, and a battle to be fought and won, a critical issue for countries concerned about having the population necessary to fuel industry and maintain a strong military.

In the United States, the American Academy of Medicine held the Conference on the Prevention of Infant Mortality in New Haven in November 1909. The president of the academy, who organized the conference, was a doctor named Helen Cordelia Putnam. She had been educated at Vassar and before medical school had done a stint there as director of physical education, which was to be one of her lifelong causes. After getting her medical degree at the Women's Medical College of Pennsylvania, and then training in Boston at the New England Hospital for Women and Children, she moved to Providence and practiced gynecology, advocating early on for better prenatal care for the poor and taking part in the movement to bring safer milk to cities.[11] In 1907, she attended a conference in England on school hygiene, where she heard discussions about the infant mortality problem; she was particularly inspired by George Newman's assertion that "it becomes clear that the problem of infant mortality is not one of sanitation alone, or housing, or indeed of poverty as such, *but is mainly a question of motherhood.*"[12]

At the 1909 New Haven conference Putnam directed, infant mortality was addressed as a multifaceted social problem, one that needed the attention of medical professionals, philanthropists, government institutions, and social workers; those were the four sections of the program, but the overarching theme was that the key to prevention lay in education for mothers.[13] The meeting ended with the formation of a new organization, the American Association for the Study and Prevention of Infant Mortality, or AASPIM. Josephine Baker tells the story of the mayor of Boston counseling her to change the organization's name, because it was much too long, and adding, "Nobody is going to write anything as long as that on a check. By the time they get halfway through, they will change their minds."[14]

The society held its first meeting at Johns Hopkins a year later, in November 1910. The president, J. H. Mason Knox, was a pediatrician who had been deeply involved in the effort to clean up the milk for the city of Baltimore.[15] His presidential address at that first meeting stressed the importance of collecting accurate data; the registration of births in the United States was still far behind what was being done in Europe, and without reliable numbers, it was impossible to calculate infant mortality. In America, infant mortality was being formulated as an institutional deficiency: babies needed maternal and child health centers, health bureaus (and bureaucrats), multidisciplinary conventions, and research meetings. Like all such societies, this one was almost immediately in the business of perpetuating itself, but the message was clear: supporting mothers and getting babies through infancy safely was not a simple goal; lots of structure needed to be in place at the local and state levels, and lots of expertise needed to be brought to bear.

The emerging social recipe for taking on this persistent problem of infant mortality involved a mixture of medical science and social science, including the bureaucracy required to track populations and count births and deaths, and a new set of services to be provided directly to families to ensure healthier pregnancies and healthier homes. What we think of as modern prenatal care was beginning to take shape, in an attempt to safeguard maternal health; Baker herself was involved early on in the question of licensing and regulating midwives. There was also a strong element of social engineering in the discussion, and along with the drumbeat of anxiety about military readiness, especially in Europe, there were also sometimes chilling elements of race purification and eugenics. Even as the experts insisted that many babies could and should be saved, some of the baby savers were concerned that certain babies should never be conceived or born in the first place. Rousseau himself, back in the eighteenth century, had written, "Fix your eyes on nature, follow the path traced by her. . . . Sickness and danger play the chief part in infancy. One half of the children who are born die before their eighth year. The child who has overcome hardships has gained strength. . . . This is nature's law; why contradict it?"[16]

It was a relatively new idea, after all, that babies who would otherwise die could be saved, and there were those who worried that saving babies meant preserving the weak, the ones nature had "intended" to weed out, and thereby damaging the community—or the nation—or "the race." Darwin's ideas about evolution and natural selection had offered a new perspective on Rousseau's "natural laws," and had been taken up by others in the second half of the nineteenth century and applied to human societies as social Darwinism, again suggesting that a society that took too much trouble to support its "least fit" members might weaken itself in the great struggle for existence. In 1883, the British scientist Francis Galton had coined the term "eugenics" to describe improving humanity by systematically selecting for desirable inherited characteristics. Galton was especially focused on the need to encourage worthy and able couples to marry and procreate, though the term also came to encompass discouraging—or even preventing—others.

The incoming president-elect of the new American Association for the Study and Prevention of Infant Mortality for 1911 was a sociologist, Charles R. Henderson, a professor at the University of Chicago who had a past career as a social activism–minded minister in Detroit. He had helped arbitrate a streetcar strike there in 1891 and was widely regarded as sympathetic to workingmen. He was also the author of an 1893 book, *An Introduction to the Study of the Dependent, Defective, and Delinquent Classes,* in which he had written, "The evolution of the race, the victory over evil, the prospect for the entire disappearance of the defective stock . . . indicate that we are moving toward an age when it will be easier to hold unquestioning and unclouded faith in the absolute and eternal truth, love, and beauty of God."[17]

In a section of the book called "Social Arrangements for the Education, Relief, Care, and Custody of Defectives," he was profoundly concerned with preventing certain groups from reproducing. He was especially worried about those he termed "feeble-minded," a group that would certainly include people with what we would today call intellectual disabilities and developmental delays but also encompassed those with epilepsy and numerous other conditions. Among other measures, he advocated strongly for the forced removal of all "feeble-minded" children from their families—for the families' own good, whether they knew it or not: "The defective child injures the family to which it belongs, if it is kept at home. It is a source of constant humiliation, annoyance, often of physical danger, loss of time and energy, weakness of the mother, and vicious example to other children."[18] If the parents were themselves "defective," he explained, not only should the child be taken away, but the parents should be separated "to prevent more mischief"—that is, to prevent them from having more children. To prevent the "feeble-minded" from reproducing, Henderson argued, it would not be enough to enact laws against their marriage or their sexual activity, since "many of this class do not understand morality, law, or penalty any more than animals." He invited his readers to imagine an ideal system in which these "feeble-minded" children would live happily "in isolated agricultural colonies, held in gentle and safe custody, enabled to produce their own food, and so to live happy and contented lives, without becoming the irresponsible progenitors of a miserable posterity."[19]

Epilepsy, he argued, was hereditary and "makes the person unfit for marriage and parenthood."[20] And again, the most stringent measures would be necessary: "It has been recommended to enact legislation making the marriage of epileptics illegal; and medical men are unanimous in advising against the union of persons afflicted with this disease. . . . But, as in the case of the insane and the feeble-minded, it is not enough to make such unions illegal; they must be made impossible by segregation and strict custody by officers of the state."[21]

Eugenic thought was very much in the mix in the early twentieth-century Progressive movement, and it was also an important element in the discussions of "national deterioration" that were taking place in Europe. The British, for example, worried about the high proportion of their young men who could not pass the physical examination certifying them as fit to be soldiers. For many of the reformers, in Europe and in America, the pseudoscience of eugenics appeared to be a plausible modern approach to moving humanity forward, improving the physical and mental status of the human race as a whole, and building better babies to build better adults. George Newman had brought it up in *Infant Mortality: A Social Problem* when he wrote, "The 'unfit' appear to marry more frequently than otherwise, and not infrequently both parents are 'unfit.' . . . Whilst it may be impossible, or indeed undesirable, to arrange marriage purely on a basis of physical fitness, we must not lose from sight the fact that physical unfitness is the source in many cases of infantile disease in the offspring."[22] Those working to decrease infant mortality had to answer the pseudo-Darwinian objections of those who believed that infant death was a cruel but necessary part of natural selection. Henderson saw it as a challenge; crusaders against infant mortality would have to make their desire to save lives go hand in hand with a "scientific vision of the progress of the race."[23] Infants needed to be saved, he said, even if they were feeble and unfit, and yet caring for increasing numbers of those feeble and unfit people would be a problem for the nation; thus certain groups should be prevented from bearing children in the first place.

L. Emmett Holt, the distinguished pediatrician from New York, responded to this same concern in his 1913 presidential address, as the argument echoed back and forth throughout the early years of the association and its work. Holt argued that many healthy babies were killed or disabled by disease, so fighting disease among the young would actually work to increase those who could grow up strong, healthy, and productive. Yet he acknowledged that in the battle against infant mortality, some unfit children might indeed be spared to grow up, and he offered a highly eugenic solution to the problem: "We must eliminate the unfit by birth, not by death. The race is to be most effectively improved by preventing marriage and reproduction by the unfit, among whom we would class the diseased, the degenerate, the defective, and the criminal."[24] These ideas, so distasteful to the modern ear, were actually seen as forward-thinking and progressive in their time; Abraham Jacobi himself, an outspoken and definitely left-leaning pediatrician of strong social conscience, was in favor of preventing marriages that would propagate the unfit.

In 1911, the AASPIM passed a resolution urging states to enact laws that would stop the propagation of the unfit, including surgery— that is to say, forced sterilization. The eugenics movement in the United States would be increasingly prominent in the 1920s, and it would take on an increasingly racist anti-immigrant tenor with the publication, in 1916, of the best-selling book *The Passing of the Great Race*. Politicians and others warned of "dilution" of the American population with too many southern and eastern Europeans. The idea of sterilizing certain groups of medical "undesirables" gained political traction, and starting with Indiana in 1907, thirty states passed laws allowing compulsory sterilization. As many as thirty thousand adults, many from poor and marginalized populations, were sterilized during the 1920s and 1930s in government programs directed at people with epilepsy, at "degenerates," and at the "feeble-minded."[25]

Preventing unfit children from being born was an important focus for Charles Henderson as an academic sociologist and criminologist, but it was essentially a side issue for most of those who were actually dealing with babies and dedicated to bringing down infant mortality. Yet they, too, tended to resort to social Darwinism in acknowledging that not all babies could—or should—be saved. It was worth battling summer diarrhea, a preventable problem that struck down otherwise healthy, "fit" babies who had already survived the newborn period. The ones who could not (and perhaps should not) survive, they believed, were the babies who died in the first month of life. Neonatal mortality reflected congenital anomalies, or prematurity, or just a general condition of weakness; these were the babies born without the wherewithal to live. Newman discussed a range of social problems (including mothers who were undernourished or badly overworked during pregnancy) that might exert a prenatal influence on these babies: "In spite of the tendency of nature on behalf of the new-born child, poor physique and ill-nutrition of the mother exerts, in a considerable percentage of cases, an injurious effect upon the infant."[26] But the prevailing opinion was that when such injured infants were born, medicine had little to offer. William H. Welch, the founder of the Johns Hopkins School of Hygiene and Public Health, and one of the most prominent physicians in the United States at the time, told the AASPIM that mortality in the first month of life was not preventable. Of the three major causes of infant mortality, they should focus their preventive energies on deaths from gastrointestinal disease and from respiratory disease and leave congenital problems alone, for there was nothing to be done about them. So spoke the "dean of American medicine," and one of the founding fathers of public health, in the year 1910.

The United States Children's Bureau was established in 1912, and its chief, Julia Lathrop, was the first woman ever to head a federal bureau. Her own life and her family history reflected very strongly that array of "good causes" that Mary V. Cook, one of the founders of the National Association of Colored Women, said owed their success to "the push of women." Julia Lathrop had been born in Rockford, Illinois, a few years after the Civil War ended; her mother had been an abolitionist, as well as a suffragette. (To be fair, her father, who was in politics, was also in favor of votes for women.) The young Julia's own causes included women's rights and the treatment of the mentally ill; after she heard a presentation by the founders of Hull House in Chicago, she left her job in Rockford to go and live at Hull House, where her experiences included home visiting and inspecting residential facilities for the mentally ill and disabled, including poorhouses and juvenile jails. She was a reformer through and through, and her experiences made her suspicious of official incompetence and corruption; it was after twenty-two years at Hull House that she was asked to take the position in Washington at the Children's Bureau.

Lathrop disagreed with those who thought that health advice should be written by the usual pundits—male doctors, in this case. Instead, she hired Mary Mills West, a widow with five children, to write pamphlets about child care—the first, *Prenatal Care,* was followed, logically enough, by *Infant Care*—and to reply by mail to the questions readers sent in (her name was printed in the pamphlet as "Mrs. Max West" to emphasize her married status). "There is a real strategic advantage," Lathrop said, "in having them come from a woman who has herself had the experience of bringing up a family."[27]

Establishing the federal Children's Bureau had been one of the recommendations of the first White House Conference on Children and Youth, convened by President Theodore Roosevelt in 1909. Because the child welfare movement had focused on the issue of child labor, the new bureau was situated within the Department of Labor, but it had a much broader mandate, ranging from infant mortality to juvenile justice—and it was also charged with gathering good statistics.[28] Therefore, researchers carried out a detailed study of Johnstown, Pennsylvania, in 1913, interviewing the mothers of all children born in 1911. They collected a tremendous amount of detail, showing that the infant death rate went up among babies of mothers over forty, for example, and that it was higher among babies born to new immigrants or to illiterate parents. They were also able to document a strong correlation between family income and infant mortality rate.

The Children's Bureau did a study of infant mortality in eight cities between 1911 and 1915; it showed that the death rates for children who were not breastfed were three to four times as high as for those who were. This was the first careful statistical measurement in the United States of a truth that had been clear to anyone working with infants.[29] The study also provided some reliable numbers as to how many women, and which ones, were breastfeeding: 57 percent of babies were exclusively breastfed for their first nine months of life, 25 percent were exclusively bottle-fed, and 18 percent got a mixture. Foreign-born women were more likely to breastfeed, especially Italians, Poles, and Jews. Rural mothers, Black and white, tended to breastfeed longer than urban mothers. In Baltimore, at the age of six months, legitimate children were twice as likely to be breastfed as illegitimate children, whose mothers were presumably more likely to have to work or to place the child in an institution.

The milk stations and dispensaries in New York were thriving by 1915; the baby health stations operated by the city alone were caring for more than thirty-seven thousand children under a year of age, which represented 26.9 percent of the total infant population of the city. As an International Health Board report stated: "When we add to this number the infants reached by municipal home-visiting nurses, private milk stations, and private home-visiting nurses, as well as by other organizations, it will be seen that under existing conditions a very large proportion of the infant population of the city annually comes in touch, for a varying period of time, with the educational influences of the Bureau of Child Hygiene and affiliated infant-welfare agencies."[30] The stations provided what we would now call well-child care; sick infants were transferred to hospitals or doctors. After carefully correcting for as many epidemiologic variables as possible, the mortality rate among the children "enrolled" at the baby health stations was 41.26 per thousand. "The rate among those

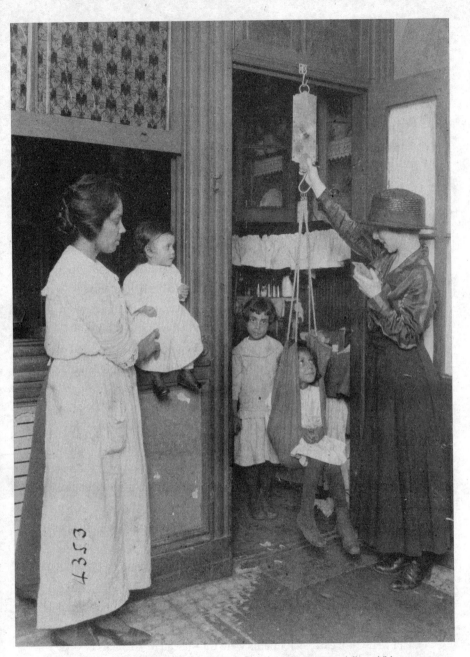

The nutritionist at the Mulberry Health Center in lower Manhattan weighs a child as part of a weekly check on growth and general health, while the mother and siblings look on. *CSS Photography Archives, Weekly Weighing of Children, 1920, #4353. Courtesy of Community Service Society of New York and the Rare Book & Manuscript Library, Columbia University.*

not cared for," noted the report, "but belonging to the same age group and living under conditions approximately similar, was found to be about 84.1."[31]

In 1915, the U.S. Children's Bureau reported that there were 539 such stations in 142 cities; they were being operated by 205 different agencies, some municipal and others philanthropic. (Another reminder of the ways health care in the United States has always been and continues to be a kind of patchwork quilt, delivering care by bringing together public, private, and philanthropic entities in a way that people in other countries find almost impossible to understand.) The milk stations and the agencies supporting them were also more consciously trying to promote breastfeeding, whether by sending nurses to visit new mothers or by asking for medical certification that a mother could not nurse before providing milk. Educating mothers, in many cases, meant emphasizing the dangers of bad food or impure milk: "DON'T KILL YOUR BABY!" read a 1910 poster in seven languages (English, Polish, Yiddish, Bohemian, German, Lithuanian, and Italian) created by the Chicago health department. It advised the use of clean milk from a clean bottle but insisted, "MOTHER'S MILK IS BEST OF ALL."[32]

By emphasizing education for mothers while offering what we would now call well-baby care to their infants, the stations were also making it clear that their goal was something beyond giving handouts to the poor, or what was then referred to as "outdoor relief" (as opposed to the "indoor relief" of institutionalization). American philanthropy was supposed to build self-reliance and, ultimately, to reduce dependency. By teaching mothers to prepare formula, to keep the milk clean, and in general to meet higher standards of health and hygiene, the milk stations could strengthen families. Lillian Wald, the social reformer who founded community nursing in the United States, called it "our principle of building up the homes."[33]

Anything like state-supported medicine in the United States has always brought opposition from some elements of the medical profes-

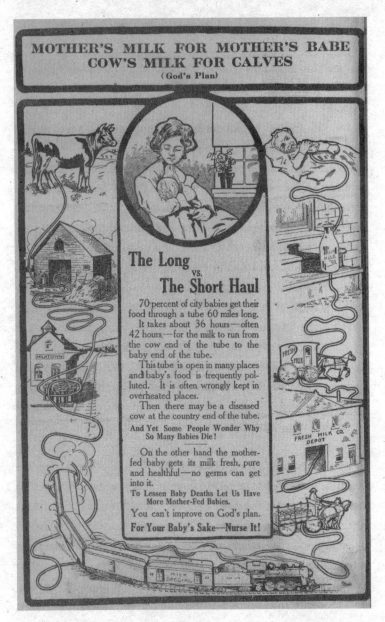

"To Lessen Baby Deaths Let Us Have More Mother-Fed Babies." This 1911 poster from Chicago promoting breastfeeding made a strong appeal to religion, but it also reminded mothers, with a graphic illustration, of the long, often tortuous, and perilous road that milk had to follow to get from cows to urban babies. *From the* Bulletin, *June 3, 1911, Chicago School of Sanitary Instruction. The Oak Street Library, University of Illinois at Urbana-Champaign.*

sion, and there were certainly physicians who resented or felt threatened by these milk stations, especially as they began to provide more and more infant care. The centers and clinics were also used, right from the beginning, as places to train young doctors. This linked them to academic medicine, where elite doctors tended to look down on their colleagues in private practice in the tenements, who were sometimes viewed as profiteering off the poor. By 1915, most of the more than 790 doctors participating at the stations were volunteers who came for a few hours every week, many of them young doctors (overwhelmingly male, because that was the face of the profession) eager to gain experience at a time when most hospitals did not offer the kind of postgraduate medical training that teaching hospitals do today.

But the nurses—900 of them working full-time—were the true front line. Lillian Wald, the founder of the Henry Street Settlement, which had grown into the New York Visiting Nurse Service, had started out as a visiting nurse herself, working in the tenements on the Lower East Side. She had raised support for the service by describing the details of her routine practice: "My first call was on the Goldberg baby whose pulse and improved condition had been maintained after our last night's care. . . . After luncheon I saw the O'Briens and took the little one, with whooping cough, to play in the back of our yard. On the next floor, the Costria baby had a sore mouth for which I gave the mother borax and honey and little cloths to keep it clean."[34] The nurses practiced in the stations, but they also went out into the neighborhoods to find the babies—Jewish, Irish, Italian—and to bring care to them directly, in the crowded buildings where the immigrant families were living.

The Lincoln School, founded in 1898 in the Bronx, with a mission to train African American women for nursing, graduated its first class of six nurses in 1900. Lincoln School nurses would play a prominent role in addressing tuberculosis in the Black communities of New York and Philadelphia, later in the twentieth century.

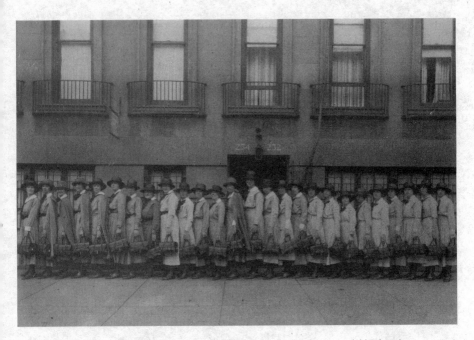

Nurses were the front line in caring for children and families in poor neighborhoods, and the social reformers at the Henry Street Settlement in New York City pioneered new roles for school nurses, and for visiting nurses as well. *Courtesy of the Visiting Nurse Service of New York.*

Elizabeth Tyler, who had finished a course of training at the Lincoln School, was hired as the first African American visiting nurse at Henry Street, by Lillian Wald, but when Tyler faced prejudice from the patients at the settlement, she moved her practice uptown, to San Juan Hill, an area on the West Side of Manhattan, near Columbus Circle, with a large Black population. At Stillman House, a new settlement house she helped found on Sixty-Second Street, Tyler, along with other pioneering African American nurses like Edith Carter and Jessie Sleet Scales, provided health care to a community with very high rates of tuberculosis, malnutrition, and infant mortality.

Many of the innovations put in place by the New York Bureau of Child Hygiene were picked up by other cities around the country, including sending nurses to visit mothers immediately after they

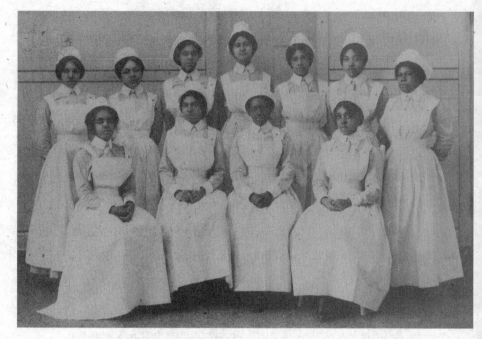

In 1898, when institutional racism made it difficult—or impossible—for Black women to train at white nursing schools, the Lincoln School for Nurses was founded in the Bronx. It graduated its first class in 1900 and continued to train nurses until 1961. *Photographs and Prints Division, Schomburg Center for Research in Black Culture, The New York Public Library.*

gave birth and using school nurses in the summer. Josephine Baker also pioneered clubs for poor and immigrant girls of twelve and up, who were often left to take care of their younger siblings. According to John Spargo's highly influential 1906 book about child labor, *The Bitter Cry of the Children*, these "little mothers" were doing their best, and "many of them show a wonderful amount of courage and precocity in dealing with the babies intrusted to their care." But they were also dangerous to the babies, so "inexperienced and ignorant" that their infant charges often died, and they were themselves the victims of "a great social crime," he wrote, since their own childhoods had been taken away from them in the service of providing care to their younger siblings.[35] His proposal was that mothers should not be allowed to work in those early months but should receive financial "pensions"; if mothers did have to work (since those pensions were not available), the babies should be placed in nurseries, or *crèches*, which, though less than ideal, he argued, "are far better for the children than the neglect or the ignorant handling of 'little mothers' from which they now suffer."[36]

But the *crèches* were not available, any more than the pensions. "We could not afford the luxury of saying things should or should not be," Baker wrote. "Since thousands of poor families were in an economic situation which made the little mother necessary, we had to turn her into something that suited our purpose." Baker decided to teach the young girls how to take care of their younger siblings, she organized a Little Mothers' League in New York City, held classes, and gave out badges (this was all happening right around the same time as the founding of the Girl Scouts, in 1912). "These youngsters," she reported, "were among our most efficient missionaries, canvassing tenements for us, cajoling mothers of their acquaintance into giving the baby health stations a trial, checking up on mothers who had backslid in attendance at the stations, telling every mother they met all about what they were learning." With her usual good humor, Baker described the dramatic plays the Little Mothers put on in which inconsolable babies were comforted and errant nutritional habits corrected by the knowledgeable twelve-year-olds. When the girls were asked to provide a list of "don'ts" for mothers of young children, she wrote, the answers included "Don't give the baby herring," "Don't give the baby beer to drink," and "Don't leave the baby sit on the stove."[37] Again, other cities and states picked up the Little Mothers' League idea.

Just as the initial formulation of the infant mortality problem in the United States had centered on immigrants in cities, so the outreach that happened in the second and third decades of the twentieth century was very variable by city and state. Rural children had initially received very little attention, with the focus on cities and their tenements, but when the federal Children's Bureau put out its *Infant Care* pamphlet, in 1914, which became the most popular publication ever issued by the Government Printing Office, it was particularly in demand among rural women, many of them far from other medical expertise.[38] While the pamphlet emphasized the importance of seeking medical advice when a baby got sick, the author acknowledged that "many mothers are so situated as to be unable to command the services of a physician at once," and, further, that "in all cases of illness the discretion and self-control of the mother are of infinite assistance to the doctor, and when the physician's services are not immediately available the life of the child may depend on the coolness and wisdom of the mother."[39]

The pamphlets were sent out by the tens of thousands from the bureau to women all over the country, distributed by legislators to their constituents, and passed around from mother to mother. The bureau had trouble keeping enough in stock to meet the demand. By 1921, almost a million and a half copies of *Infant Care* had been disseminated, and in June 1929 the bureau estimated they had affected half of the babies in the country. More than 125,000 letters a year came back to the bureau in return, asking for help and advice: "He looks to be anaemic but I really don't know what to feed him. . . . If it is possible for you to send me a prescription for a good tonic to build him up and give him an appetite I would be very thankful to you for same."[40] "I would like to know is it now too late to train him not to cry after me. . . .. Please send me some advice as to how I can wean him & to stop him from clinging to me so."[41] "My baby is breast-fed and now two months old. [He] is gaining in weight about half a pound a week, but his bowels are not normal. . . . He is very cross and seems to be in pain before his bowels move."[42] The pamphlet stressed the importance of hygiene—fresh air and sunshine, clean water, breastfeeding and purified milk—and warned against the dangers of flies, which could spread diarrhea germs. The author acknowledged the dangers of a long list of diseases, from measles to hookworm to trachoma to tuberculosis, which was described as "one of the common and fatal diseases of childhood."[43] When I read

Infant Care, I am struck by the very strong emphasis on producing "a properly trained baby," though it also encouraged gentle care with such comments as "Harsh punishment has no place in the proper upbringing of the baby. A baby knows nothing of right or wrong, but follows his natural inclinations." In fact, if the baby did not behave well, the pamphlet suggested, the problem could probably be traced to "physical causes" that might well be the mother's fault: "Babies who are fussy, restless, and fretful are usually either uncomfortable in some way because they have not been properly fed and taken care of, are sick or ailing, or have been indulged too much."[44]

The federal Children's Bureau was not the only evidence of new and stronger government interest in the health and well-being of children. In 1921 Congress passed the Sheppard-Towner Maternity and Infancy Protection Act, with bipartisan sponsorship, which provided funding to thousands of child and maternal health centers working with state departments of health. This act was fought strenuously by the American Medical Association (fearing "socialized medicine") and by the political Right, and in June 1929, funding was allowed to lapse. "Asserting that mother love was all women needed to raise healthy children, Sheppard-Towner opponents called the bill's emphasis on scientific childrearing information an insult to American motherhood," wrote historian Molly Ladd-Taylor, who studied mothers' letters to the Children's Bureau; its opponents described the act as "an 'invasion of the castle of the American citizen' . . . and accused the Children's Bureau staff of being spinsters and Communists."[45] Economists looking at the effects of the act in retrospect, comparing states that participated with states that didn't, have estimated that Sheppard-Towner funds and the health centers they supported were responsible for between 9 and 21 percent of the decline in infant mortality over the period during which the act was in effect. Most of the impact was on mortality among the non-white population.[46]

In the activities of many other reformers working to bring down infant deaths, urban or rural, there was much less attention paid to deaths in the African American population, despite the fact that Black babies were dying at twice the rate of white babies in several southern cities. And in the rural South, there had been very little effort made to reach the Black population by the public health reformers, with few health stations or visiting nurses. Some areas were served by African American physicians, and the local teaching hospitals, like Freedmen's Hospital in Washington, D.C., associated with Howard University College of Medicine, were important sources of health care for Black families during the era of segregation. There were 1,465 African American doctors in 1905, and 85.5 percent of them had been trained at the eight Black medical colleges, all but two of which closed in the years after the 1910 Flexner Report, which set high professional standards that many smaller and poorer schools could not meet; the report also led to the closing of many of the women's medical colleges. Of the Black medical colleges, only Howard and Meharry Medical College qualified, and many of the medical schools that remained after the Flexner Report would be slow to open up to African Americans and women.[47]

Diarrheal diseases were still taking a terrible toll on the rural African American population as late as 1920. With funds from the Sheppard-Towner Act, some southern states did begin trying to reduce infant mortality among Blacks. There were certainly Progressive reformers who viewed racial equality as part of the agenda—Ida B. Wells, the anti-lynching activist, founded a Chicago settlement house to serve the Black community, and the NAACP was founded in a 1909 meeting at the Henry Street Settlement—but there were also racist assumptions by many experts who believed that excess Black infant mortality indicated that the babies represented an inferior, weaker stock or who attributed greater infant mortality in the Black population to less competent Black midwives. Even in northern cities with large Black populations, the focus of the reformers' work was often European immigrants, and there was less outreach into Black neighborhoods.

Meanwhile, despite all the most correct hygienic practices, as well as state-of-the-art nursing care, half the babies in the New York City foundling hospitals that cared for orphaned and abandoned infants died. Josephine Baker was called in to inspect the facilities and could find no deficiencies: "By that time I had acquired a flair for hospital inspection and there was apparently absolutely nothing wrong. Intelligent, well-trained nurses carrying out the last technique to the letter, absolute spotlessness and sanitation, approved feeding; nothing was wrong except that the babies were dying like flies, poor little wretches." She began to wonder, though, as she thought about those unfortunate foundlings, whether there was a connection to be made to another puzzle: while reformers' efforts to inculcate principles of hygiene and nutrition seemed to be bringing the death rate way down in the tenements, the infant death rate in the wealthy districts was proving harder to move. "Sometimes," she wrote, "it really looked as if a baby brought up in a dingy tenement room had a better chance to survive its first year, given reasonable care, than a baby born with a silver spoon in its mouth and taken care of by a trained nurse who knew all the latest hygienic answers."

So Baker's team tried an experiment, not quite believing that it would work, with those foundling babies, half of whom would otherwise be expected to die in the foundling hospitals. They sent them to live with the mothers in the tenements, "actually removing them from the admirable conditions of the hospital and exposing them to the hazards of slum conditions. Poor mothers, who had already had experience in raising families under supervision of the Bureau of Child Hygiene, were paid ten dollars a month to become foster mothers of foundling babies until they were well started on the problem of staying alive." And it worked: "In four years we had only one foundling in three dying where one in two had died before, and the decrease would probably have been much sharper if we had had funds and facilities for boarding them all out." Accordingly, the program was extended to include babies from the "hopeless ward" of the foundling hospital, where premature and "obviously moribund" babies were given good care, albeit in the gloomy expectation that all would die: "Any scrawny, bluish, half-alive baby that went there, to be wrapped in cotton wool and fed with a medicine dropper, was morally certain to fade out after a little while, and through nobody's fault at all." So there was no harm to be done by boarding them out: "We began moving these poor little potential ghosts out of this ward where everything was light and sterile and spick and span, into tenement rooms on Hester and Orchard streets. Offhand it sounds like murder."

But instead, some of these doomed babies thrived: "the foster mothers worked miracles. We reduced the death rate among these hopeless cases from practically one hundred percent to a little over fifty percent in one year." In the era before antibiotics and before routine childhood immunizations, there were plenty of hazards, perhaps especially in the crowded conditions of the tenements, to which these babies would be exposed when they left the hygienic conditions of the hospital. And yet they were surviving in much greater numbers. Again, Baker reflected on the high mortality rates among wealthy infants: "There were the rich children, beautifully taken care of by white-starched professionals, dying with uncanny readiness as soon as something went wrong with them. There were the slum children who, given halfway proper feeding and care, could stand up under diseases that would have killed the rich children. There were the wretched little foundlings dying wholesale under fine hygienic conditions and flourishing, relatively anyway, when conditions were much worse—but, very significantly, when they began to get personal care from a maternally minded woman." In both situations, the babies had paid caregivers, but the tenement mothers were doing better than the trained nurses.

Baker went on to speculate that growing up in the tenements necessarily exposed children to a wide variety of diseases, strengthening their immune systems, which made it easier to keep those children healthy, once their basic needs were met. In addition, perhaps it was the love and affection and regular handling by that "maternally minded woman" that made all the difference. "That was why," she wrote, "I became and still am a firm believer in mothering for babies: old-fashioned, sentimental mothering, the kind that psychologists decry. . . . There is little doubt in my mind that many a baby has died for lack of it." Babies needed that, she concluded, even more than they needed "butterfat and fresh air and clean diapers."[48]

Baker's observations on institutionalized infants were prescient; the emerging evidence over the twentieth century would show that even when many of the medical problems had been solved, babies did not thrive and develop well in institutions.[49] Clearly, she also wondered whether some of those wealthy babies, being raised by trained nannies, were suffering from some of the same deficiencies, perhaps in maternal affection, perhaps in contact with other children and a certain microbiologic rough-and-tumble that left a child better able to withstand illnesses. Today, we would probably look to developmental evidence about the importance of close interactions early in life, from skin-to-skin contact (which we now suggest should begin in the delivery room), to the "language bath" that surrounds young children as they grow, to the "serve and return" back-and-forth that shapes babies' brains, in which a young child communicates with a parent and gets back an immediate response. We talk about those interactions now as a foundation of early brain development, for language, for cognitive growth, and also for social and emotional development. The foster mothers in the tenements could not keep all the foundlings alive, of course, any more than they could keep all their own children alive; then again, several decades into the twentieth century, though the shamefully high infant death rates in the tenements had been brought down, even wealthy parents could not feel confident that their children were safe.

Infant mortality was, of course, not the only issue on the world stage in those years: World War I raged from 1914 to 1918, with the United States joining in 1917. The dark notion that saving babies

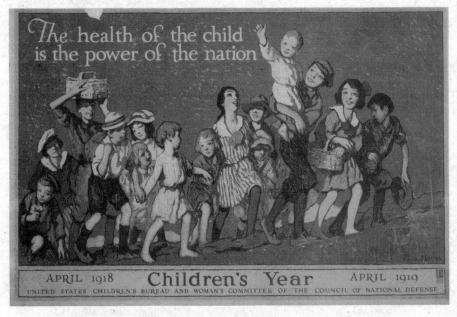

The health of the child
is the power of the nation

APRIL 1918   Children's Year   APRIL 1919

UNITED STATES CHILDREN'S BUREAU AND WOMAN'S COMMITTEE OF THE COUNCIL OF NATIONAL DEFENSE

Wartime meant shortages of nurses, of milk, and of nutritious food, and also made it more likely that mothers—and children—would enter the workforce. The Children's Year campaign—involving 17,000 committees and eleven million women—emphasized keeping children in school and out of the workforce, providing more opportunities for recreation and exercise, and educating parents about child health and nutrition. As Josephine Baker acknowledged, war cast a dark shadow on efforts to bring down infant mortality and promote children's health; the physically active, well-nourished children shown here were meant to provide the country with its future soldiers. *Library of Congress, Prints and Photographs Division, LC-USZC4-9867.*

was partly about providing cannon fodder had come to seem both true and tragic, as millions died on both sides. In many ways, Josephine Baker wrote, the terrible waste of human life that took place in the First World War helped draw attention to the value of children. Nations looked to them as the future, as replacements for the soldiers who were dying, to fill out the population, and also, of course, as potential soldiers for future conflicts.

When the war ended, dignitaries from all the combatant nations came to New York to look at the Bureau of Child Hygiene and learn how to replicate it: "enthusiastic Frenchmen; peering, solemn and intelligent Germans; voluble Russians; close-mouthed and sharp-eyed Englishmen; smiling delegations from China and Japan."[50] It was all very flattering at the time, but when Baker looked back in 1939, as the world was going to war again, she saw those visits as far more sinister and considered how "the piling up of corpses in the trenches of the western front forced them to speculate, subconsciously perhaps, as to how many recruits would be available for conscription in 1939."[51]

She also marveled at the willingness with which Americans, during the postwar period, donated to new charities promising to aid starving children in Belgium and Armenia, and even in Russia, Germany, and Austria. Save the Children was founded in Britain in 1919, and the American Red Cross was particularly active in helping the civilian European population after the war—and certainly the need was great in the devastated countries of Europe.[52] But Baker couldn't help wondering why such causes appealed "far more successfully to the American pocketbook than the equally miserable and rickety little people on Washington Street, Manhattan Island." And yet, she wrote, all of that attention to the starving children of the world did, in the end, draw money and attention to the conditions of children in America. One after another, cities and states duplicated the office to which she had given her professional life, the New York City Bureau of Child Hygiene. There had been only five other states with such offices in 1914; in the postwar period, they spread throughout the country. Baker promised herself that she would retire as soon as all forty-eight states had them, and in 1923, she was able to keep that promise. "It is a rare privilege to have been present at the birth of a great and new idea and see it grow to maturity, even though some of its growth must be credited to a world disaster."[53]

In 1923, the American Association for the Study and Prevention of Infant Mortality merged with the Child Hygiene Organization of America, which addressed the health of school children, to become the American Child Health Association. In 1935, the organization voted to dissolve, passing along its educational activities to the National Education Association and its health activities to the American Public Health Association. The initial, more narrow mission of the AASPIM had been subsumed into the larger projects of education and health, first for children more generally, not just babies, and then for the entire population.

Other attitudes about children were changing as well; 1938 would see the passage of serious legislation regulating child labor as part of Roosevelt's New Deal. And by 1935, real progress had been made in the narrower mission of getting babies to their first birthdays. Antibiotics and immunizations were still to come, but babies were no longer dying in the kinds of numbers that had horrified reformers in the nineteenth century and had persisted as an embarrassment and a reproach into the twentieth. The summer diarrhea plagues had ended. There were no longer cities where 20 to 30 percent of the children born died before their first birthdays. Infant mortality in the United States overall had fallen from around 100 deaths by the first birthday for every 1,000 live births at the turn of the century to 71.7 per 1,000 live births in 1925, to 55.7 in 1935.[54] From 1900 to 1940, deaths by the age of five among Black children in America declined sharply, from 264 out of every 1,000 live births—more than one child in four—to 90. While this represented a dramatic number of lives saved, it also indicated persistent racial disparities.[55] Many of the deaths, Black or white, were of newborns, and were still thought to be inevitable.

Josephine Baker believed that parents were important, but she never lost sight of the larger social context. Parents could not do it alone; they needed support and help from the society around them. Although parent education was important, so were health care and immunizations; so were adequate nutrition and good care for expectant mothers; so were decent living conditions, and the clean air and clean water that the sanitarians had started campaigning for a century earlier. As far as she was concerned, the persistent high mor-

tality of newborns was not due to their weakness or their parents'
failures but to the practical failures of society—above all the failure
to provide proper prenatal care to pregnant women. "We have done
nothing about it—and we could," she wrote in 1939. "There is still
much work to be done in the field of child hygiene."

What Baker was proposing—and working toward—was a revised
vision of the human infant. Instead of accepting that many babies
would inevitably be born only to die, she was asserting that the right
to live and thrive is there from birth, and so is the government's
responsibility to protect and preserve. "Every baby can have a chance
for life," she wrote. "This cannot be given by the mother and father
alone; it needs more help than that. Our goal will be reached only
when public health officials, social welfare agencies, doctors, nurses
and parents work together." Children, she emphasized, could not
be reduced to statistics, however useful statistics might be in public
health. "We are dealing with little Susan and John and Mary and
Thomas. They are our children. Each one carries all the potential
possibilities of all humanity. Whatever the statistics say, each has a
right to live. And each *can* live."[56]

CHAPTER 5

"The Plague Among Children"

Diphtheria and the Doctors

have never seen a case of diphtheria. I studied the disease in medical school, in the 1980s, in microbiology, along with smallpox, for which the last human case had been recorded a decade earlier. Diphtheria was by no means extinct—it still isn't, with thousands of cases every year in Asia and Africa, and two hundred thousand cases and five thousand deaths in the nations of the former Soviet Union between 1990 and 1998—but it's not a concern in an American clinic or emergency room. Still, medical students learn the basics: the disease is caused by bacteria, *Corynebacterium diphtheriae,* and it's an infection of the throat and tonsils, starting out as a sore throat and a low-grade fever. Its famous hallmark, its pathological signature (the thing you might be asked about as a medical student), is a "pseudomembrane," a thick gray sheet of murderous tissue that can form in the throat. The pseudomembrane develops because this particular bacterium produces a potent toxin, the result of the bacteria harboring a virus, which destroys the cells that line the mucous membranes of the mouth and pharynx. The debris of those dead cells forms part of the pseudomembrane, which sticks to the other structures, making it difficult and even impossible to breathe. Just as young children's smaller bodies are more vulnerable to dehydration, the smaller tubes of their respiratory systems are more precariously vulnerable to anything that inflames them or obstructs them. The diphtheria wards of the nineteenth century were full of children who were being slowly suffocated. That same potent toxin can travel through the body and attack different organs, and do great harm to the heart, to the kidneys, to the muscles—or it can cause a generalized severe infection that results in the shock and death that we call bacterial sepsis, dangerous to adults as well as to children.

Recognizable descriptions of diphtheria infection go back to classical times, and the French doctor, Pierre Bretonneau, who named the disease in 1826 called it *diphtérite,* deriving the name from the Greek word for "leather," to evoke the membrane (and putting in place the silent *h* that makes the word so often fatal to spelling bee contestants). Although Bretonneau had no knowledge of bacteria, he knew that the infection was in some way contagious, and he blamed the disease, retrospectively, for the 1814 death of Empress Joséphine; he believed she had caught it from her daughter Queen Hortense, who had, in turn, contracted it from her own firstborn child, who had died of the disease.[1] Bretonneau was also the first to treat the disease by performing a tracheotomy, cutting a hole in the patient's throat and inserting a tube into the airway, a drastic treatment in those days, and one that the patient would not necessarily survive. His description of the disease called forth a certain amount of controversy from other doctors, over the course of the nineteenth century, including arguments about different systems of classifying the various kinds of croup—respiratory infections that cause inflammation in the upper airway—and debates about whether there could be a diphtheria infection in the absence of a pseudomembrane. (What we call croup nowadays is a viral infection, more technically called laryngotracheobronchitis, in which inflammation and swelling in the child's trachea produce a characteristic barking cough—and sometimes respiratory distress; when diphtheria was around, people thought in terms of two different forms of croup, with "diphtheritic croup" the more deadly.)

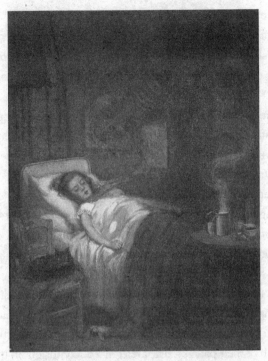

In this 1912 watercolor by British graphic artist Richard Cooper, the specter of a skeleton, representing diphtheria, is strangling a child as she lies in bed. *Wellcome Collection. Attribution 4.0 International (CC BY 4.0).*

Before it was called diphtheria, epidemics of the disease swept through eighteenth-century Europe and colonial America. It was especially savage on children, who died at very high rates—as many as 40 percent of those infected. In his 1800 book, *A Brief History of Epidemic and Pestilential Diseases*, Noah Webster, the famous grammarian and lexicographer, described the terrifying advent of the disease in colonial New England: "In May 1735, in a wet cold season, appeared at Kingston, an inland town in New-Hampshire, situated in a low plain, a disease among children, commonly called the 'throat distemper,' of a most malignant kind, and by far the most fatal ever known in this country. Its symptoms generally were, a swelled throat, with white or ash-colored specks, an efflorescence on the skin, great debility of the whole system, and a tendency to putridity." He went on to trace the epidemic, as it moved through one town after another, "almost stripping the country of children." Writing sixty-five years after the epidemic, he noted that those fortunate children who survived the disease did not generally live to old ages, as if the sickness had done some damage even to the survivors (we would probably understand this now as related to the lasting damage the diphtheria toxin can do to different organs, including the heart and the nerves), but he concentrated most on the devastation of the young. "It was," he pronounced, "literally the plague among children."[2]

Though there were epidemics in a few European countries early in the nineteenth century, it was not until 1856—when a diphtheria pandemic struck both Europe and North America and lasted for two years—that diphtheria began to claim the lives of thousands of children in American cities.[3] Of those who got sick, mortality could run as high as 70 percent. The doctors of the New York Academy of Medicine who debated it in 1860 had no way to explain the illness and death of their patients. They referenced "confusion" in the medical journals of Europe. Severe cases were relatively easy to diagnose, but milder cases could be very difficult to distinguish from other types of sore throats. And there were other infections that caused children to have trouble breathing; the relatively narrow airways in those small throats and chests make any kind of respiratory infection much more dangerous. The academic doctors spent a good deal of time and energy trying to separate one kind of croup from another scientifically, but all doctors who cared for children worried about anything that caused inflammation and swelling in the throat or the airways.

Dr. Abraham Jacobi's cause was scientific pediatrics, the idea that the diagnosis and care of children ought to be studied and taught and practiced as distinct from the care of adults. "Pediatrics does not deal with miniature men and women, with reduced doses and the same class of disease in smaller bodies," he wrote, in words still regularly cited in discussions of pediatric pharmacology.[4] The phrase came up again and again in my own training more than a century later: children are not small adults. And tied to that interest in children's health was a strong connection to what would today be called the social determinants of health. True to the revolutionary ideals of his student days in Germany, Dr. Jacobi believed that poverty and malnutrition were the enemies of children's health, and he felt a particular calling, personally and professionally, to reduce the horrific levels of childhood disease and death among the poor.[5]

In 1873, he married another doctor, Mary Putnam, who was from a very different background; she had grown up as the brilliant oldest child in a well-off intellectual Protestant family in New York City. (Her father founded the publishing company that still bears his name.) Mary herself was a talented writer who was desperate to train as a doctor and a scientist. She received her MD from the Female Medical College of Pennsylvania but argued that medical education should be coed, and later went for further medical training in Paris. Her admission to the Sorbonne's École de Médecine required an order from the ministry of education; she was the first female student and was required to use a separate entrance. As a trainee in Paris, she recorded in detail the various responses of her male fellow students, professors, and social circle to the strange project of a woman studying medicine.[6] Like Abraham Jacobi, she too was caught up in the revolutionary politics of that era in Europe, sending back vivid reports of the French defeat in the Franco-Prussian War, the proclamation of the Republic, and the Paris Commune of 1871. She obtained her degree that same year with brilliant marks at the Sorbonne, writing home to her mother, "I have passed my thesis, and am now *docteur en médecine de la Faculté de Paris*. Considerably to my astonishment, my thesis was a success,—even decided success; for I received the highest note,—*extrêmement satisfait,*—and a good many compliments during the argumentation."[7]

Returning to New York City, she took up her career in medicine and was promptly elected to membership in the Medical Society of the County of New York. Dr. Abraham Jacobi, the newly installed president of the society, noted her election approvingly in his inaugural address at the subsequent meeting on December 4, 1871: "Let it not be forgotten in this history of this Medical Society of the County of New York, that we have opened our doors to worthy members of the medical profession, male or female, white or colored, and thus granted reality to the gospel of American citizenship, the Declaration of Independence, according to which we are all created free and equal."[8] (The American Medical Association, at the time, accepted neither African Americans nor women.) Mary Putnam and Abraham Jacobi began their courtship in the question-and-answer sessions after the scientific presentations, which yielded intense conversations that continued when Dr. Jacobi escorted Dr. Putnam back to her family's home on East Fifteenth Street.

The two doctors settled into a married life centered on the practice and teaching of medicine. Abraham had been married twice before. His first wife, Fanny, who had come with him from Europe, had borne a son, Julius, who had died at the age of one day, from what his father diagnosed as "meningitis"; Fanny herself died a year later. Jacobi's second wife, Kate, who was apparently never in very good health, had given birth four times, twice to stillborn children and twice to babies who died almost immediately, and had also lost a number of other pregnancies. She died from the complications of a miscarriage in 1871. Abraham signed the death certificates of his children, diagnosing both of the children who died with "debility"— that is, with weakness. He had thus lost two wives and five infants by the time he married Mary Putnam. Reading this story today, it's hard not to marvel at the sheer courage of the women who embarked upon the enterprise of reproduction, even with a personal physician in attendance.

The first child of Abraham and Mary Putnam Jacobi was born

alive but died on the first day of her life, with a diagnosis recorded by her father of "atelectasis pulmonum (from intrauterine respiration)." Reading this now, I wonder if it denotes meconium aspiration, a problem we worry about in the delivery room, when a distressed fetus excretes meconium—the thick, tarry stool that normally is passed after birth—into the amniotic fluid before delivery. If the newborn inhales the meconium on the way out of the uterus, it can cause severe pulmonary disease; nowadays, we routinely suction out the baby's trachea when meconium has been passed before birth, ideally before the umbilical cord is cut and the baby inhales for the first time, often when only the head has emerged. I also wonder if the child was premature—born eight months after the wedding, she was either premature or conceived before the marriage—and a somewhat premature infant might have been at risk for what we now know as hyaline membrane disease, in which the immature lungs are stiff and inflexible. I can come up with another several possible diagnoses that today would require respiratory care, and possibly a ventilator, treatment that was a full century away—but I pause here only to note that this particular baby, fathered by the man who is generally credited with fathering my entire profession, the pregnancy carried by a woman who was an expert on the capabilities of the female body and the female reproductive system, almost certainly would not die today.

Abraham Jacobi believed it was part of the mission of American medicine to reject what he considered the unhelpful European medical tradition of high-flown academic rigmarole and aim instead for therapeutic effect—for actually helping patients. He believed—and based much of his life on the belief—that taking proper care of children, saving their lives even if they started out sickly and weak, as he had himself, and training their mothers in the importance of proper nutrition would make the world better. And yet, that day there was nothing he could do but once more sign his own baby's death certificate.

Mary Putnam Jacobi became pregnant again; her second child

was born a year after the first, at their upstate New York summer home on Hiawatha Island in Lake George. The family story was that Abraham had just decided to go—by boat—to fetch another doctor to help with the labor when he heard the baby cry. The child was a boy, and he lived and thrived. His father almost immediately began to collect medical articles and research papers in anticipation that Ernst would grow up to follow him into medicine. Mary wrote to her brother, "The loss of our first baby, last year, makes this one, if possible, all the more precious. I always felt that my first baby would not live,—I can scarcely know why, except that a great misfortune so often precedes a great happiness. But now, the doctor at least, has had so many misfortunes that it seems as if the time had come for him to be perfectly happy,—or rather to stay as happy as he is at present."[9] She tracked her son's development with great pleasure: "He has four teeth and should have eight. He is backward with his teeth but with nothing else."[10] Two years later, the Jacobis had a daughter, Marjorie.

In 1880 Abraham Jacobi, who wrote prolifically on pediatric topics, published a lengthy essay, *A Treatise on Diphtheria*. In this volume, he pulled together his own enormous clinical experience with an extensive review of the literature. Diphtheria, he reminded his readers, was "pre-eminently a disease of early life."[11] The previous decade had seen a burgeoning of research on bacteria, especially in Germany, with the discovery of new stains and other techniques for identifying and classifying microorganisms; a few had been linked to specific diseases, though not yet to diphtheria, and the overall relationship of these microorganisms to human health was still unclear. In Jacobi's preface, he considered the question of whether bacteria might be the cause of diphtheria and expressed his doubts: "The safest verdict of the sober critic is still: 'not proven.'"[12] Diphtheria, he felt, was clearly infectious, contagious—but there were so many aspects of the disease and its variability that he did not think could be explained by the presence of one of the bacteria recently identified in the German scientific literature. Sometimes the affliction seemed to linger or recur, almost like a chronic illness, and his recurrent cases may well have included other illnesses. Other times it flared as an epidemic, and the epidemics had grown more deadly since the early nineteenth century.

Jacobi's *Treatise* is both exhaustive in its account of the manifestations of the disease and disheartening in its acknowledgment that many of the therapies then available were of dubious benefit. What comes through vividly is that he had personally presided over many fatal cases and found himself unable to save the young patients. He expressed his frustration, and even his despair, writing, "I cannot refrain from stating that, in proportion to the increasing severity of the diphtheritic epidemics, the results of tracheotomy in my hands and in those of others have grown worse and worse. Of sixty-seven tracheotomies which I published twelve years ago, twenty per cent recovered; about two hundred tracheotomies performed by me since that time, brought down the percentage of recoveries to such a low figure that only the utter impossibility of witnessing a child's dying from asphyxia has goaded me on to the performance of tracheotomy."[13] In an era of untreatable infections, a senior and committed pediatrician found himself repeatedly performing a dangerous surgery he knew would probably not save a suffocating child.

In 1883, three years after the publication of the *Treatise,* both of the Jacobi children came down with diphtheria. Ernst Jacobi died on June 10; his sister was also sick, but she recovered. The death notice in the newspaper gave his age as "7 years 10 months and 7 days." The paper on diphtheria in adults that his father published a year later actually contained in it an account of diphtheria in the Jacobi family, though he presented it as a case study:

> In the family of a physician, there were two children—a boy, in good health otherwise; a girl, robust and vigorous. Both suffered from diphtheria repeatedly for many years, until the girl came near dying and the boy died. . . . Almost every

time when the children were sick the old, trusted, and trust-
worthy nurse was also affected with diphtheria, sometimes
seriously. What, however, was not known at that time, and
was discovered later—indeed, too late—was that the woman
had concealed many an attack of throat disease, fever, difficult deglutition [trouble swallowing], out of a sense of
duty. . . . In the early part of the summer of 1883 the boy
died; the surviving girl was sent to the country. . . . Then
the nurse was discharged; that was the end of diphtheria in
that family.[14]

As a pediatrician and a scientist, and most particularly as an expert
in this disease, Jacobi needed a theory of causation that would satisfy
science; in fact, he was correct that some adults can carry the diphtheria germ in their nose and mouth without themselves getting sick,
and can spread the disease to others. But as a parent, he may have
needed a theory that made it clear that he himself could not possibly
have brought this disease back from his practice and into his house.

Whatever the source of the infection, the two doctors had not
been able to keep their son safe, or to cure him when he got sick, and
they both went on replaying the medical—and parental—decisions
of 1883. Fifteen years later, when Mary Putnam Jacobi wrote a letter
to the man who married her daughter, Marjorie, she recalled having
had some worries that her husband had dismissed, perhaps related to
exposures: "And I having naturally a great confidence in his professional opinion and knowing his great love for our little son, did not
sufficiently urge the different precautions about his health, which I
now think might have sufficiently increased his power of resistance
when the trial came."[15]

Over the years after her son's death, Mary Putnam Jacobi embraced
the new microbiological discoveries, and eventually the husband and
wife, both prominent physicians, publicly took somewhat different
positions. New ways of staining and examining bacterial cells had

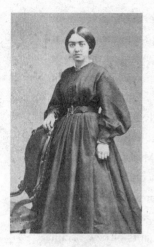
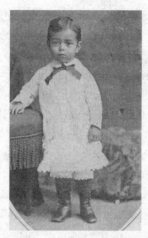
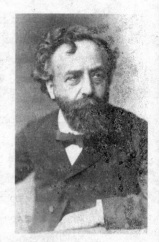

Ernst Jacobi (center) at the age of three or four, with his parents, Dr. Mary Putnam Jacobi and Dr. Abraham Jacobi. His mother blamed herself, as a physician and as a mother, for his death: "I feel sometimes as if the whole world must stand and hoot at me for my inability to retain this lovely child, when he had once been entrusted to me." *(Mary) Library of Congress, Prints and Photographs Division, LC-USZ62-138374; (Ernst) Library of Congress, Prints and Photographs Division, LC-USZ62-138373; (Abraham) Alamy Images.*

been developed, and in the 1880s, especially in Europe, the new science of bacteriology was advancing rapidly, with different bacteria being discovered and theories developed about infection and disease. Diphtheria was a focus for many of these investigators, but Abraham Jacobi continued to express doubt about the idea that a single microbial cause had been identified and could account for all the many manifestations of the disease. Both parents returned to Ernst's death in their different ways, assigning blame, creating causal narratives, reproaching themselves. They may well have blamed themselves or each other—for letting their child get sick, for failing to save him, perhaps even for infecting him. It divided them, though it's possible that it also held them together. They knew as much as there was to know about the disease, and they had not been able to protect their child.

As a pediatrician, I often find that when I read the accounts of children's illness, I want to intervene, to yell across the years that there is a way to hold off death. I imagine offering antibiotics in a world where they didn't yet exist or insisting on aggressive oral hydration to save a child dying of cholera. But I never feel that illogical impulse more strongly than in reading the story of Ernst Jacobi and his parents.

When the diphtheria bacterium was initially identified, Mary Putnam Jacobi reported on the discovery at an 1884 meeting of the Clinical Society of the New York Post-Graduate Medical School and Hospital. A few months later, when Abraham Jacobi gave his inaugural address as president of the New York Academy of Medicine, he spoke much more negatively about the bacteriological studies: "Have we not had enough yet of the monthly installments of new bacilli which are invariably correct and positive sources of a disease, and replaced by the next man who comes along? . . . The very nature of diphtheria is said to be revealed again, as several times before; still, the discoverer admits there are cases without the bacterium. . . . The matter is becoming ludicrous."[16]

The diphtheria bacterium was finally identified in 1883 by Edwin Klebs, a pathologist working in Switzerland. A year later, Friedrich Loeffler, a German bacteriologist, succeeded in culturing the "Klebs-Loeffler bacterium"; he confirmed that it caused diphtheria by injecting it into guinea pigs, rabbits, horses, and dogs. He and other scientists were also able to show that it produced a toxin—that the fluid in which the bacteria grew was still dangerous, even when there were no bacteria in it.

In 1888, two researchers at the Pasteur Institute in Paris, Émile Roux and Alexandre Yersin, definitively showed that it was the toxin, not the bacteria, that did the damage in diphtheria; this led directly to the next huge step in treatment. In 1890, a German doctor, Emil von Behring, and his Japanese colleague Shibasaburo Kitasato developed what they would ultimately call antitoxins to diphtheria and tetanus—not antibiotics to attack the bacteria but antibodies that neutralized the toxin the bacteria produced. To produce the antitoxin, guinea pigs were first immunized with diphtheria toxin that had been heated to inactivate it. Because the toxin was inactivated, the guinea pigs did not get sick, but their immune systems still recognized the poison and reacted, making the antitoxin. And the serum extracted from the blood of those immunized animals, with all the cells removed, could then be injected into humans with diphtheria. Von Behring supposedly used his antitoxin to save a child, an eight-year-old boy who had severe diphtheria, on Christmas Eve 1891, in Berlin. The holiday "miracle" became part of the legend of the triumph of bacteriology, though the story was not verified. Von Behring and his associates continued to use the antitoxin in humans, with dramatic results; in 1901, he would win the first Nobel Prize in medicine for his work.

Meanwhile, in Paris, Roux and Louis Martin had independently developed a technique to get antitoxin from horses, and they treated a series of 448 children with it, all the diphtheria cases at the Hôpital des Enfants Malades. More than three-quarters recovered; meanwhile, at another hospital, the Hôpital Trousseau, no antitoxin was given and more than half of the patients with diphtheria died. Roux presented his work at the Eighth International Congress of Hygiene and Demography, a scientific meeting in Budapest, in September 1894. An American physician in attendance reported, "Hats were thrown to the ceiling, grave scientific men arose to their feet and shouted their applause in all the languages of the civilized world. I had never seen and have never seen since such an ovation displayed by an audience of scientific men."[17]

The New York City Department of Health had already been targeting diphtheria when the antitoxin was produced. In the 1890 census, diphtheria was the sixth leading cause of death in New York City, responsible for 15,199 deaths over the course of six years, a large number of those deaths involving children under five, and the new scientific discoveries made it possible to imagine new ways to bring those numbers down.

By 1892, the New York City Department of Health had established a new division—Pathology, Bacteriology, and Disinfection—with bacteriologic laboratories on Bleecker Street. The laboratory director, Dr. William Hallock Park, developed a culture kit, which allowed doctors to swab throats with a sterile cotton swab and then transfer the bacteria into a tube of solidified blood serum where bacteria could grow. The city provided the culture kits to doctors and established thirty-four depots where they could drop off their cultures. The health department collected them and reported the results the next day—"a most radical proposition for the State to step in and offer to become the diagnostician of disease," as a medical journal noted, with the state in this case being the city.[18]

Historian Evelynn Hammonds has traced the ways that battling diphtheria drew the government into public health work. (The federal CDC would not be founded until 1946.) Such intervention made it possible to chart the occurrence and spread of diphtheria so that sick people could promptly be quarantined or hospitalized. Still, more rigorous diagnosis alone would not stop the disease.[19]

Howard Markel, a pediatrician and historian of science, tells the story of how Dr. Hermann Biggs, the chief inspector of the New York City Board of Health, had been in Europe for the antitoxin announcement and was so impressed by "essentially human history's first effective treatment against a devastating infectious disease" that he and a colleague put up the money themselves to buy horses to be used to make antitoxin for New York City.[20] By 1895, antitoxin was being produced in the United States by the New York City Department of Health and by a Philadelphia company that would later become Merck Sharp & Dohme. Another major pharmaceutical company, Lederle Laboratories, was built on diphtheria antitoxin. In New York City, the thirteen horses kept at the New York College of Veterinary Surgeons, on East Fifty-Seventh Street, were constantly in the news, always described as heroes. The public was assured that they were treated tenderly, fed well, and cared for like hospital patients, in gratitude for their humanitarian role. The New York City Department of Health stayed in the business of manufacturing anti-toxin for decades, making medication available to doctors throughout the city and providing free serum for the poor. There was initially no way to gauge the strength of the serum, however, and contamination was a problem—in 1901, in St. Louis, thirteen children died from being given serum from a horse that had contracted tetanus. Bacte-riologic advances helped researchers learn how to purify serum and dose it more accurately, while contamination problems drew increas-ing attention to the need for government standards and regulation.

And so, by the early 1900s, a diphtheria treatment was available. It was not universally available, or universally used, and when it was used, it had to be dosed according to the severity of the symptoms. Thus the efficacy of the treatment depended heavily on the experi-ence and skill of the doctor. A 1927 Canadian Public Health Associa-tion article reflected on what caring for children with diphtheria had been like in the past, quoting a physician who had taken care of a little girl, five or six years old, who "literally choked to death, remain-ing conscious till the last moment of life." The doctor was quoted as saying that he felt, "as did every physician of the day, as if my hands were literally tied and I watched the death of that beautiful child feel-ing absolutely helpless to be of any assistance." A decade later, when the doctor's own daughter came down with diphtheria, he was able to treat her with antitoxin and to "watch the choking dreadful mem-brane melt away and disappear in a few hours. . . . [It] was one of the most dramatic and thrilling experiences of my professional career."[21]

The miracle therapy also had some unintended consequences: in 1905, a new disease called "serum sickness" was identified by two doctors, Clemens von Pirquet and Béla Schick, who noted that chil-dren who were treated with large amounts of horse serum developed fever, rash, and joint pains—symptoms we now see as an immune system response to all the alien substances in the horse serum.

The horse serum could help a child fight off the disease by neutralizing the toxin, but giving those antibodies to a child who had never had diphtheria would not have made the child immune going forward, because the protective antibodies don't last long in the child's bloodstream. And even with the antitoxin available, many children didn't receive it, and many of those who did still died. The final conundrum of fighting diphtheria was to find a way the disease could be prevented, rather than treated. It was Emil von Behring who, in 1913, announced that he had developed a vaccine from diphtheria toxin mixed with antitoxin, to prevent the toxin from doing damage while triggering an immune system response. The first major vaccination campaigns using von Behring's formula took place in New York City in 1921 under the direction of Dr. Park. Some 180,000 schoolchildren were involved; half were tested for immunity to diphtheria using a test developed by Dr. Schick (that is, the Schick test); those who were not immune got vaccinated. The 90,000 children who were neither tested nor vaccinated developed four times as many cases of diphtheria. By 1929, a strong citywide immunization plan had cut New York City's death rate from diphtheria in half.

But there was no national program of mandatory universal vaccination, and diphtheria continued to kill children in the United States and around the world. The most famous incident in the conquest of diphtheria was the 1925 sled dog journey to Nome, Alaska, to combat a developing epidemic. The nearest fresh antitoxin was in Anchorage; it was sent by train to Nenana, which was still 674 miles from Nome. Twenty sled dog teams took the antitoxin across Alaska, stopping at intervals to warm it as they traveled through the frozen landscape. This played out as a public and dramatic rescue, with people throughout the country—and the world—cheering on the heroic mushers and their valiant Siberian husky dogs. The story of the journey across Alaska is evoked every year when the Iditarod is run, and a statue of Balto, one of the lead sled dogs on that original trip (fans of Togo, another lead sled dog, point out that he ran a much longer and more difficult part of the route), stands in Central Park in Manhattan and is probably the most beloved and most popular souvenir of the fight to conquer diphtheria.

Dr. Park's early New York vaccination campaign targeted children in the public schools and their younger siblings and paid particular attention to immigrants, with cards printed up in Yiddish and Italian to obtain parental permission. And though diphtheria could strike the children of the rich and powerful, it was often identified as a disease of poverty. In Harriette Arnow's novel of the Depression *The Dollmaker,* a heroic Kentucky mother performs an emergency tracheotomy on her own child because there is no doctor near. And it plays an essential role in the plot of the famous short story "The Use of Force," by William Carlos Williams, the great American pediatrician-poet. Once again, the diagnosis is associated with fear, but also with shame. In the story, published in 1934, a doctor goes to a poor family's apartment to examine a sick little girl. He is concerned that she may have diphtheria, because there have been several cases recently, and he needs to check her throat to see if the membrane is present. When the girl resists him, he battles her, trying to force her mouth open first with his tongue depressor, then with a spoon. He becomes angrier and angrier, as the parents fail to hold her, and as she bites right through his tongue depressor, and he mixes his anxiety about her diagnosis with the more brutal emotions called up in him by this protracted battle: "I have seen at least two children lying dead in bed of neglect in such cases, and feeling that I must get a diagnosis now or never I went at it again. But the worst of it was that I too had got beyond reason. I could have torn the child apart in my own fury and enjoyed it. It was a pleasure to attack her." Finally, in a passage that has been cited for its sexual imagery and brutality, the doctor forces the child's mouth open, using the heavy silver spoon: "And there it was—both tonsils covered with membrane. She had fought valiantly to keep me from knowing her secret."[22]

Perhaps she was just a sick child who didn't want to open her mouth when told to do so—a very familiar scenario in any pediatric examining room. But it is also true that in the early twentieth century, the diphtheria diagnosis often meant quarantine, with warning placards put up on apartment buildings and children taken to hospitals regardless of their families' wishes. Fear of such a separation could certainly make a child stubborn.

In the 1940s, a new vaccine was developed that was effective against both diphtheria and tetanus, a terrifying bacterial infection that sometimes got into wounds and caused "lockjaw" and death. The two inactivated toxins, or toxoids, were combined with a vaccine against pertussis, or whooping cough, in the earliest version of the DTP vaccine. As vaccination campaigns became more successful, with vaccines mandatory for school entry and support from the government—and from international health organizations—all three bacterial diseases became much rarer in the United States, and eventually around the world. There are only about thirty cases a year of tetanus in the States, mostly in people who have not kept their tetanus booster shots up to date. Pertussis continues to show up much more often, again usually in adults whose immunity from the vaccine has worn off. (It's a very unpleasant disease—I caught it in the line of pediatric duty, before there was an adult booster shot, and it was a cough beyond all other coughs—but it isn't actually dangerous in adults.) Diphtheria, however, is essentially gone; between 2004 and 2017, there were only two cases reported in the United States.

If you read the obituaries of people who have died in recent years in their eighties and nineties, you see the almost forgotten traces of diphtheria. In 2015, Bess Myerson's obituary said that the former Miss America had been born in 1924 as a "substitute" for a brother who had died of diphtheria.[23] Sherwin Nuland's obituary mentioned that the prominent surgeon and author had been hospitalized at the age of three for diphtheria.[24] Peter Rodino, the former chair of the House Judiciary Committee who had presided over the Nixon impeachment hearings, died in 2005; his obituary described how, as a child, he had practiced speaking with pebbles in his mouth, like Demosthenes, to overcome the raspy voice that was an after-effect of his childhood diphtheria.[25] Doctors and parents of my generation have no memory of that world in which diphtheria wreaked regular havoc.

In 1895, thirteen-year-old Pablo Picasso's seven-year-old sister, Conchita, died of diphtheria; the family, in Spain, had waited in vain for serum to arrive from Paris. Pablo had drawn her when she was healthy, and he drew her when she was sick. He also promised God that he would give up painting if Conchita could be saved, and then immediately began to worry that the promise would be too great a sacrifice. "He did paint again and the serum failed to come in time," wrote Picasso's biographer John Richardson in an article called "Picasso's Broken Vow."[26] Picasso would live all his life with a sense of guilt and responsibility, confiding the story of his vow to the women in his life (partly as a warning that they too would be sacrificed to his vocation), painting Conchita into many different works, including *Guernica,* and choosing a bronze statue of his sister to mark his own grave in Provence.

In 1899, in Atlanta, diphtheria killed W. E. B. Du Bois's eighteen-month-old son, who is remembered in *The Souls of Black Folk,* in a piece called "Of the Passing of the First-Born." Du Bois could not connect with one of the few African American doctors in the city; nor could he find a white doctor in Atlanta who was willing to treat his son. "Ten days he lay there,—a swift week and three endless days, wasting, wasting away. . . . Then we two alone looked upon the child as he turned toward us with great eyes, and stretched his string-like hands,—the Shadow of Death!" Du Bois went on to write that at least by dying so young and so innocent, by living such a perfect life, his son had been spared the evils of racism and preju-dice: "My soul whispers ever to me, saying, 'Not dead, not dead, but escaped; not bond, but free.' No bitter meanness now shall sicken his baby heart till it die a living death, no taunt shall madden his happy boyhood. . . . Well sped, my boy, before the world had dubbed your

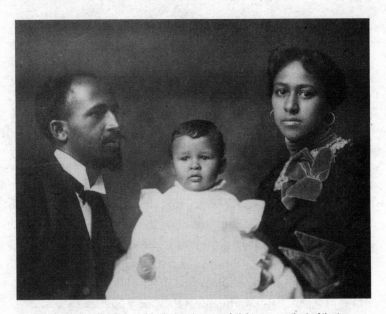

Burghardt, the first Du Bois child, died at the age of eighteen months in Atlanta, where his father, W. E. B. Du Bois, the sociologist, historian, and civil rights activist, was working as a professor. When he looked at his new son, he wrote, he "saw the dream of my black fathers stagger a step onward in the wild phantasm of the world." *W. E. B. Du Bois Papers (MS 312). Special Collections and University Archives, University of Massachusetts Amherst Libraries. Reprinted with permission of the Permissions Company, LLC, on behalf of the David Graham Du Bois Trust.*

ambition insolence, had held your ideals unattainable, and taught you to cringe and bow. Better far this nameless void that stops my life than a sea of sorrow for you."[27] And yet, Du Bois continued, his son might have borne this burden more bravely than he did himself, and might have lived to see a better society. He insisted that the child's body be carried back to Great Barrington, Massachusetts, where it was buried far from the unfriendly red earth of Georgia.

It did not necessarily help to have doctors. Five years later, in January 1904, Ruth Cleveland, the first child of President Grover Cleveland, was diagnosed with diphtheria, a few days after coming down with what the doctors had said was a mild case of tonsillitis. Ruth, born in 1891, between her father's two terms as president, was a celebrity child, nationally known as Baby Ruth. Cleveland wrote in his diary on January 6, 1904, "Dr. treated us all with antitoxin and reported that Ruth was getting on well. Dr. Carnochan came at 2:30 and Dr. Wykoff at 3:30. We had been excluded from Ruth's room, but learned that dear Ruth died before Dr. Wykoff came, probably about 3 o'clock A.M., Jan. 7th."[28]

Part of this book was written at Yaddo, the artists' colony in Saratoga Springs, New York, that was established on the beautiful estate of a very wealthy financier, Spencer Trask, and his wife, Katrina. In 1880, after the couple's first child died suddenly of meningitis at the age of four, Mr. Trask wanted to take his wife away from the scene of the loss, and bought the property in Saratoga Springs, a town they knew from the fashionable racing seasons. They built a lavish mansion there and had two more children, Christina and Spencer Jr. In 1888, Katrina came down with diphtheria, and, so the story goes, the doctor allowed the children to come see her—or, in some versions, to come kiss her good-bye.[29] She survived, but both children got sick and died, and with no descendants, the couple made their estate into a refuge for artists and writers.[30] Two large portraits of the children hang in the music room, and inevitably, there are stories about their ghosts inhabiting the mansion.

CHAPTER 6

"Most Dreaded of All the Diseases"

Scarlet Fever, Strep, and Antibiotics

Back in the 1990s in my Boston health center, I once told a grandmother from Mexico that her young grandchild had scarlet fever, which I could see by the very distinctive rash ("red and sandpapery," you memorize as a medical student). In fact, I was able to retrieve the Spanish word for scarlet fever, *escarlatina*, because "scarlatina" is also one of the terms we sometimes use in English for this rash, which we sometimes see in children with streptococcal infections, most often strep throat. Confident that penicillin would take care of the problem, I was proud of having made the diagnosis, and of even having known the Spanish name.

To my surprise, the grandmother looked terrified and began to cry, and I realized that she probably had memories of scarlet fever as a frightening disease that regularly killed children of all ages, toddlers and school-aged children and adolescents. And indeed it once was. The bright red rash of scarlet fever brought death to the families of some of the most famous scientists, writers, and artists of the nineteenth century—and to so many other families all over the world. Lingering aftereffects in damage to the kidneys or the heart crippled and killed for years after the fever had abated. Houses used to be quarantined for scarlet fever, with signs posted on the door.

Like diphtheria, scarlet fever was a standard childhood disease that could wipe out an entire family.

Scarlet fever was behind one of the most famous death scenes of nineteenth-century children's literature, the death of Beth March in *Little Women*—and also behind the death of the real person behind the character. Louisa May Alcott based *Little Women* on the story of the four Alcott sisters growing up together in Concord, Massachusetts, at the time of the Civil War. She cast herself as Jo, the willful and indecorous tomboy who longs to be a writer, and she modeled Beth, the shy, musical, quiet angel of the house, on her younger sister Elizabeth, who died at the age of twenty-two. In the novel, Beth also dies in her early twenties, no longer a child, though she dies because of the far-reaching effects of a childhood disease. *Little Women* was an international hit in the nineteenth century, and it continues to be read and loved as a childhood classic around the world. Like Stowe's Little Eva, Beth March has died over and over and over, on the stage and the screen as well as on the page; her deathbed provides the tragic moment in several different movie versions (she's been played most recently by Eliza Scanlen to Saoirse Ronan's Jo, and before that by Claire Danes to Winona Ryder's Jo, by Margaret O'Brien to June Allyson's Jo, and by Jean Parker to Katharine Hepburn's Jo), in a 1958 TV series, in a 2017 PBS miniseries, and in plays, a musical, a ballet, and an opera. The medical details are not always as clear on the stage as they are in the original book, and people often come away with the vague sense that Beth dies of tuberculosis, like Little Eva. But, in fact, Alcott gives an excellent case history for scarlet fever and its complications as she describes the facts of the illness and death.

Beth March's travails in *Little Women* begin with an act of Christian charity. The March sisters have interested themselves in the fortunes of a family of poor German immigrants, the Hummels.[1] Louisa May Alcott's mother, Abigail May, whom she made into Marmee in the book, was in fact an early social worker, not to mention

a passionate abolitionist, and though they were not well off themselves, she and her daughters certainly did charity work. But when
Marmee goes away to Washington to nurse her army chaplain husband, fourteen-year-old Beth is the only one who keeps up the visits
to the poor Hummels, where the baby is sick. She comes home to
tell her sister Jo that the baby died in her lap. "'My poor dear, how
dreadful for you! I ought to have gone,' said Jo, taking her sister in
her lap as she sat down in her mother's big chair, with a remorseful
face." Jo's reaction is not shock or horror but just a kind of mild guilt
that she let her little sister do an unpleasant job she should have
done herself. And Beth herself is saddened but by no means trau-
matized: "It wasn't dreadful, Jo, only so sad! I saw in a minute that
it was sicker, but Lottchen said her mother had gone for a doctor, so
I took baby and let Lotty rest. It seemed asleep, but all of a sudden
it gave a little cry and trembled, and then lay very still. I tried to
warm its feet, and Lotty gave it some milk, but it didn't stir, and I
knew it was dead." When the doctor arrives and discovers that the
baby's siblings have sore throats—what we now call strep throat—
he instantly diagnoses scarlet fever and tells Beth, she relates, to "go
home and take belladonna right away, or I'd have the fever."[2] Though
the doctor feels that he should have been called earlier, it's not clear
what he would have been able to offer. Certainly, if his best recommendation for treatment is belladonna, it's unlikely that would have
saved the baby. Belladonna is a potentially toxic herbal remedy that
can produce hallucinations and may be useful as a painkiller, but it
is not an antibiotic.

Thus begins the long story of Beth's slow death, which won't actually occur for another five years or so (and twenty-two chapters).
The main concern on everyone's part is the contagious nature of the
disease—before Beth will let Jo hear the story, she needs to verify
that Jo herself has had scarlet fever (Jo and Meg had it years before).
When Beth gets sick, the fourth sister, Amy, is sent to live at a relative's house so she won't be exposed.

The real Beth, Louisa May Alcott's younger sister Elizabeth Sewall Alcott, did indeed contract scarlet fever while providing charitable help to a poor German immigrant family. She recovered but was never fully strong again, and she died two years later, at the age of twenty-two, in 1858, probably from the aftereffects of scarlet fever, in particular damage to her heart.[3] Among the pallbearers who carried Elizabeth's coffin to the Concord, Massachusetts, cemetery were the Alcott friends and neighbors Henry David Thoreau and Ralph Waldo Emerson. In 1842, Emerson had lost his own first son, Wally, to scarlet fever, and had buried him in that same cemetery.[4] The boy was five when he died, and in the poem "Threnody," Emerson wrote, "I mourn / The darling who shall not return." This was the child he went on to describe as

The hyacinthine boy, for whom
Morn well might break and April bloom,—
The gracious boy, who did adorn
The world whereinto he was born.[5]

The cemeteries of nineteenth-century America, like the cemeteries of nineteenth-century Europe, were full of headstones marking the terrible virulence of scarlet fever in that century, a common childhood disease which could surge in deadly epidemics.

The virulence of scarlet fever seemed to wax and wane; at the beginning of the nineteenth century, it was mostly appearing in a milder form. And then, starting around 1825 or 1830, doctors noticed increased severity of disease and more deaths, both in Europe and in America, presumably reflecting the prevalence of bacterial strains with stronger toxin. An Irish physician noted that the disease had undergone "a notable alteration in its character" around 1831, and was causing occasional deaths, but that in 1834, scarlet fever "spread far and wide, assuming the form of a destructive epidemic." It was especially deadly in certain households, he observed: "The contagion seemed to act as a more deadly poison on the individuals of some families than upon those of others, and, consequently, when one member of a family had died, there was always much reason to fear for the others when attacked."[6] In the spring of 1856, the archbishop of Canterbury lost five of his six daughters to scarlet fever. In 1840, a British epidemiologist called it "the leading cause of death among the infectious diseases of childhood."[7]

And so it would remain until the end of the nineteenth century, a disease always present—that is, endemic—in the population, but sometimes inexplicably erupting with greatly increased numbers of cases and greatly increased fatality; these cyclic epidemics could have death rates as high as 55 percent for children under two years old, and 20 to 30 percent for children under five, all through Europe, Great Britain, and the United States.[8] In adults, it was generally a less serious disease, though they were not completely immune—everyone knows that you can get strep throat more than once, but the more serious systemic infection of scarlet fever confers some protective immunity against that specific toxin-producing strain and probably helps defend you against other strains as well. The mortality rate from the disease varied widely from year to year in the nineteenth century, probably reflecting different strains of streptococci with different levels of virulence moving through the population. An 1894 pediatric compilation, *An American Text-Book of the Diseases of Children by American Teachers,* described scarlet fever as "the most dreaded of all the diseases of children."[9]

And then the virulence shifted again; starting in the 1880s, without benefit of antibiotics or vaccination, the death rate from scarlet fever began to fall. Case fatality rates—the likelihood of dying from the disease, if you had it—would plummet, over several decades, from around 15 percent or higher to around 1 percent or lower, in England and America. Russia still had a death rate of over 20 percent up through 1915, and China saw a horrible outbreak in 1921–22 that killed around fifty thousand people in Kunming, mostly children (it was less lethal to newborns and infants, perhaps because some of them had antibodies from their mothers). The children who died had a devastating form of the disease, with shock, hemorrhagic symptoms, and death within twenty-four hours[10]—it must have been a particularly virulent strain of strep, producing a particularly potent toxin. On the other hand, less dangerous strains had clearly come to predominate in America and many parts of Europe.

The great scientists of the nineteenth century had no names for the microorganisms that threatened their own lives and took their children. In 1849, when Charles Darwin had returned from his voyages on the *Beagle*, settled down, started his family, and begun writing scientific papers, his three daughters came down with scarlet fever, in the midst of an epidemic with high fatality rates. The two younger girls recovered, but Annie, who was eight, never fully regained her strength, and two years later, in the spring of 1851, she went into a decline. Some sources attribute her final illness to tuberculosis, others to the aftereffects of the scarlet fever; she also became ill with what is described as "influenza," which would have been particularly dangerous to her if scarlet fever had left her with a weakened heart or if she already had TB. Darwin's wife, Emma, was very pregnant with their ninth child (one had died as a young infant) and could not travel, but Darwin brought his daughter to the spa town of Malvern (where Catherine Dickens was taking the waters during the same month of April, when her daughter died suddenly in London) to consult an expert, Dr. Gully, who practiced hydrotherapy. The worried father hovered closely over the sick child. On April 21, he wrote to his wife in detail: "In the night she rambled for two hours & became considerably excited . . . when the Dr. came at 11.30 he pronounced her decisively better." Darwin kept almost a nursing record, updating the letter every couple of hours, documenting every change, every medical intervention, every bodily function, as, for example, when Annie could not urinate: "At 10 oclock the surgeon failed to draw the water, but in the dead of the night her bladder acted of itself

& has again, & so have her bowels. . . . I was in wonderful spirits about all this & no doubt it is very good, but I have just now been a good deal damped (8. A.M.) by the Dr. finding her pulse tremulous & his strong dislike to her bowels having acted loosely."

Darwin's tender care for the child comes through from all his careful charting and the domestic details of tending a sick child: "Poor Annie is in a fearful mess, but we keep her sweet with Chloride of Lime; the Dr. said we might change the under sheet if we could, but I dare not attempt it yet. We have again this morning sponged her, with vinegar, again with excellent effect."[11] The author of the theory of evolution, whose thinking underlies all of modern biology, was fighting disease with vinegar and chloride of lime—an effective disinfectant, but not much use here since Annie already had the disease.[12] Darwin wrote a second letter later that same day, updating his wife yet again, worried but hopeful.

Nevertheless, two days later, on April 23, it was all over, and he wrote again to Emma: "She went to her final sleep most tranquilly, most sweetly at 12 oclock today. Our poor dear dear child has had a very short life but I trust happy, & God only knows what miseries might have been in store for her."[13] Charles and Emma Darwin would lose another of their children to scarlet fever, their young son Charles Waring Darwin, seven years later. He was eighteen months old, and his father was clearly worried about the propensity of scarlet fever to spread within families; he wrote to the Reverend William Darwin Fox, his second cousin, on July 2, 1858: "Our poor Baby died on 28th at night. One of his nurses has caught Fever. We had resolved not to move the others, after consultation & taking all sorts of precautions; but . . . this very day they all go to Sussex to their Aunt. . . . You may believe we are terribly anxious, but fear has almost driven away grief."[14]

The anniversary of a child's death was acknowledged to be very difficult; it was hard for Mary Lincoln, with her spiritualist tendencies, and it was hard for those Victorian men of science who did not

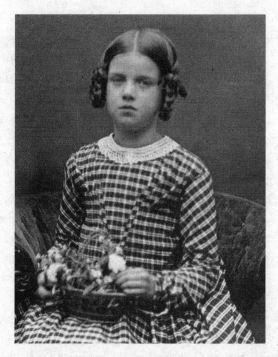

A week after his daughter's death, Charles Darwin wrote, "The Daguerrotype is very like her, but fails entirely in expression: . . . she often used to go before pirouetting in the most elegant way, her dear face bright all the time, with the sweetest smiles." *Alamy Images.*

believe in the spirit world but still found themselves haunted on those memorial occasions. A year after his six-year-old daughter's death, Darwin's closest friend, Joseph Dalton Hooker, a great British botanist, wrote to Darwin about his trip to the meeting of the British Association for the Advancement of Science: "I go to Bath tomorrow for 2 or 3 days, I am glad to do so though I go with a very heavy heart—on principle I think we should not keep anniversarys of great sorrows, but as the day draws nearer I feel all the misery of last year crawling over me & my lost child's face & voice accompany me everywhere by day & by night."[15]

Nine years after Annie Darwin's death, as controversy raged over the publication of *On the Origin of Species*, the English biologist Thomas Henry Huxley, who was one of Darwin's greatest defenders, lost his son Noel: "Our first-born, after being for nearly four years our delight and our joy, was carried off by scarlet fever in forty-eight hours. This day week he and I had a great romp together. . . . On Saturday night the fifteenth, I carried him here into my study and laid his cold still body here where I write." Darwin wrote to Huxley in sympathy, advising him that "time, & time alone, acts wonderfully. To this day, though so many years have passed away, I cannot think of one child without tears rising in my eyes; but the grief is become tenderer & I can even call up the smile of our lost darling, with something like pleasure."[16]

Try to imagine them, these prosperous, bearded Victorian fathers, deep in their voluminous scientific correspondence—many of these letters also include comments on articles they were reading or writing—but noting, as they go, the vulnerability of their children and the natural history of loss and grief. What they do not say, these men of science, is that there must be some way to prevent or avert such deaths; they are, in their way, as accepting and fatalistic about it as any pious and uneducated person might be. Even in an era when the death of children was an unavoidable concomitant of parenthood, it was also a life-changing tragedy and an inescapable grief. It marked the lives of parents in ways that we can recognize in their words and art and music.

Fifty years after Annie Darwin's death, the same year the Rockefeller Institute was founded, Gustav Mahler began writing the music for his song cycle *Kindertotenlieder,* or "Songs on the Death of Children." He had not yet actually lost a child, but the poems he was setting to music were by a German poet, Friedrich Rückert, who had lost two of his children to scarlet fever in the 1830s.[17]

Mahler had certainly seen children die—he was the second child in a family of fourteen children, but only six of his younger siblings lived to grow up. When he was fourteen, he was particularly distressed by the protracted illness and death of his younger brother Ernst and began to write an opera about him as a memorial. Some scholars have suggested that Mahler was drawn to Rückert's poems because they also involved the death of a child named Ernst. Of the first songs, Mahler wrote, "It hurt me to write them and I grieve for the world which will one day have to hear them, they are so sad."[18] "Often I think they have just gone out," one poem begins. "Soon they will come home again." Another addresses a dead daughter directly:

> When your dear mother comes in at the door and I turn my
> head toward her, my gaze does not fall on her face at first,
> but on the place closer to the threshold, there where your
> lovely face would be when bright with joy you would have
> entered with her, as once, my dear little daughter.[19]

As Gustav Mahler worked on music to accompany such lines only a few weeks after the birth of their second daughter in 1904, his wife, Alma, expressed anxiety: "I found this incomprehensible. I could understand setting such frightful words to music if one had no children, or had lost those one had. . . . What I could not understand was bewailing the deaths of children, who were in the best of health and spirits . . . hardly one hour after having kissed and fondled them. I exclaimed at the time, 'For heaven's sake, don't tempt Providence!' "[20]

When biographers or critics write about this song cycle and how it fit into Mahler's life and work, they often suggest some kind of uncanny premonition or some terrible artistic irony, forgetting that the experience Rückert wrote about was still so very common in Mahler's time. During the summer of 1904, Mahler spent a great deal of time playing with his older daughter, Maria Anna, nicknamed Putzi; his biographer notes that "a 'strange' and powerful bond seemed to unite father and daughter."[21] She was clearly his favorite

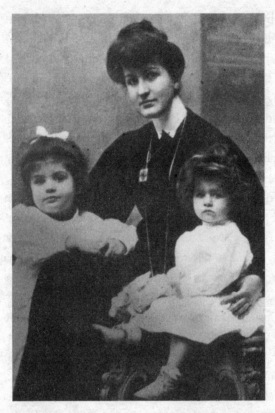

Alma Mahler, shown here with her two daughters, Maria (left) and Anna, was an aspiring composer when she married the older Gustav Mahler. This photo is from around 1906, the year before both girls got sick and Maria died. *Wikimedia Commons*.

of his two daughters, and the one who resembled him; Alma Mahler described her as "every inch his child. Wonderfully beautiful and defiant. . . . Black curls, big blue eyes!"[22]

In 1907, the two Mahler daughters came down with scarlet fever and diphtheria. The younger, Anna, recovered, but Maria Anna died after being sick for two weeks. She received the best possible medical attention, including a last-ditch tracheotomy to try to keep her airway open during a "terrible night," as Alma Mahler recalled it, "in which my English nanny and I set up an operating table and put the poor, poor child to sleep. During the operation I ran along the shore screaming loudly though no one could hear me."

But the "heroic" surgical intervention was no use: "I saw the beautiful child lying with eyes wide open, gasping for breath, and so we suffered another day—until it was over. . . . Mahler ran back and forth weeping and sobbing outside her, or rather my bedroom door, for with a sort of death wish I had put her in my bed. He fled so that he would not have to hear her. He could no longer bear it."[23]

Alma and Gustav Mahler were much more "modern" parents than Charles and Emma Darwin; when Darwin's daughter was dying, her scientist father had no science-based understanding about what was killing her, and the doctor could do little more than check her pulse. When the Mahlers' daughter was dying, fifty-six years later, they understood that their daughter was sick because she was infected with bacteria, and the doctor hoped—though vainly—to save her with a dramatic intervention, though there was still no medication that would specifically treat scarlet fever. Alma herself was later to think of her husband's "Songs on the Death of Children" composition as a warning, or shadow, of the death to come.[24] Mahler himself did not discuss his feelings about his daughter's death, though his assistant, Bruno Walter, wrote, "He is a broken man: outwardly one notices nothing, but those who know him can tell that inwardly he is at the end of his tether."[25] Gustav and Alma spent the following winter in New York City, where he was conducting at the Metropolitan Opera for the first time. Alma wrote that he would not allow the child's name to be mentioned, and that "Mahler and I were, for the time being, strangers to each other, estranged by suffering. Without knowing it, he blamed me for the death of the child."[26]

Later in his life, speaking of the *Kindertotenlieder*, Mahler is supposed to have told Guido Adler, "I placed myself in the situation that a child of mine had died. When I really lost my daughter, I could not have written these songs any more."[27] Mahler died in 1911 at the age of fifty, possibly of complications from the same disease that killed his daughter; he had suffered for years from bacterial endocarditis, a slow-smoldering bacterial infection of the heart that is particularly likely to prey on heart valves that have been damaged—as they can be in the aftermath of streptococcal infections. At his request, he was buried beside his daughter Maria Anna, in the small suburban cemetery of Grinzing. When Bruno Walter made his celebrated recording of *Kinder-totenlieder* in 1949, scarlet fever was already a curable illness. The song cycle remains an artistic monument to an age of child mortality.

Over the second half of the nineteenth century—in the time between the death of Darwin's daughter and the death of Mahler's daughter—scientists figured out that microbes were causing infections and identified the specific organism, the streptococcus, that was responsible for scarlet fever. Much of the figuring out begins with two gentlemen who hated each other, Pasteur and Koch.

It was Louis Pasteur himself who first isolated the organism we know as Group A strep, in 1879, from the blood of a woman with puerperal fever, the dangerous postpartum bacterial infection of the uterus that has also been called "childbed fever." The medical profession had been slow to recognize that this infection was often carried on the hands of doctors and medical students, some of whom went directly from dissecting cadavers in the anatomy lab to attending women in labor. Pasteur recognized this new bacterium as the organism causing the highest mortality among women and their newborns, and he told a medical audience at the French Academy of Sciences in Paris in 1879 that "it is the nursing and medical staff who carry the microbe from an infected woman to a healthy one."[28]

A few years later, German scientists were able to grow the streptococci in culture and to find them in the throats of patients with scarlet fever. One of these scientists named the organism *Streptococcus pyogenes*, which means "pus-causing streptococcus." As bacteriologic techniques improved, researchers realized that this same organism could cause a wide variety of infections and diseases. The female reproductive tract after the trauma of childbirth was particularly susceptible, but so were the tonsils and the throat, giving rise both to simple sore throats and to scarlet fever, which can develop from those sore throats.

Bacteriology thrived in Germany; meanwhile, American scientists were taking note as well. John D. Rockefeller, the oil magnate, was America's first billionaire. He had been thinking about funding a biomedical research institute for some time (he had helped found the University of Chicago in 1890), but it was the death of his three-year-old grandson, John Rockefeller McCormick, from scarlet fever in January 1901 that sent him into action. Like the death of his own thirteen-month-old daughter, Alice, back in 1870, it must have been another reminder that even if you were literally the wealthiest man in America, you were helpless to protect your children and grandchildren against the standard childhood diseases. The new Rockefeller Institute for Medical Research, established in 1901, was to take its place alongside the Institute Pasteur and the Koch Institute. (In Europe, the biomedical institutes were named for the scientists; in the United States, the money would, at least at first, all be private, and the institute would be named for its donor.) The child who died was the son of John D.'s daughter Edith and her husband, Harold Fowler McCormick; Edith Rockefeller McCormick was a lavish-living socialite, and there was a rumor in circulation that when the news of her son's death was brought to her—in the middle of a dinner party—she nodded and went on entertaining her guests. This story brings to mind Mary Lincoln and her tragic White House gala, but it was not true—Edith Rockefeller McCormick was with her son at the family estate when he died, and a year later, she and her husband established a medical institution of their own, the John McCormick Institute for Infectious Diseases in Chicago.[29]

As bacteriology advanced in the early twentieth century, the streptococci were analyzed and carefully classified into types, with specific links to disease syndromes. The organism that killed the fictional Beth, and the real Elizabeth Alcott, is the Group A beta-hemolytic streptococcus, a common human passenger. We now recognize it under the microscope in short chains of round bacterial dots, usually colored purple, since they are gram-positive—that is, their cell walls pick up a particular purple stain. Charles Darwin, who loved all aspects of biology, especially taxonomy, would have found all that of interest, but he was a little too early for microbiology.

In 1922 Margery Williams published *The Velveteen Rabbit*, the story of a stuffed bunny who belongs to a child known only as "the Boy," and who dreams of being "Real." A wise old toy, the Skin Horse, tells him that it will happen when he is truly loved by a child, and sure enough, eventually the Velveteen Rabbit rejoices to hear the Boy say that his rabbit is real. Then the boy gets sick, quite suddenly. "His face grew very flushed, and he talked in his sleep, and his little body was so hot that it burned the Rabbit when he held him close." The rabbit stays close, hidden under the bedclothes, and when no one is around, he whispers in the Boy's ear about all the wonderful things they will do together when he is well. And finally, the fever "turns," and the Boy recovers, and the plan is to send him to the seaside, presumably to regain his strength. But then the doctor sees the old rabbit and says, "Why, it's a mass of scarlet fever germs!—Burn it at once. What? Nonsense! Get him a new one. He mustn't have that any more!"[30] And so the Velveteen Rabbit is placed in a sack and carried off to be burned, while the Boy is provided with a beautiful new stuffed bunny to take to the seaside. Scarlet fever was clearly understood to be a contagious illness by 1922, and the word "germs" was so familiar that it could appear in a book for children.

The rash of scarlet fever is caused by one of several toxic substances, technically erythrogenic (meaning it makes things red) toxins, more specifically streptococcal pyrogenic (meaning it makes things hot) exotoxins. What that means is, many symptoms of the disease are not caused directly by the bacteria doing damage to the cells and organs but because the microbes produce a toxin molecule, a kind of poison that acts in a distinctive way on the host's body. Some strains of Group A strep can cause strep throat but are less likely to produce the toxin that causes scarlet fever, which acts not just in the throat—where the bacteria are actually multiplying, where you can pick them up with a throat swab and grow them in culture—but all over the body. The disease gets its name from the rash, which I was so proud to identify in my young patient in Boston, a rash that, every medical student learns, is bright red—it looks like a sunburn—and has a sandpapery texture. It usually starts on the face or the neck but then extends down over the trunk and the arms and the legs, covering most of the body, with distinctive red lines where the skin folds occur, at the groin or the armpits or the elbows. The rash is warm to the touch, and it can be significantly itchy. The face is flushed, with a pale area around the mouth, and there's a characteristic "strawberry tongue" appearance, bright red with little bumps on it. A high fever is evidence that the immune system has recognized the infection and is trying to fight it off. And a few days in, the skin begins to peel.

Scarlet fever was largely a children's disease, but even for those who recovered, any infection with Group A strep could have after-effects that reached into adulthood. Elizabeth Alcott's death, like Beth March's death (and Gustav Mahler's), was probably the long-delayed result of rheumatic fever—an inflammatory condition that comes on after some strains of strep infection. The symptoms are very variable and can include fever, rash, fatigue, joint pain or swelling, especially in the knees or ankles, and uncontrollable jerking movements in the hands and feet (Sydenham's chorea).[31] Children can get rheumatic fever, which is sometimes fatal, but if they survive it, after having also survived that initial strep infection, they often live with permanent damage to the heart muscle and to the valves, especially the mitral valve, located between the left atrium and the left ventricle, leaving it either too tight for blood to get through or too weakened to close properly, ultimately leading to arrhythmias or failure in the weakened heart. That is why we are so vigilant about treating strep throat with antibiotics; most people can fight off the throat infection, but strep, left untreated, can harm the kidneys or cause rheumatic

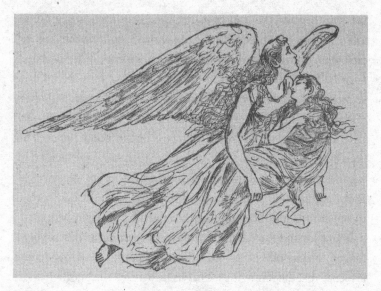

Beth March is carried up to heaven by an angel in this illustration by Frank T. Merrill
for the *Little Women* chapter that contains her death. Louisa May Alcott meant it
to be a beautiful and instructive death. But Beth suffers: "Ah me! Such heavy days,
such long, long nights, such aching hearts and imploring prayers, when those who
loved her best were forced to see the thin hands stretched out to them beseechingly,
to hear the bitter cry, 'Help me, help me!' and to feel that there was no help." *General
Research Division, The New York Public Library*.

fever, which can leave lasting pathology in the heart.[32] So Beth March
recovers from scarlet fever but is left with a badly weakened heart.
After a good deal of pain and distress, she dies peacefully, in her
sleep. In the most famous death in American children's literature, "in
the dark hour before dawn, on the bosom where she had drawn her
first breath, she quietly drew her last."[33] This is the saddest final duty
for a mother, to cradle the head of the dying child, to see her out of
life with tenderness, as she had seen her into life.

Rheumatic fever and subsequent rheumatic heart disease have
always been particularly dangerous for people living in crowded conditions and repeatedly exposed, since new streptococcal disease can
kick off another bout of rheumatic fever in anyone who has had it
once, and recurrent episodes increase the risk of serious damage to

the heart. Rheumatic fever has declined markedly over the past fifty years, in the United States and other developed countries, which may largely be due to better living conditions and better nutrition, and also to those "rheumatogenic" strains becoming less common, though there have been some well-documented small outbreaks of those strains in the States. However, as of 2016, there were 470,000 new cases a year of rheumatic fever in the developing world, in children and in adults, and about 60 percent of those people will go on to develop heart disease. There are 15 million people in the world today with rheumatic heart disease, nowadays largely a disease of poverty and crowding, most common in low-income countries.

Group A strep is also still capable of causing bad infections—those toxins can precipitate a form of toxic shock syndrome. But for the most part, the advent of antibiotics took the danger out of strep throat and scarlet fever; that's why, in the 1990s, I looked at the rash and saw it as something easily treated, easily cured. Antibiotics treat the acute infections, and they also prevent the later complications; although rheumatic fever is now rare in the United States, we still prescribe antibiotics—usually some form of penicillin—for all cases of strep throat, for just that reason.

As the new science of bacteriology developed at the end of the nineteenth century and into the beginning of the twentieth, and as bacteria were definitively implicated in more diseases, researchers dreamed of finding substances that could be used against them, to stop those diseases. Many cases of puerperal fever could be prevented with good hygiene, but if a woman got sick after childbirth, she needed something more. Like puerperal fever, many other diseases that regularly caused great suffering and death—diphtheria, tuberculosis, pneumonia, skin and wound infections—were painstakingly traced by science to specific bacteria, but in 1922 the doctor in *The Velveteen Rabbit,* though he knew that germs caused scarlet fever, had nothing more to offer than Beth March's doctor had in the 1860s.

Calvin Coolidge Jr., the younger son of the president, was known as a regular, unspoiled kid. The story goes that the day his father went from being vice president to being president, because of the death of Warren Harding, Cal Jr. was working a summer job on a tobacco farm in Connecticut, and one of his coworkers said, "If my father was President I would not work in a tobacco field." Cal Jr.'s response: "If my father were your father, you would." On June 30, 1924, he was a sixteen-year-old playing lawn tennis on the White House lawn with his older brother, John, wearing tennis shoes without socks, and he developed a blister on the third toe of his right foot. Soon he had a fever, as well as clear signs of "blood poisoning" (that is, bacteria in the blood, also known as sepsis), and on July 4, his father wrote to his grandfather, back in Vermont, "Calvin is very sick, so this is not a happy day for me." He continued: "Of course he has all that medical science can give but he may have a long sickness with ulcers, then again he may be better in a few days."[34]

But despite the attention of numerous doctors, and admission to Walter Reed Army Medical Center, he was dead by July 7. Coolidge, who refused to seek reelection in 1928, would write in his autobiography, speaking of his son, "When he went, the power and the glory of the Presidency went with him."[35] The culprit was *Staphylococcus aureus,* a common skin bacteria, though it could also have been strep, the source of many wound infections. And there was nothing that the power of the presidency, or the assembled medical expertise, or the might of the military hospital could do against those common bacteria, once they had gotten in through a wound in the skin of the boy's third toe and started to multiply in his blood.

———————————//———————————

There was exactly one antibiotic available when Calvin Coolidge Jr. was dying, but it was useless against those common skin bacteria like strep and staph. Salvarsan was a miracle drug in its day; it had been around since 1910 and was used to treat syphilis, another long-time scourge. But that such a substance existed—that it had been searched for and found by a determined scientist—meant that by the 1920s, a systematic hunt was underway, one that would yield the great pharmaceutical boon of antibiotics and would tame scarlet fever, along with skin infections and many other diseases.

The syphilis drug, that first "magic bullet," which would attack the infecting microbe without hurting the cells of the host, was developed by Paul Ehrlich, a German doctor born in 1854, a few years after the death of Darwin's daughter. The German schools in which Ehrlich trained were part of the best educational system in the world at the time, especially for scientific research, and his dissertation topic concerned the dyes that are used to stain and identify different kinds of cells—including bacterial cells. In 1891, he went to work at Berlin's Royal Prussian Institute for Infectious Diseases, which was headed by Robert Koch; Ehrlich was trying to understand how the immune system worked so that those who survived smallpox, for example, would never get it again, even if they were exposed. He was involved in the first great victory of antibacterial therapy, the production of an antitoxin to diphtheria, when his techniques were used by von Behring to produce clinically useful serum. Ehrlich won the 1905 Nobel Prize for developing a theory of the immune system that suggested that side chains, very specific components of cell membranes, "recognized" invading bacteria and then locked onto them, stimulating production of many more identical side chains, which then went into the bloodstream and could lock onto more matching bacteria.

In the late nineteenth century, Dr. Ehrlich began looking for compounds that could attack the bacteria causing a disease but not in any way harm the host. It was he who called them, in German, "magic bullets."[36] The compounds Ehrlich was using came out of the large and important German dye industry, which had done a great deal to foster the development of modern chemistry. Systematically, Ehrlich's lab tested compound after compound after compound, looking for something that would kill the protozoan parasite that causes African sleeping sickness, a trypanosome. But when they found their compound, arsphenamine, it killed not only trypanosomes but also the bacteria that cause syphilis, one of the most feared diseases all over Europe. Earlier treatments were generally futile and often highly toxic (the expression "A night with Venus, a lifetime with Mercury" conveys the general idea). Here now, in 1910, was a drug that actually worked; within a year, it was more widely prescribed than any other medication in the world.[37]

The world went to war in 1914, but when the war ended, the German chemists continued the hunt for more magic bullets. Germany also merged its eight largest chemical firms into one entity, IG Farben (the name stands for Interessen-Gemeinschaft Farbenindustrie, or Community of Interests of Dye Businesses), which was large enough and powerful enough to start working through possible therapeutic compounds, many derived from dyes that Ehrlich had determined had affinities for particular cells. A researcher named Gerhard Domagk had isolated a strain of streptococci that was consistently fatal to lab mice, and each new compound was tested against that strain of strep to see if it could save the mice, but the range of drugs did not really increase in the 1920s. And then, in 1932, researchers tried a new kind of chemical, also brought over from the dye business, linked to a sulfa molecule. Twenty-six mice were infected with the "superstrep," and twelve were treated with the compound, sulfanilamide-azo. The fourteen untreated mice all died; the twelve who got the sulfa compound survived.

The discovery was announced in 1935. Bayer, the pharmaceutical division of IG Farben, patented the drug and named it Prontosil. In December 1935, Dr. Domagk's daughter, Hildegarde, age six, was carrying an embroidery needle when she tripped, and the needle went deep into her hand. Although it was removed at the hospital, she developed a high fever and swelling, with the red stripes of severe skin infection spreading up her arm, and blood tests showed streptococcal bacteremia. The doctor recommended amputating the arm.

"A year earlier," writes William Rosen in *Miracle Cure,* "she would very probably have lost her arm, and possibly her life. But this was the year of Prontosil." Although it had not been thoroughly tested in humans, Domagk gave it to his daughter, and it worked: A week after starting the therapy, Rosen reports, "her infection was beaten."[38] Domagk, however, left that story out of his report on the drug, waiting for the formal clinical trial results.[39]

In 1936, only twelve years after the death of Calvin Coolidge Jr., another presidential namesake son, Franklin Delano Roosevelt Jr., twenty-two, contracted a serious streptococcal throat infection, with sinus complications. He was treated with Prontosil, prescribed for him by the White House medical staff. When he recovered, the front-page headline of the *New York Times* of Thursday, December 17, 1936, read, "YOUNG ROOSEVELT SAVED BY NEW DRUG."[40] "Franklin D. Roosevelt Jr. faced death from a throat infection last week," the article began. "Dr. Tobey revealed he employed the new chemo-therapeutic agent to ameliorate the streptococcus infection. The patient responded 'beautifully,' he said." Roosevelt's highly public case did a great deal to publicize the new sulfa drugs; by the time that article appeared, the company had already been besieged with calls from people with sinus complaints. The message was clear enough: the world had changed. The best you could do for the president's child, when he had a life-threatening infection, was dramatically more than anyone had been able to do for a president's child in the decade before. The new era had started, at the top.[41]

After Prontosil had gone on the market, in 1935, many other companies had begun to develop their own sulfa drugs. Bayer wouldn't send samples to the Pasteur Institute, but Pasteur managed to make its own version, as did numerous other companies, eager to get in on the antibiotic gold rush. By the end of 1937, a hundred companies were selling a hundred different versions of sulfanilamide, in countries around the world. It was highly effective against puerperal fever—mortality from the disease fell from 20 to 30 percent to 4.7

percent when women were treated with the new drugs. There was also a sulfa drug disaster: a company in Tennessee decided to create a liquid form of sulfa but chose to mix it with a very toxic chemical, diethylene glycol (a component of antifreeze). When they put it on the market in 1937, 108 people died from drinking Massengill's Elixir Sulfanilamide, mostly children. The existing drug laws were so lax that the only crime the company could be charged with was incorrect labeling.

The next year, 1938, President Roosevelt signed the Federal Food, Drug, and Cosmetic Act, legislating that ingredients be listed on packages, that warnings accompany drugs that might be dangerous, and that the government would henceforth regulate all new drugs. Even so, sulfa drugs continued to boom. Larger quantities were being produced, the pharmaceutical companies were marketing them aggressively, and when the Second World War came, they played an important role, with all American soldiers being issued packets of sulfa powder to sprinkle on wounds.[42]

We still use sulfa drugs today, but they are by no means the most common antibiotics; they turned out to have a number of side effects, including relatively common allergic reactions, and they can be difficult to administer. Starting in the late 1940s and early 1950s, a new set of wonder drugs arrived with the commercial availability of penicillin. In one of the most famous discovery stories in science, Alexander Fleming observed that a mold had contaminated a staphylococcal culture plate, in his lab at St. Mary's Hospital in London, and stopped the bacteria from growing. He had been away on vacation in August 1928, he said, and had left the petri dishes unattended. On his return in September, he found that one had been invaded by a fungus that had come in through a nearby open window. The zone around the contamination was clear of staphylococci; they had been killed by whatever was in the fungus. In his Nobel banquet talk, Fleming said, "I isolated the contaminating mould. It made an antibacterial substance which I christened penicillin. I studied it as far as I could as a bacteriologist. I had a clue that here was something good but I could not possibly know how good it was and I had not the team, especially the chemical team, necessary to concentrate and stabilise the penicillin."[43]

This famous story has been subjected to a good deal of analysis and doubt. (Did that window really open? Do the dates in the story line up with the dates in his lab notebook? Does it make sense that the mold would have killed established colonies of bacteria when we now know that penicillin kills bacteria only when they are dividing?) Whatever the exact origin story, Fleming did realize that what he called "mould juice" was killing staph, and he did a number of experiments to find out what other bacteria it killed (strep) and did not kill (typhus). Unfortunately, it was very unstable stuff, and very difficult to make. He published a report in 1929, but nobody took much notice, and his lab went on to other things.

Two other researchers would share the 1945 Nobel Prize with Alexander Fleming for their work on penicillin. One was Howard Florey, an Australian physician who came to England on a Rhodes Scholarship in 1922, followed that up with a fellowship from the relatively new Rockefeller Foundation, which took him to study in America, and in 1935 became director of the Dunn School of Pathology at Oxford. The chemist Ernst Chain, the third scientist who would share in that penicillin Nobel, was another immigrant to England, a Jew from Germany who'd left when the Nazis came to power; he was the chemist son of a chemist father, who had himself emigrated from the Pale of Settlement in Russia and opened a factory in Berlin. Ernst Chain had been a piano prodigy, and his superb control over his hands, together with what was apparently something close to a perfect photographic memory, made him a powerful force in the lab.[44]

Working together in Oxford, either Florey or Chain found Alexander Fleming's little-read and rarely referenced paper from 1929— Florey always said he gave it to Chain, and Chain always said he gave it to Florey. In May 1940, Howard Florey chose *Streptococcus pyogenes,* the scarlet fever bacterium, for the first animal tests of this promising substance. He infected eight lab mice and treated four of them with penicillin. The untreated mice died overnight. But all of the mice who got penicillin did fine. As Florey and Chain ran more experiments, they learned that penicillin was far more powerful than the sulfa drugs; it could be diluted way down and would still work against bacteria. In a famous story, as their financially hard-pressed lab continued its research, they "borrowed" bedpans from the hospital to use as vessels for growing penicillin.[45] And in the *Lancet,* on August 24, 1940, their article appeared: "Penicillin as a Chemotherapeutic Agent." The seven authors were listed in strictly alphabetical order, to avoid having to settle who deserved how much credit. On September 2, Alexander Fleming came to visit their lab—and to establish his own claim for credit, asking what had been done "with my old penicillin."[46]

It was still the era before clinical trials were in any way systematized or regulated. To see if it was safe to inject into humans, the Dunn lab group asked Charles Fletcher, an academic medical doctor affiliated with the team, to find them a patient with a fatal disorder who might be willing to help. Dr. Fletcher wrote, "There were no ethical committees in those days that had to be consulted, so I looked around the wards and found a pleasant 50 year old woman with disseminated breast cancer who had not long to live." This was Elva Akers; Dr. Fletcher told her that he "wanted to try a new medicine that could be of value to many people, and asked if she would agree to a test injection of it. This she readily did."[47] She developed fever and seizures, which turned out to be due to impurities in the penicillin. The scientific team found a new way to purify it and the doctors reinjected the same woman, and this time she had no reaction.

They then tested it on a policeman named Albert Alexander, who had scratched his face on a thorn and developed terrible infections, first in the skin and later in the lungs. The penicillin brought dramatic improvement, but to keep treating him, they needed more of it than they had, so they had to collect his urine, run it over to the lab, purify out the excreted penicillin, and give it back to him using an IV.

The British researchers next took their discovery to America, where it became a project of the USDA's Northern Regional Research Laboratory in Peoria, Illinois. One of the bacteriologists there, Mary Hunt, was sent to find moldy fruit and vegetables from all over Peoria; in 1943 she would turn up a cantaloupe with a penicillin strain so strong that it would basically become the source of all future versions of the drug. American pharmaceutical companies began trying to make penicillin, and a disaster brought the new drug to the attention of the public. In November 1942, the crowded Cocoanut Grove nightclub in Boston caught fire (the blaze began in one of the artificial coconut trees). That night, 492 people were killed, and many more were badly burned. The Merck Pharmaceutical Company sent over thirty-two liters of penicillin broth from New Jersey, which the doctors used to try to ward off infections in the burn patients. That got penicillin into the newspapers, and soon people were clamoring for the drug.

The War Production Board got involved, as did the new Office of Scientific Research and Development (which would, among other things, direct the Manhattan Project) and its Committee on Medical Research. The CMR provided funding, pulling together an array of universities, pharmaceutical companies, and hospitals, all directed to work on the penicillin project. They found ways to manufacture and purify the drug more efficiently; they tested it and sent it out to soldiers to treat wounds and also to cure gonorrhea, another military scourge.

The Germans lagged in the penicillin race, probably because they had set their massive chemical industry to the task of producing fuel. Many of the American companies that participated in the effort, and were able to keep the patents on any new processes that they developed, would grow into pharmaceutical giants. Thus, the production

of penicillin became in part a wartime story, of great strategic importance, just like the race to build an atomic bomb—two very different expressions of human ingenuity. Albert L. Elder coordinated the
penicillin program for the War Production Board, ultimately pulling
together twenty-one manufacturing plants, rationing civilian use,
and working to stockpile ample stores of the drug for the military
in time for D-Day, in June 1944, and the invasion of Europe. (They
had three hundred billion units of penicillin ready.) The rush toward
penicillin was driven in large part by the need to treat the injuries
inflicted by military technology, even as scientists were working to
develop and enhance that technology.

Eventually, there were Nobel Prizes for many of the researchers
who had developed antibiotics. Inevitably there were hard feelings
about who got what credit, and sometimes worse than hard feelings:
Gerhard Domagk was awarded the 1939 Nobel Prize for his discovery of sulfanilamide, but he ran afoul of the Gestapo for accepting it
and was jailed for being "too polite to the Swedes." He was forced to
send a letter turning down the prize, though he did finally get his
medal in 1947.[48]

In 1903, scientists had classified the streptococci into three
groups, one of which was hemolytic—it dissolved red blood cells
and produced toxin. But the hemolytic streptococci and the role they
played in human disease were not well understood at all, including
their connection to scarlet fever and rheumatic fever. Some of the
most important answers would come from the research institution
established in memory of the Rockefeller grandson. Rebecca Lancefield, a young bacteriologist, took a job there in 1918 because, she
said, "it was the only place that answered my job letters," and began
studying how to classify the streptococci. She was to work there until
1980 when she broke her hip and retired, at the age of eighty-five.[49]
Her first paper, identifying four different serological types of bacteria,
"represented," the geneticist Maclyn McCarty wrote, "a record of the

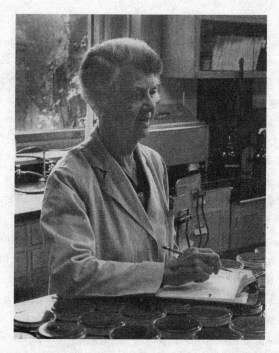

Dr. Rebecca Lancefield in her laboratory, with clipboard and petri dishes. Working with samples from military medical facilities, she classified beta-hemolytic strepto-cocci, meticulously sorting out their chemical properties and propensity to cause disease, and collected more than six thousand different strains in a bacteriological "library" still maintained at Rockefeller University. *Courtesy of Rockefeller Archive Center.*

first encounter between these microorganisms and the investigator who was destined over the next five decades to become the master of their diversity."[50]

Lancefield had grown up in an army family. Before and during World War II she ran a laboratory that worked with bacterial cultures from military patients, investigating contagious diseases. The lab was often called the "Scotland Yard of streptococcal mysteries."[51] Their research led to a system of sorting the streptococci according to car-bohydrate molecules—distinctive bacterial markers—on their cell walls. Although some aspects of the classification system have now been superseded by new bacteriologic techniques, this represented a great step forward in identifying and understanding the clinically virulent forms of strep and teasing out the different kinds of damage they could do. Every time I have identified the organism that causes scarlet fever (and strep throat, and puerperal fever, and wound infections) as Group A strep, I am using what we still refer to as a "Lancefield grouping," under a system laid out by Lancefield in the 1930s.[52] During the 1920s and 1930s, as this research was going on, scarlet fever had again undergone a transformation, and it was no longer the terrifying killer it had been; from 1926 to 1937, there were plenty of scarlet fever cases in the United States, but mortality was low, with only twenty-five hundred deaths a year. In 1937, when the first antibiotics, the sulfa drugs, were introduced, deaths plummeted.[53] But strep infections from those years before antibiotics left a long shadow of post-streptococcal rheumatic disease. From 1925 to 1950, rheumatic fever was the leading cause of death in American children five to nineteen years old, and the leading cause of heart disease in those under forty. Fortunately, in 1951, researchers showed that by treating strep infections with penicillin, you could dramatically reduce, perhaps even eliminate, the likelihood of rheumatic fever later on.

We now live in an era of worry over the overuse of antibiotics, in humans and also in domestic animals. These days, pediatricians try to prescribe antibiotics only when they are clearly necessary—a sore throat gets penicillin only if the test is positive for strep; ear infections are often managed with "watchful waiting," as long as the child doesn't seem to be seriously ill. This is because using antibiotics too freely contributes to the development of resistant strains of bacteria, and also because more recently we have come to understand that there may be serious consequences to the kinds of changes that antibiotics bring about in the microbiome, or bacterial population, of the human gut. Some parents now worry when their children are given antibiotics, although other parents feel dissatisfied when the doctor holds the line and won't prescribe antibiotics for a bad cold or runny nose, even after the doctor explains that those infections are more likely to be viral and will get better by themselves. We've been trying for years to regard antibiotics with a little more care and circumspection, recognizing their power and trying to preserve it by preventing overuse and slowing the development of resistance. We need these drugs to stay potent for us, and it's important to remember what game changers they were when they were first developed.

Penicillin was used to treat—and probably save—tens of thousands of soldiers during World War II. The first medical report about a child treated with penicillin described a seven-year-old girl in the United States who got a dose on July 11, 1942, because of what her doctor thought was a severe blood infection caused by staphylococci. At the American Academy of Pediatrics meeting in November 1944, in St. Louis, Dr. Wallace Herrell from the Mayo Clinic presented a paper titled "Penicillin: Its Use in Pediatrics." In the very first paragraph, you can hear the announcement of a new era beginning, as the doctor and his colleagues describe the first series of fifty-four children at the Mayo Clinic to be treated with the brand-new drug: "With the introduction of penicillin in the treatment of susceptible bacterial infections, it would appear that a new chapter is being written in the chemotherapy of diseases affecting not only adults but patients in the so-called pediatric age group."[54] The most dramatic case they reported on was that of a ten-day-old infant who had accidentally been mildly injured on the chest after delivery, with an abrasion that turned into a superficial skin infection, which then spread to the front and back of the torso and to the stomach, with staphylococci in the baby's blood as well.

The doctors had given the infant sulfa drugs, but they had not helped. They then began giving the baby shots of penicillin every three hours. Penicillin was easier to administer, and it worked against organisms that the sulfa drugs did not affect. "Blood cultures became negative and the cellulitis subsided as penicillin therapy was contin-

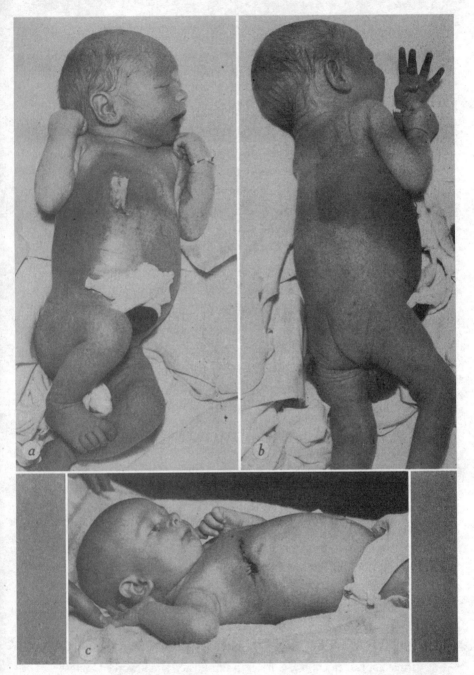

Before penicillin, this virulent bacterial skin infection would have consumed and killed the child; the "after" photograph at the bottom of this image attests that such infections were now treatable, survivable, and curable. *Reprinted from Wallace E. Herrell and Roger L. J. Kennedy, "Penicillin: Its Use in Pediatrics,"* Journal of Pediatrics 25, no. 6: 505–16. *Copyright 1944, used with permission from Elsevier.*

ued," the article said; it was accompanied by rather dramatic before and after photos of the infant. In the before photos, even in black and white, the substantial discoloration of much of the baby's chest wall is clearly visible, showing the extent of the angry skin infection, as he lies on his back with his arms and legs flexed tightly after the fashion of a newborn, eyes tightly closed, mouth slightly open, as if in distress. In the after photo, one month later, he lies on his back looking rather relaxed, eyes open, with a scar to show where the abscess was, and a facial expression suggesting calm contemplation. The postwar era of Kodak baby pictures was about to begin, and the after photo somehow suggests the happy safety of the babies whose pictures would illustrate the baby boom.

"In view of the extensive nature of the cellulitis present and in view of the overwhelming generalized sepsis as indicated by the blood cultures, it seems likely that penicillin was responsible for changing an almost hopeless situation into a recovery," wrote the doctors from Mayo, in language that, for a medical journal, gives a strong sense of the medical drama that had taken place. "During the period before administration of penicillin was begun the infant was rapidly losing weight and strength," the authors wrote. "It is further interesting that this infant within a few days after penicillin therapy was started began to gain weight and to progress in a fashion not unlike that expected of a normal infant of this age."[55] The antibiotic age had begun, and many previously hopeless situations would become recoveries.

PART III

"What Marvellous Days"

CHAPTER 7

"Strides of Modern Medical Science"

Preventing Polio, Treating Tuberculosis

The decades after World War II in the United States, as the baby boomers were born, were a time of increasing prosperity and medical progress. Parents and physicians were moving toward the idea that no child should die—or that, at least, it should be possible to protect any child who was born mature enough to survive the neonatal period. Diseases were problems to be solved, and science and medicine were publicly vowing to solve them, with scientist heroes making promises, with dramatic press conference reveals—and with activist parents playing a leading role in campaigns to defeat the diseases which threatened their families.

By the end of the 1950s, both tuberculosis and polio would be medically "solved": polio with the development of not one but two successful vaccines, and tuberculosis with the arrival of several successful antimicrobial drugs. (It turns out that to treat TB successfully, you need to administer multiple drugs at the same time.) By the time I was growing up, in the 1960s, polio figured in our lives only as a vaccine—and in our parents' vivid memories of polio epidemics in the 1930s and 1940s. TB seemed more remote and less terrifying, though we were all familiar with the annual ritual of the skin test, the little injection of a derivative of TB bacteria carefully placed in the tender skin of your forearm, to be checked for a positive reaction two days later by the school nurse. (The danger sign would be a red swelling at the site of the injection, suggesting that the immune system is revved up because it has already been exposed to these bacteria.) A positive skin test doesn't mean that you're sick with tuberculosis; it tells you that you've been exposed and that the bacteria have taken up residence in your lungs, where they may wait quietly for years—but eventually wake up and cause disease—so preventing the illness ideally means finding and treating that "latent" infection.

Neither polio nor TB would admit of simple solutions: both are still very much in the headlines, both inside and outside the medical literature. As I write this in 2019, we are finally on the brink of eliminating polio altogether—but it's a difficult brink, and we have been hovering near it for a long time, with the infection hanging on in just a few countries, most recently Pakistan, Afghanistan, and Nigeria. Both the oral live attenuated polio vaccine and the killed injectable one are still in play, and issues of which vaccine to use and the rare complications of vaccination have combined with complex political situations in some parts of the world in ways that have meant that children are still left dead or paralyzed by polio. Meanwhile, though tuberculosis is now a treatable disease, it requires a long and not necessarily pleasant course of medication. TB bacteria continue to infect a very large proportion of the world's population, especially in poor countries, and with the emergence of AIDS, tuberculosis among that immunocompromised population has meant a whole new category of disease and treatment conundrums. Tuberculosis bacteria in different parts of the world have evolved resistance to many of the first-line drugs. In 2013, in the United States, there were 485 cases of TB among children under fifteen years old, and the CDC estimates that there are a million such cases worldwide every year.

Both the polio virus and the tuberculosis bacterium were identified long before they could be treated or prevented, tuberculosis at the end of the nineteenth century, polio at the beginning of the twentieth. The polio virus is spread by the fecal-oral route—that is, the virus is excreted in the stool and transmitted when someone swallows it, usually in contaminated food or water. The tuberculosis bacterium is most often transmitted through inhalation (though there is another type that infects cows; you can get that one from drinking contaminated milk). Both diseases were sometimes identified with poverty and dirt and crowded slum conditions, but both were also very publicly claiming victims from the families of the richest and most powerful people in the world, some of whom threw themselves and their money into medical research. There was a large and very visible charitable effort aimed at defeating polio by the March of Dimes, and a similar effort aimed at defeating tuberculosis through the international Christmas Seals campaign, but when World War II ended, polio epidemics were still a threat, and tuberculosis remained what it had been for centuries: a silent and slow killer that sometimes moved faster in children.

The efforts against both diseases captured the popular imagination, and people bought Christmas Seals or supported the March of Dimes as small-scale, day-by-day popular efforts to protect children from these dangers that could interrupt or end a life. The March of Dimes pioneered other public relations and fundraising strategies; that organization was the first to use celebrities to raise awareness—and money. In 1938, Judy Garland and Mickey Rooney were filmed sending their dimes to "President Franklin Roosevelt, the White House, Washington D.C.," to help fight infantile paralysis. In 1954, it was Lucille Ball and Desi Arnaz and their children; Lucy talked about parents who live in fear of polio, saying, "I know I do." But, she added, within a year, there might be a vaccine—so send money to help with large-scale testing. And a year later, in 1955, Sammy Davis Jr., performing in front of a March of Dimes banner, was asking for money to buy the "Dr. Salk polio vaccine."

Polio epidemics and polio research played out in the context of midcentury American realities, including racial prejudice—but the

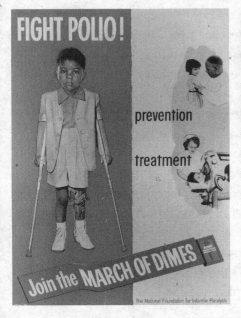

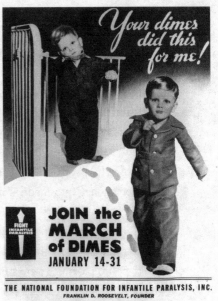

Along with other innovative fundraising strategies (like sending dimes to the White House), the March of Dimes pioneered the idea of the "poster child." *March of Dimes.*

times were changing. In 1944, the National Foundation for Infantile Paralysis, recognizing that African American children were not receiving services (and were barred from segregated treatment centers) hired Charles H. Bynum, an educator who had been working at the Tuskegee Institute, to lead its "Negro Activities," and he formulated polio—and differential care—as a civil rights issue, increasing interracial fundraising and making better treatment available to African American polio victims.[1] Even so, as rehabilitation was extended, and as the poster children campaigns continued to draw attention to the needs of survivors, the goal—and the promise to parents—went beyond rehabilitation. The promise was prevention.

But in the meantime, both diseases created populations of sufferers and survivors who needed help. In addition to those highly public charities—and supported by them—specialized institutions had developed for people suffering from both diseases. Children who had been left paralyzed after polio could get physical therapy and hydro-therapy in rehabilitation centers funded by the March of Dimes; one such was the Warm Springs Institute for Rehabilitation, founded and patronized by Franklin Delano Roosevelt. The late nineteenth and early twentieth centuries saw the development of sanatoriums where people with tuberculosis could breathe outdoor air of a particularly salutary variety (mountain air, for example), follow a set regime of rest or gradually increasing exercise, eat a special diet, and hope to regain their health.

Evidence of tuberculosis infection has been found in skeletons from ancient and classical times, from both the Old World and the New, and bacterial DNA has been cultured from Egyptian mum-mies. Humans have known TB as an enemy and a killer for millen-nia and have tried all through history to understand it according to their evolving knowledge of disease and debility. TB is mentioned in Deuteronomy and Leviticus, and may claim the dubious honor of having killed more human beings than any other microbe in history. It was certainly a major cause of child mortality. Medical historians have argued convincingly that improved nutrition, liv-ing conditions, and hygiene had already brought down death rates from TB long before the medical discoveries—the combinations of specialized antimicrobials—that made it possible to cure individual cases. When we talk about improved nutrition helping child survival rates, tuberculosis is probably one of the areas where it was most helpful. Around the world today, TB remains much more likely and much more dangerous in circumstances of poverty, overcrowding, and malnutrition.

In literature and music, TB has often been treated as a sanctifying, etherealizing, and operatic exit, with plenty of time for last speeches (or last arias) and no unpleasant gastrointestinal effluvia. Little Eva, that petted, cherished, saintly darling, was not atypical as a wealthy, beloved, medically attended child, dying because the tuberculosis bacteria were too much for all the world's best doctors. Tad Lincoln, who had survived the typhoid infection that killed his brother, would grow up—or not quite grow up—to succumb to tuberculosis at the age of eighteen.[2] Frances Hodgson Burnett, best remembered now for her children's books, including *Little Lord Fauntleroy, The Secret Garden,* and *A Little Princess,* had a son named Lionel who contracted TB; she took him all over Europe, searching for a cure, accompanied by her own private doctor and nurse. But all the medical treatments failed, and he died at the age of sixteen, in 1890, leaving his grieving mother to write him one letter after another ("They make for heartbreaking reading," comments her biographer), as she lapsed into depression. Looking back, Burnett felt she should have known about his sickness from his lovely fair complexion: "That fine ivory tint was only a sign in Lionel that strong and splendid as he always was, there was really in his blood that deadly taint of the disease which killed him."[3] Thus, like Little Eva, he was marked for death by his ethereal pallor. It has been suggested that the figure of the crippled Colin in *The Secret Garden,* which Burnett published in 1911, was based on this lost son, a bereaved mother creating a fictional boy whom everyone supposes to be fatally ill but who recovers, as tuberculosis patients were supposed to do, with fresh air and healthy outdoor living.

Tuberculosis bacteria, after they are inhaled, are often walled off in the lungs by the body's efficient immune system. Inside the little walled-off nodules, or tubercles, the bacteria can lie dormant for years—or, indeed, forever. This latent infection—what we look for with a TB test, either a skin prick or a blood test—is capable of waking up again, perhaps when you are elderly or your immune system is weakened; if we discover it we treat it prophylactically with antibiotics designed to wipe out the bacteria before they can cause disease. When the bacteria are active, they can cause all different kinds of infections, from that classic lung disease in which people cough up blood, to bone and joint infections, to meningitis. Hard to diagnose, hard to grow in culture, and hard to treat, TB bacteria are notoriously slow-growing. Once bacteriology had discovered and identified the strep that cause scarlet fever, for example, you could swab someone's throat and know in twenty-four to forty-eight hours whether or not those bacteria would grow from your sample. But TB is finicky and difficult; even if someone has active pulmonary TB and is coughing up sputum, the bacteria can be tricky to identify.

By the early nineteenth century, TB was killing enormous numbers of people all over Europe and North America.[4] More than 25 percent of all the deaths recorded in New York City between 1810 and 1815 were from TB.[5] It was chiefly identified as a killer of young adults, but TB has also always been a deadly childhood disease, though it was harder to recognize in children, where it often did not look like standard pulmonary tuberculosis. This was especially true in younger children; TB was rarely listed as a cause of death in babies, although at the beginning of the twentieth century, some autopsy studies in American cities showed that more than 10 percent of all the infants who died were infected with tuberculosis, and infants born to mothers with TB had a mortality rate more than two and a half times as high as that of other babies.[6]

By the end of the nineteenth century, the massive epidemic of the early 1800s had begun to recede. Many theories as to why have been proposed, including improved hygiene, public sanitation, isolation of the sick in treatment institutions and sanitoriums, and improved nutrition, but there is no single clear explanation.[7]

Right through the first half of the twentieth century, before there were effective drugs, trips to healthier climates continued to be recommended, with wealthy patients sent to luxurious sanatoriums, for rest and mountain air—which did indeed often slow the progress of the disease. TB infection, severity, and mortality all decrease with higher altitude. The first American sanatoriums were in Asheville, North Carolina, and in the Adirondacks, where Dr. Edward Livingston Trudeau opened a sanatorium at Saranac Lake in 1885. His brother had died of TB, and he had expected to die of it himself after he contracted the disease, a year out of medical school. He had gone to the Adirondacks to die; when, instead, he apparently recovered, he developed a regimen of diet and outdoor exercise, which he believed could cure others. Life in a sanatorium isolated TB patients, and probably had some protective effect on the general population, but it's hard to tell whether the treatments actually extended many lives that would otherwise have ended—TB in adults is often a prolonged disease that waxes and wanes.[8] Dr. Trudeau did survive, and he became the first president of the National Association for the Study and Prevention of Tuberculosis. The sanatorium treatments and the public health efforts to control TB were in large part funded by a new kind of charity. In 1904, the first Christmas seal was issued in Denmark, with a picture of the Danish queen. The campaign was the inspiration of Einar Holboll, a postal clerk who had dreamed up the idea of selling a special stamp for holiday cards, and the proceeds built a sanatorium for children with TB. The idea spread throughout Europe and was brought to the United States in 1907 by Emily Bissell, where it grew into a large program administered by the National Tuberculosis Association.

In the Betsy-Tacy books, a series of stories for girls by Maud Hart Lovelace set in the idyllic small town of Deep Valley, Minnesota, around the turn of the century, the piano teacher, Miss Cobb, is a town heroine for having taken in her sister's four children to raise, after the sister died. By 1908, "the little girl had followed her mother and the youngest boy had followed his sister. One of the two remaining boys was delicate."[9] Leonard, the "delicate" boy, "a slender fifteen-year-old boy with sandy hair and vivid cheeks," is clearly sick with TB, which has already wiped out three members of his family, and in due course, he is sent off to a sanatorium in Colorado, where he dies. Nobody in the book thinks that there is anything to be done to retard the inevitably fatal progress of the disease, beyond the possibility of mountain air, and interestingly, no one has any worries

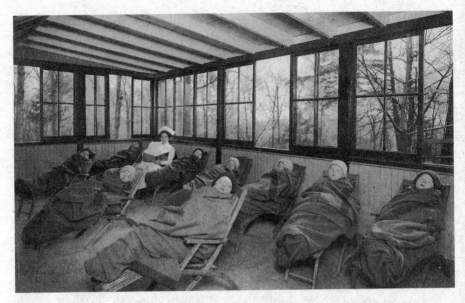

The sanatorium ideal was a mix of fresh air—usually cold air—and some blend of rest with mild, carefully controlled outdoor exercise. Here, a nurse reads to a group of children who are bundled up against the cold, fresh air. *Alamy Images.*

about sending children to take their piano lessons in a house where there is a boy dying of TB, who often reclines on a couch to hear the music. TB is an unremarkable presence in a middle-class home in a middle-class town.

Friedrich Franz Friedmann used bacteria from turtles in the Berlin zoo and claimed to have developed a curative turtle serum. He brought it to New York in 1913, hoping to make his fortune, and created a furor: "Crowds gathered at the entrance to a hospital with their tuberculous children in carriages. A mother threw herself in the path of his car desperate for treatment for her 9-year-old son."[10] Ultimately, the New York City Board of Health ruled against the turtle cure, and Friedrich Franz Friedmann went back to Europe, having made some money, though not as much as he had hoped.

Early in the twentieth century, two scientists in France, Albert Calmette and Camille Guérin, set out to create a vaccine against tuberculosis. They developed a strain of bovine tuberculosis and made it into a vaccine in the 1920s, testing it first on an infant born to a mother who was dying of pulmonary TB and cared for by a grandmother who also had the disease. The child survived. Unfortunately, early on, there was a disaster in which 250 German infants were given the live TB bacteria, rather than the weak vaccine, and more than 70 died. But the research continued, and the modern BCG vaccine, named for that strain of bovine tuberculosis (which was, in turn, named for its discoverers), bacillus Calmette-Guérin, is still used today to vaccinate children against TB in many countries around the world, although not in the United States. It does not offer perfect protection against infection, but it lowers the risk. (Different studies have shown widely ranging rates of efficacy and immunity.) It does not, however, help a child who is already sick.

In the United States, there were particularly high rates of TB in urban African American communities, made worse by crowded living conditions and the underlying poverty and malnutrition. Access to care was limited, and there was well-founded distrust about what treatment would be like in sanitoriums.

Jessie Sleet Scales, considered the first Black public health nurse in the United States, was actually born in Ontario. She trained in Chicago and was initially unable to find work in New York City because of racial prejudice. When she was hired in 1902 by the Charity Organization Society, her job involved making home visits to Black families with TB and convincing them to get medical treatment; her reports were so exemplary that they were published in the *American Journal of Nursing*, under the title "A Successful Experiment"; they offer a glimpse of her heavy caseload and her high level of dedication:

> I beg to render to you a report of the work done by me as
> a district nurse among the colored people of New York
> City during the months of October and November. I have
> endeavored to search out the families in which there was

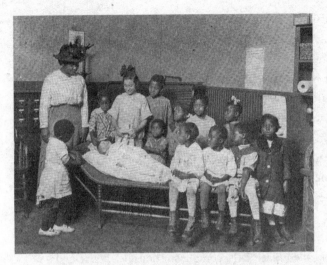

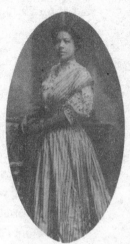

Two of the pioneering African American nurses who battled tuberculosis in urban Black communities, where mortality was high. At left is Elizabeth Tyler in south Philadelphia, where her work expanded beyond tuberculosis care to other areas of health and education; she is shown here with the "Little Mothers" club. At right is Jessie Sleet Scales in New York City. *(left) Whittier Centre Annual Report (Philadelphia, 1914), image courtesy of the Special Collections Research Center, Temple University Libraries, Philadelphia, PA; (right) image was published in Marie O. Pitts Mosley, "Satisfied to Carry the Bag,"* Nursing History Review 4 (1996) *with permission of Dr. Mary Elizabeth Carnegie.*

sickness and destitution. . . . I have visited forty-one families and made 156 calls in connection with these families, caring for nine cases of consumption, four cases of peritonitis, two cases of chickenpox, two cases of cancer, one case of diphtheria, two cases of heart disease, two cases of tumor, one case of gastric catarrh, two cases of pneumonia, four cases of rheumatism, and two cases of scalp wound. I have given baths, applied poultices, dressed wounds, washed and dressed newborn babies, cared for mothers.[11]

Mortality from TB for Black Philadelphians was two and a half to three times higher than for non-immigrant whites in the early twentieth century. In seeking to engage the trust of members of the Black community, the Henry Phipps Institute for the Study, Treatment and Prevention of Tuberculosis hired Elizabeth Tyler, the public health nurse who had been the first African American nurse at the Henry Street Settlement in New York City. In this endeavor, the Phipps Institute was working cooperatively with the Whittier Centre, a private association with a mission to help the Black community of Philadelphia with health issues and social problems. Elizabeth Tyler had studied at the Freedmen's Hospital Training School in Washington, D.C., and worked at Smith College and A&M College in Alabama before undertaking her postgraduate course at the Lincoln School in New York City. When she moved to Philadelphia, Tyler worked chiefly in the so-called Black Belt, going from house to house and assessing families, recommending clinical treatment for TB. Inspired by her success, the institute hired a Black physician, Dr. Henry Minton, who became well known as a tuberculosis expert, and remained on the staff until 1946. In part through this strategy of hiring African American clinicians, the institute was able to attract increasing numbers of patients from the Black community; the outreach strategies included a church campaign. Dr. Minton reflected later that "the success of these clinics is largely dependent upon the efficiency and faithfulness of the nurse."[12]

Dr. Edith Lincoln started the Children's Chest Clinic at Bellevue Hospital in New York City in 1922. She had been born right at the end of the nineteenth century, in 1899, and had studied medicine at Johns Hopkins. She was one of the first women to be accepted as an intern at Bellevue; later she recalled insisting on eating with the other interns, though she had been told to sit with the nurses. Children who ended up on the tuberculosis ward at the hospital did not necessarily know they had the disease when they came in; everyone got a TB skin test on admission. So in evaluating children, Edith Lincoln had available to her that test and X-ray technology to see what was going on in children's chests. But there was not a tremendous amount

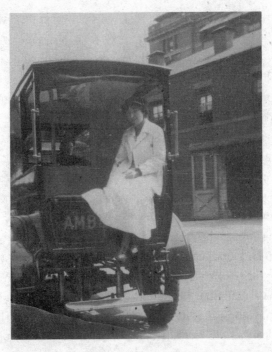

Dr. Edith Lincoln at the beginning of her studies at Bellevue Hospital, sitting on an early ambulance. *Image courtesy of the Lillian and Clarence de la Chapelle Medical Archives at NYU.*

of information available to interpret what those skin test results and those X-ray findings meant for any given child.

The patients Lincoln was taking care of at Bellevue were mostly poor, the children of those crowded New York slums. She started a long-term study, planning to sign up one thousand children with chest X-ray evidence of primary tuberculosis in their lungs and follow them until they were twenty-five years old. (Ultimately, she would study more than twenty-five hundred children.) She had no effective medication to offer them, and almost a quarter of the children with recent primary TB infections in their lungs died, 90 percent of them within a year after diagnosis. Of the babies diagnosed when under six months old, 55 percent died; for those one to two, 28 percent died;

and for those who were four to nine years old when they were diagnosed, the fatality rate was 15 percent.[13] Meningitis was a particularly
fearful—and fatal—course the disease could take; more than half of
the children who died had developed this slow, progressive infection of
the central nervous system, which, over the course of days and weeks,
rendered them groggy, semiconscious, and finally comatose. Another
very dangerous pathway, much more common in children than adults,
was the general spread of the tuberculosis bacteria in the blood—called
"miliary" disease because it resulted in tiny nodules of disease, once
thought to resemble millet seeds, throughout the lungs. And 25 percent of the children died eventually of disseminated disease, bacteria
spreading through their bloodstreams, or of progressive pulmonary TB.

In 1943, a drug called streptomycin was made from a fungus,
building on research by a scientist at Rutgers, Selman Waksman,
who was actually the first to start calling these new antibacterial
drugs antibiotics, and his graduate student Albert Schatz. It caused
tuberculosis lesions to heal, almost miraculously. Unfortunately, it
then turned out that a few months later, those same patients were
sick again, this time with drug-resistant strains of TB. The next drug
to be developed was the first oral anti-TB medication, isoniazid, still
a mainstay of anti-TB therapy today. Used in combination, these
two drugs could actually eliminate the TB bacteria before resistance
developed. Patients needed to take both drugs for many months, but
for the first time, medicine could wipe out the infection.

In 1944, the children who were being treated for tuberculosis
at Bellevue Hospital were given medicine; until then, there had
been nothing to offer them. The first drugs were not very effective,
but soon, with streptomycin and then isoniazid, survival rates for
children with miliary tuberculosis went up to 96 percent. Selman
Waksman won the 1952 Nobel Prize for the work that had led to
streptomycin. (Albert Schatz, who had sued for a share of the commercial royalties, felt that his own essential role in the discovery was

not properly credited.) Dr. Lincoln reviewed her results in 1954, ten years after she had been the first to use drugs to defeat tuberculosis in children. With combination drug therapy, 98.5 percent of her cases had been cured and even tuberculous meningitis could be cured 85 percent of the time, if it was diagnosed early. But she was already finding that some of the bacteria were resistant to one of the drugs. Another new drug—rifampin—was developed in the 1960s, and the new combination shortened the treatment from eighteen to twenty-four months to six months. Although therapy was now available, Dr. Lincoln wrote in 1961, "the pediatrician must continue to be aware of the possibility of tuberculosis. Wherever there are tuberculous adults there are infected children. . . . No child will be even relatively safe from tuberculous infection and some of its dread sequelae until tuberculosis is diminished to the point where it is no longer a public health problem."[14]

When I finished my own medical training and started out in practice, we were still doing the skin tests I'd received as a child, to discover latent infections that now were treatable. We were also giving the live polio vaccine. At the two-, four-, and six-month routine pediatric checkups, and again with the preschool boosters, in addition to giving the DTP shots, I would take a little plastic ampule out of the vaccine freezer. I would warm it slightly with my fingers, twist off a tiny plastic piece, and squeeze sweetened pink liquid into the baby's mouth. It always seemed like a gift—one fewer shot at the visit, four needles less over the child's first four years of life. When the word came down in 1997 that we would need to change over to giving the injectable killed-virus polio vaccine, many of us felt at first that it was a bad idea, an overreaction to very rare problems with the oral live-virus vaccine. But with the elimination of polio as a contagious disease in this hemisphere, the only cases of polio to be seen were the few instances, every year, of polio that developed from the live but weakened polio virus in those little plastic ampules—no

longer an acceptable risk. (The oral vaccine, which is so much easier to administer, requiring neither clean syringes nor specialized
training for health care workers, is still used in many parts of the
developing world.)

Plenty of adults around today, people in their sixties and older,
had polio as children or can remember friends and family members
who did. David Oshinsky, in *Polio: An American Story,* tells the tale
of its conquest as a combination of immigrant scientific achievement
and postwar civic mobilization. The March of Dimes collected money
and raised awareness through the use of poster children, and parents
across the nation mobilized, contributing to the cause but also very
definitely looking to science to fulfill the promise of protection and
prevention, which was made over and over again in the March of
Dimes appeals. And we still remember Franklin Delano Roosevelt,
the much-beloved president who was struck by polio at thirty-nine
years old and went on to lead the country to victory in World War II,
from his wheelchair.

Polio, Oshinsky writes, was the last of the truly terrifying epidemic diseases. Smallpox had been defeated; sanitation had taken
care of cholera and typhoid and plague. Polio had probably been
around in occasional individual cases for centuries; there had been
a few small outbreaks in Europe in the nineteenth century. And yet,
in the twentieth century in the United States, polio emerged as a
relatively new and wholly terrifying disease, capable of producing
summer outbreaks that left some victims paralyzed for life and killed
others by paralyzing the respiratory muscles they needed to breathe.
The first recorded outbreak in the country happened in Vermont in
1894, with 123 cases of the disease, 18 deaths, and 50 people permanently paralyzed.

Subsequent epidemics in the United States were increasingly frequent, and increasingly severe as the twentieth century progressed.
The virus was isolated in 1908 by Karl Landsteiner, an Austrian scientist, and then targeted, only a few years later, by Simon Flexner,

the first director of the new Rockefeller Institute, who was quoted in the *New York Times* in 1911 as saying, "The achievement of a cure, I may conservatively say, is not now far distant."[15] In fact, the research at the Rockefeller Institute would prove to be a wrong turn in more ways than one, but polio, Oshinsky argues, became an American research problem. The virus might have been identified in Europe, but it would be taken on and solved in the United States, establishing and strengthening American research institutions, building on and enhancing civic ties, and adding up to a midcentury victory for the scientists, politicians, parents, and children.

In 1916, there was a major polio outbreak in Pigtown, a poor part of Brooklyn, among Italian immigrants. Although foreigners and squalor were initially blamed for the disease, it turned up in neighboring states as well, and a fairly intense public health effort to quarantine infected children and improve sanitary conditions among the immigrants did not seem particularly effective. In vain were stray cats rounded up and killed; in vain were increasingly intense quarantine measures implemented, until at one point, all children leaving New York City had to have public health certificates showing that they were not infected. Wealthy families in Pennsylvania and Connecticut with, as one newspaper put it, children who were "well nourished and cared for" were also suffering, and though some people blamed this on servants who carried disease, polio remained mysterious, terrifying, and not obviously linked to poverty and dirt.[16] Fearful parents worried about different pieces of information; there was a theory that the disease, a summer infection, often came on after swimming, and children were kept away from pools and lakes and beaches.

The protected and more intensely "hygienic" life of more well-to-do children may have left them more vulnerable to polio. Poor urban children who made it through the first couple of years of life— and many of them did not—were probably immune to a wide range of viruses and bacteria; their immune systems were fully primed.

It was the child who grew up in relative solitude, with servants to scrub every surface and cooks to boil the water, who might end up vulnerable to polio as an older child or an adult. Franklin Delano Roosevelt had grown up in that kind of isolation at his family home in Hyde Park, New York, and he kept his wife and five children at their summer home on a Canadian island to avoid the 1916 polio epidemic. Five years later, in 1921, after almost dying of pneumonia in the great influenza epidemic of 1918–19, he came down with polio at that same summer home, after a swim in the cold water of the Bay of Fundy.

FDR plays a complex if iconic role in the history of polio. Crippled by the disease, he threw tremendous support and influence behind the campaign to conquer polio, and he spoke repeatedly about the value of those who were disabled or hurt by disease, "that large part of humanity which used to be pushed to one side or discarded."[17] He thus played a very public role as a prominent polio patient, and he did a great deal to pull money and effort into research on vaccines and programs of care and rehabilitation. But he also regarded the details of his own disability as something to be minimized, especially in the context of his political career. In 1938, he founded the National Foundation for Infantile Paralysis, which was later renamed the March of Dimes; that organization, by raising money and funding both research and therapy, revolutionized medical research and also made it possible for polio survivors to get care and rehabilitation.

In the campaign to raise money for polio research, the March of Dimes would invent the poster child. FDR, in a larger sense, would be the poster child for overcoming polio and its disabilities, though he has been faulted by modern disability activists, for example, for refusing to be photographed in his wheelchair, or even while being helped in and out of his car. Earlier in that statement about those who used to be pushed to one side, he promised, "Today, through the fine strides of modern medical science, the great majority of crippled children are enabled . . . to get about and, in many cases, find complete or practically complete cures."[18] He himself was able to walk short distances with the help of leg braces, often leaning on a companion, but when not in public, he relied on a wheelchair. It was a complete, or at least practically complete, cure that he claimed for himself, and he put tremendous effort into preserving that illusion, emphasizing his own strength and stamina to an electorate that was all too familiar with the disease he had survived, and with which he continued to identify himself in the search for prevention and cure.[19]

In 1927, at the age of two, Carol Rosenstiel came down with polio. She was a child who had just won a beauty contest, her daughter Anne K. Gross writes in her book *The Polio Journals: Lessons from My Mother,* and her parents would later destroy all the photographs recording her as she had been. Carol's mother blamed herself for the polio because she had let her daughter go swimming.[20] What comes through clearly in the memoir is that for the family, there was something shameful about polio—a persistent conviction, against the evidence, that it was somehow related to squalor, poverty, and flies, and perhaps as well, for Carol's first-generation Jewish parents, an association with the immigrant tenements of the Lower East Side, though they themselves were well-to-do, cultured people who lived on the Upper West Side.

In 1928, Carol went off with her aunt to Warm Springs, the Georgia sanatorium FDR had bought and turned into the world's first center for the rehabilitation of polio victims. "We must get these people out of the back rooms," Roosevelt said. "All over the country there are polios, crippled, stuck away in back bedrooms by their families to spend their days in frustration and misery."[21] Certainly for three-year-old Carol, the pools of Warm Springs were a relief and a physical joy. "I remember the experience of freedom, no longer confined by my braces or wheelchair, no longer confined by my crippledness—a glorious feeling of mastery, of being in full charge of my body which responded magically, miraculously to every motion I wanted to make," she wrote.[22] She also met FDR and developed a friendship that passed into "family legend"; he cheered her on in swimming races. "Roosevelt was my hero," she said, "as indeed he was to all children (and undoubtedly adults as well) who were crippled."[23]

When World War II ended, there was still no way to prevent polio. But in 1948, researchers in Boston, led by John Enders, found a way to grow the polio virus in a laboratory, for which they won the 1954 Nobel Prize. When I trained in pediatrics at Boston Children's Hospital, the Enders Building was one of the laboratory buildings, and the shadow of John Enders, the leader of this project, did not seem so very far away.

Jonas Salk had been excused from military service in World War II because he made the case that his research on influenza was of national importance, and much of his early work on using killed virus to create vaccines was done on influenza, in the laboratory of his mentor, Tommy Francis, at the University of Michigan.[24] When Salk moved to the University of Pittsburgh, he began to use the tissue culture techniques developed in the Enders lab, and by 1953, his group had developed a killed polio vaccine. In 1954, the large vaccine trials began.

The early 1950s saw major polio epidemics, a last generation of children in the United States and Canada stricken right before the vaccine became available. Marc Shell, now a professor of English at Harvard, wrote in his book *Polio and Its Aftermath,* "As for me . . . Salk's polio vaccine came too late. *September 1953:* I was beginning first grade at Van Horne School in Montreal. *October 14:* I contracted polio. It was the same day that the foundation backed Jonas Salk's proposal to test his vaccine."[25] Dr. Moses Grossman, a pediatrician working on the infectious diseases ward at San Francisco General Hospital right after the war, recalled insisting that his trainees take a turn in the famous iron lung: "Polio was very prevalent in 1953–54. There were big epidemics and if you were rich, you were provided all the supplies and equipment. If you were poor, you went to San Fran-

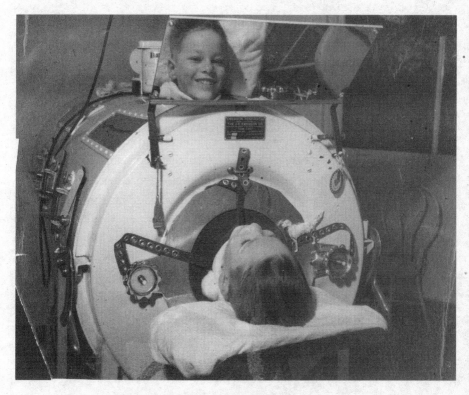

After the iron lung was invented in 1928, polio-stricken children who had lost the ability to breathe independently might spend decades in the machine. This child was photographed at the Herman Kiefer Hospital in Detroit around 1955, when polio could finally be prevented, though not cured. *New Contributed Photographs Collection, Otis Historical Archives, National Museum of Health and Medicine, NCP 4145.*

cisco General. . . . You need to know what it feels like, what it feels like to give up breathing, to let the machine breathe for you, which is very difficult. . . . When the resident came on the service, he had to go on the respirator."[26]

In 1955 Dr. Francis, Salk's original mentor, announced the success of the Salk vaccine at a press conference in Ann Arbor. The conference was held on the tenth anniversary of FDR's death and was broadcast around the world; the effectiveness of the vaccine was front-page news, and more. Polio in America had become a story of parents demanding safety for their children and scientists dramati-cally delivering. Then, paradoxically, it turned almost immediately into a story of a new kind of risk, as a number of cases in vaccinated children led to the discovery that certain batches of the new vaccine, which had been produced at one particular site, Cutter Laboratories, were contaminated with live, infectious polio virus, causing paralytic polio in 260 children. The Cutter story led to much stricter federal licensing laws, and there has never been another case of killed-virus vaccine contaminated by live virus. (The decision made in 1997 to abandon the oral polio vaccine because it did lead to rare cases of "vaccine-associated polio" was not because there was something wrong with the vaccine, as there had been in the Cutter incident, but because those pink drops contain live but inactivated virus, and, very rarely, that virus can cause infection and paralysis.)

After 1955 and the subsequent vaccination campaigns, the inci-dence of polio declined dramatically in the United States. In 1950, there were thirty-nine thousand cases; by 1962, there were fewer than one thousand, thanks to the Salk vaccine. At the same time, the rival vaccine, the oral vaccine made from weakened but living polio virus, was tested by its creator, the American researcher Dr. Albert Sabin, in the Soviet Union, in a somewhat stunning Cold War moment of medical cooperation. The FDA accepted the Rus-sian tests results in approving the vaccine in 1961—perhaps, it was speculated, because after losing the *Sputnik* race, Americans wanted to win the vaccine race. The Sabin oral vaccine was produced and marketed, and in 1962, it was adopted in the United States in place of the Salk vaccine, since it was effective, cheaper, and much easier to administer.[27]

The last case of polio caused by the "wild" virus in the United States was diagnosed in 1979; after that, all cases were either imported from other countries or traceable to that weakened vaccine virus, which caused eight to ten cases a year. Meanwhile, Dr. Salk continued to press hard for the increased safety and efficacy of his

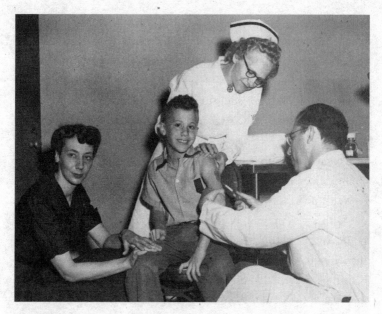

In 1953, Jonas Salk vaccinated his family—himself, his wife, and his three sons—in a public demonstration of his confidence in the safety and efficacy of his new polio vaccine. *March of Dimes*.

injectable killed vaccine, and it was adopted in many European countries. A 1981 *New York Times* story reported that he has "accused the medical establishment of following a 'live-virus dogma' that flies in the face of facts regarding immunity. 'The public,' he says, 'should be given the facts, and given a choice.'"[28]

In 1996, the CDC recommended that the first two doses of polio vaccine for every child should be the shots of killed polio vaccine, and in 1999 the schedule became all injectable killed polio vaccine. Doctors agreed that the world had changed. "In a polio-free nation, in a polio-free hemisphere, we cannot have eight to 10 individuals paralyzed every year when there are alternatives," said Dr. Samuel Katz, one of the great vaccine specialists of the twentieth century, who had done some of the pioneering work on the measles vaccine.[29] But this message had come in large part from parents as well, parents who got involved in the battle to change back from oral polio virus to injectable, parents whose children had contracted a polio infection from the vaccine. John Salamone became an advocate for changing vaccines after his son, David, developed polio in 1990 from the oral vaccine (he had a rare congenital immunodeficiency, but this was not known before he was vaccinated). Salamone told the newspaper that "doctors 'sacrifice' a handful of healthy children each year to accomplish a public health goal that was met 15 years ago in the United States."[30]

With polio, as with tuberculosis, the twentieth century started out with a certain amount of science and a great deal of scientific hope. And in both cases, those victories were substantially won in the United States in the decade after the Second World War: polio became a preventable disease (though still with no effective treatment), and tuberculosis became a treatable disease. Even so, tuberculosis, in its scariest manifestations in our new century, serves as a textbook example of the looming dangers of drug resistance and the new risks that can arise as we implement our medical miracles. The eradication of polio has been elusive because poverty and ongoing conflict continue to interfere with health care efforts in certain countries. The coronavirus pandemic in 2020 further disrupted vaccination programs, raising the specter of resurgent polio and other vaccine-preventable diseases, especially in areas without strong public health systems. Tuberculosis, which, before the coronavirus pandemic, was the leading infectious cause of death worldwide, continues to kill children in many countries, especially in Southeast Asia and Africa. TB kills, as it has always killed, in concert with poverty and malnutrition, and nowadays also in connection with HIV.[31] As causes of child mortality, then, both diseases remind us of incomplete victories and global disparities.

CHAPTER 8

The Incubator Show

Life and Death in the Delivery Room and the Nursery

According to medical student lore, if you find yourself in the delivery room yearning to follow the baby, rather than stay with the mother, that may mean that you are destined for pediatrics. I gave birth to my first child in my second year of medical school, and by the time we got to our clinical placements, in the third year, I had my own memories of being a maternity patient, and I certainly identified with the women in labor. Still, every time a new baby arrived, something in me always wanted to be over at the warming table, checking out the baby, doing what has become the pediatrician's job, and, in fact, I spent many months of my residency running to deliveries when newborns were in distress or were being born too early.

The delivery room, for most of human history, was the woman's own bedroom at home, although whether that room was in a home or a hospital, two people did not always come out, mother and baby, alive and well. If parenthood was colored by the knowledge that children might not live to grow up, pregnancy and the advent of childbirth was also shaded with danger, for both the mother and the baby. In 1872, Ellen Regal wrote of her pregnant sister, "It is not strange that she should tremble and shrink at the thought of that Valley of the

Shadow of Death which she must so soon enter."[1] All through history, women were well aware that their own deaths could come at or soon after delivery, and they worried about it, prayed over it, and prepared for it. They thought about who would rear their older children, for example, or how they would be remembered. Judith Walzer Leavitt, who collected these accounts in writing her 1986 history of American childbearing, *Brought to Bed,* discussed the ways women and their family members coped with the fear of labor and what might follow: "Young, vigorous, healthy women who should have been anticipating a long life ahead instead faced the very real possibility that their pregnancies would bring their deaths, that in creating a life they would pay with their own." Clara Clough Lenroot wrote in 1891, "I wonder if I should die, and leave a little daughter *behind* me, they would name her 'Clara.' I should like to have them. . . . I should want Mama and Bertha [her sister] to have the bringing up of it, but I should want Irvine [her husband] to see it every day and love it so much."[2]

One particularly frightening prospect was the bacterial infection of puerperal fever that doctors unwittingly spread from patient to patient right through the nineteenth century and into the twentieth. Other major causes of maternal mortality were hemorrhage and eclampsia, the malignant high blood pressure syndrome that can develop during pregnancy; both of these conditions were not effectively treatable until the twentieth century. But there were also many other reasons that a woman might die, some related to poor obstetrical practice, some to conditions that had already undermined the mother's health, such as tuberculosis or malnutrition.

So childbirth was dangerous, and the danger was recurrent, in those eras when high infant and child mortality meant that families tended to be larger. It's no coincidence that so many women were already pregnant again when their children were young (and sometimes when their young children died); childbirth was a frightening lottery for women, and a lottery that many were compelled to enter over and over. The confidence that children will live to grow up is conducive to planning smaller families—this is both historically true and true around the world today in countries where infant and child mortality have remained high. Lowering infant and child deaths helps bring women into the workforce (and lowering the incidence of serious childhood illness makes it easier for them to stay there, since they are freed from at least some of their sickbed responsibilities).

Childbirth became much safer in the twentieth century; it also moved into the hospital, and it has now been "medicalized," to the point where many women have pushed back, resisting routine medical interventions from anesthesia and cesarean section to episiotomy, and arguing that making things more intensely medical does not always make them safer. The United States continues to struggle with the highest maternal mortality rate in the developed world, one with alarming racial disparities. Still, as with child mortality, maternal mortality in this medicalized setting has now been driven down to rates that would seem reassuringly low to our great-grandmothers.

My grandmother would have thought it powerfully unlucky to make any but the most practical preparations for a new baby before it came. You might perhaps provide a place for it to sleep and a basic layette, but you certainly wouldn't give the baby a name in advance or go to a great deal of effort to prepare the nursery. The elaborate baby showers of today, with full registries and participants often advised in advance of the baby's sex, and sometimes of the baby's name, are the rituals of a generation that worries much less (and with good reason) about something going tragically wrong at the last minute for either the baby or the mother. Pregnant women may be scared of labor (although, again, part of hospital marketing is to promise them a reasonable degree of freedom from pain, according to the newest and least invasive anesthesia strategies), but they are not, for the most part, scared of dying—and again with good reason. Any mother's death now is—and should be—a "sentinel event" in a hospital, evidence that something went terribly and tragically wrong, requiring an investigation and, often, a lawsuit.

In an excellent report by the investigative journalism enterprise ProPublica, researchers lay out what they've learned from an initiative in which they have been tracking down each of the stories of the women who died in the United States in 2016 from pregnancy-related causes.[3] There are between seven hundred and nine hundred of those deaths, and the argument made by the journalists reviewing them is that many represent deaths that should not have happened or would not have happened in other developed countries. As with infant mortality, we are tantalizingly close to safety, which makes the deaths that do occur—whether of mothers or newborns—seem even more tragic, more indicative of holes in our social safety nets, racism, disparities in how we care for women and children, medical judgment calls and mistakes that occasion a lifetime's worth of regret.

Even today the first moments of life outside the womb are physiologically dramatic and often dangerous, especially for a baby who is born too soon. A St. Louis pediatrician, Dr. John Zahorsky, wrote of his experience in helping people take care of premature babies in the late nineteenth and early twentieth centuries, during the days when improvised care was provided at home by mothers, sometimes assisted by a doctor: "For many years the care of the premature infant in the home was the pediatrician's task. To keep the baby at an even temperature, all sorts of extemporaneous devices were constructed! A market basket, or a small wooden box, padded and bedded, kept warm by beer bottles or Mason jars filled with warm water, or a box with one side removed set before a radiator, or a box heated by an electric light bulb. . . . It did not cost one-third as much as hospital care and our results were even better than in the hospital."[4] He was always proud, he wrote, when he ran into an adult who turned out to have been a premature infant he had saved.

But even for full-term infants, the first days and even weeks have always represented a time of particularly high mortality, a kind of liminal zone in which an infant's hold on life might prove to be too tenuous to "take." Aristotle commented on the very early deaths of newborns: "Most of the babies are carried off before the seventh day, that is why they give the child its name then, as they have more confidence by that time in its survival." In fact, many of the celebratory welcoming, naming, and initiating rituals that different cultures and societies develop to mark births leave a deliberate perinatal firebreak, anywhere from three to eight days after birth, allowing for the death of those babies who were clearly not meant to live.[5] Thus, Jews circumcise their sons on the eighth day of life, and the Muslim naming ceremony is performed at one week of age.

As the social movement to drive down infant mortality took shape at the beginning of the twentieth century, most reformers focused first on the older babies, the six- and eight- and ten-month-olds, who had a better hold on life and who could therefore survive in larger numbers, the reformers hoped, with better air, better handling, better hygiene, better milk. But by the time I was in medical school, many of the most dramatic "saves" were happening—almost routinely—in the newborn intensive care unit. Saving newborns required coming to grips with a different set of issues, from starting a baby breathing at birth to coping with birth defects and, perhaps above all, with prematurity. And more than any other aspect of childhood death, taking on perinatal mortality, death in the delivery room or in the first weeks of life, required medical practitioners and parents and society in general to confront the issue of whether every baby was, in fact, meant to live, or whether some were simply too weak, too small, or in other ways unfit. Aristotle, after all, went on to write, "As to the exposure of children, let there be a law that no deformed child shall live."[6] This can sound very harsh to us, but there was a certain lack of sentimentality about newborns, especially those who did not seem likely to thrive.

Even so, as the twentieth century approached, some scientists and some doctors did begin to contemplate the medical challenges of systematically saving too-weak, too-small, and too-compromised infants, though it was not until the last three decades of that century that what we would recognize as modern neonatology developed the technologies we now routinely rely on. Neonatology was built on a framework of other medical advances, notably including the development of increasingly sophisticated antibiotics, but also many life-support technologies that were initially developed in the adult ICU, then miniaturized. In fact, all of the activity around perinatal mortality constituted part of the "medicalization" of childbirth, the movement of labor and the first days of infancy from the home into the hospital, but the questions of whom to save and how to save them were more complicated than the development and application of technology. Ethical issues arose at every turn, and they are still woven through neonatology today, discussed on a daily basis in all those gleaming newborn intensive care units.

In the late nineteenth century in Europe, as the incubator movement began, French physicians attempted to create a stable technological environment in which the baby born too early could safely and scientifically breathe, feed, and grow. In the early 1880s, a leading French obstetrician, Étienne Stéphane Tarnier, created a device he called a *couveuse,* meaning a brooding hen, and he reported great success in using it to care for premature infants at the large maternity hospital in Paris. Dr. Tarnier was already a famous figure, a successful crusader against childbed fever at his hospital, a hero who had cared for his patients through revolutionary violence. He claimed to have been inspired by a visit to the Paris zoo in 1878, where he saw poultry incubators. The machine he constructed was mostly a warming device, a system that kept premature babies warm by boiling water and circulating it through metal pipes in the chamber, which could hold two or more infants.[7]

Jeffrey Baker, a pediatrician and historian who has written a history of the incubator and the development of neonatology, comments, "What was most striking about the work of Tarnier and other French obstetricians in the 1880s was not so much a new invention but a new interest in the premature infant."[8] Most nineteenth-century

French doctors viewed prematurity in terms of weakness, referring to *faiblesse congenitale* (congenital feebleness), and to premature babies as *débiles*, or weaklings; the incubator ward at the maternity hospital, established by Pierre Budin, who had been Tarnier's intern, was called the *pavillon des débiles*. Babies' weakness could be quantified by their birthweight. Weighing newborns and tracking their survival helped establish weight cut-offs for what later doctors would consider a "pre-viable" infant, one that could not be expected to survive. The incubator was most effective, Dr. Tarnier found, for infants between fourteen hundred grams and two kilos (three to four and a half pounds); the larger babies tended to survive even without it, and the smaller did not survive even with the devices. None of these survival statistics reached beyond the hospital period; whether the babies did indeed go on to grow up and whether they were left with problems related either to their prematurity or to their time in the hospital would not be researched or thought about for some time to come.

Budin's own survival statistics for premature infants, using the incubators, continued to show that even with these warming machines, many premature babies and most very premature babies did not survive. Dr. Budin did look beyond infant survival in the hospital. He was deeply concerned that babies might be discharged only to die, and he played a major role in promoting breastfeeding, with his *consultations de nourrissons* clinics. Along the same lines, his hospital work in Paris would call for involving the mother in the care of the child in the incubator; he had the mothers stay in the hospital, breastfeed their children when possible, and even breastfeed other children in the nursery to keep up their milk supplies if their own babies were too weak to nurse.[9] "First, save the infant, the essential point," Tarnier wrote. "Second, save it in such a way that when it leaves the hospital it does so with a mother able to suckle it."[10]

Throughout gestation, the fetus gets oxygen from the mother's blood; birth marks the transition to breathing air, to taking oxygen from the atmosphere through gas exchange in the lungs. For this reason, helping babies breathe when they had trouble with that transition would turn out to be much more than a mechanical question. Babies can suffer oxygen deprivation before birth, such as when something is interfering with the blood supply from the placenta—maybe the cord is wrapped around the baby's neck or is pinched off by the contractions. Or they can be fine as long as they're getting oxygen through the umbilical cord but suffer oxygen deprivation after birth because something gets in the way of breathing air—meconium that's been passed too soon, for instance, or congenital anomalies of the airway or the heart. And coming out of the regulation and protection offered by the mother's body can be dangerous in other ways as well. Newborns have only limited powers of temperature regulation, and tiny preemies have none at all; they lose both heat and water across their incredibly thin skin. The initial job of the incubator was simply to keep newborns warm, and that all by itself was enough to help survival; the pediatric job in the delivery room is always done under warming lights to make sure that the babies don't get cold.

The relatively simple French warming device, the *couveuse*, really addressed only a single variable in the survival of a premature baby: it kept the baby warm. Some statistics suggested that it was more effective than what had been used before, a padded basket warmed by hot water bottles, but other studies suggested that the baskets were equally effective. When the incubator idea crossed the Atlantic, it became a more advanced piece of engineering developed to create something much closer to an artificial womb. Thomas Morgan Rotch, the Harvard professor of pediatrics and committed scientist who developed the famous (or infamous) percentage feeding method for infants, partnered with John Pickering Putnam, a Boston inventor, to develop the Rotch-Putnam brooder. This device would not only keep an infant warm but also protect it from dust and dirt, and all the newly understood dangers of bacteria and infection, and even from excess stimulation, leaving the baby in a state of "darkness, silence, and warmth," Rotch wrote, which would replicate the conditions of the mother's uterus from which it had been expelled too early.[11] Another model, the Lion incubator, which was actually developed in France but became very popular in the United States, featured an elaborate ventilation system to bring in air from outside the hospital, filter it, and then get rid of it, through exhaust pipes, so the air the baby was breathing was constantly refreshed. American sanitarians believed in the essential healing qualities of fresh air, for babies in the slums and for infants in the hospital. When the inventor of this appliance, Alexandre Lion, wanted to find a way to show off and promote his high-tech invention, he opened storefront "incubator charities" in a number of French cities in the mid-1890s, charging fifty centimes for admission and letting the public in to observe.

And then began what was perhaps the strangest and most public piece of the development of neonatology, both in Europe and America: the "incubator-baby sideshows," at fairs and exhibitions and on amusement park midways, including Coney Island. "I recall being puzzled about the 'incubator-baby exhibit' when I walked by what I thought was one of many ordinary sideshows in the amusement area of Chicago's Century of Progress Exposition in 1933," wrote William Silverman, a pediatrician who helped establish modern medical neonatology, and who traced the remarkable career of Dr. Martin A. Couney, the "incubator doctor" who immigrated to the United States in 1903 and made it his cause to show the people of his new country what incubators could do.[12]

Couney claimed to have trained in Germany, but his past is shadowy, and it has been suggested that he had in fact never actually trained as a doctor at all.[13] He had already arranged an exhibition in Berlin, backed by Lion, at the World Exposition of 1896, "borrowing" the babies from the Berlin Charity Hospital; it was called the *Kinderbrutanstalt,* or "child hatchery," and it was a big draw. As Dr. Couney told the story, the six babies were loaned to him in part because they were thought so unlikely to survive; that all of them lived was a testament to the effectiveness of the care they received in the exhibit.

Couney followed this presentation up with a show at the Victorian Era Exhibition in London, and the *Lancet*, the highly distinguished British medical journal, reviewed it, saying, "The incubators and ventilating tubes are silvered, which gives them a bright and cheerful appearance, while the infants within look clean and comfortable, so that altogether it is a pleasant as well as an interesting sight."[14] The *Lancet* would develop doubts over the next decade about whether the exhibit was in fact an appropriate venue for the newborn babies, possibly in response to the imitation incubator-baby shows, including one put on by Barnum & Bailey. The medical journal ran an editorial asking, "What connection is there between this serious matter of saving human life and the bearded woman, the dog-faced man, the elephants, the performing horses and pigs . . . ?"[15]

Couney brought his exhibitions to the United States in 1898, at the Trans-Mississippi Exposition in Omaha, and in 1901, at the Pan-American Exposition in Buffalo. The newspaper coverage of the Buffalo fair included an ode to the incubators that reached for comparison to the nearby natural wonders: "The falls of Niagara with the great system of lakes and rivers behind them; the diminutive baby in its hot-air chamber, sightless, deaf, feeble—but with the great human race, the vast sea of organized thought back of it."[16] When the exhibition closed, the Children's Hospital of Buffalo bought the incubators.

Couney was not involved with the incubator exhibition at the Louisiana Purchase Exposition in St. Louis in 1904, where a beautiful building with towers and spires and Grecian colonnades was built especially for the incubators and their occupants and their attendants. When summer brought an epidemic of diarrhea, that longtime nemesis of young babies, and the mortality rate among the infants reached 50 percent, a committee of local doctors investigated, made some changes in the management of the exhibit, and put Dr. John Zahorsky (the prominent St. Louis pediatrician who was so resourceful about rigging up baskets and wooden boxes in the home) in charge of the incubators. He took the job very seriously, writing, "I made two, more often three, visits to the baby exhibit daily." He was proud that he was able to bring the mortality rate down below 20 percent, most of the deaths occurring "in infants weighing less than two pounds." He also felt that the infection that had killed so many of the babies was "undoubtedly due to a sick, infected infant from one of the foundling homes."[17] He kept careful records and published all his data, putting together a 1905 monograph called *Baby Incubators: A Clinical Study of the Premature Infant*.

Still, between the diarrhea and the deaths and the high cost of maintaining the babies in the incubators, St. Louis discouraged most future such exhibitions. Couney settled in Coney Island and opened an exhibition there, a sideshow on the boardwalk that operated every summer until 1943. "The incubator-show became a fixture of the amusement area," Dr. Silverman wrote. "A sign at the entrance read 'All the World Loves a Baby.'"[18] Barkers called in the public— "Don't pass the babies by!" (One of them was the young Cary Grant, then still known as Archibald Leach.) Dr. Couney married a nurse with expertise in the care of premature infants, and their daughter, who spent the first months of her life in an incubator, grew up to do the same job. Periodically, Couney took his show on the road, with a particularly lavish and successful exhibit at the Panama-Pacific International Exposition in San Francisco in 1915 and another at the Chicago Century of Progress International Exposition in 1933–34. When the 1939–40 New York World's Fair was set up, a bright pink building was erected for Dr. Couney, with quarters for nurses and wet nurses, as well as a "sumptuous apartment" for the doctor. But the exhibit did not make money; the incubator babies were no longer the novelty they had been, and the health department gave him trouble.

The incubator-baby exhibitions appear to us now to straddle an uncomfortable line between educational displays of science and technology and something closer to freak shows. Certainly some people expressed doubts at the time—the Society for the Prevention of

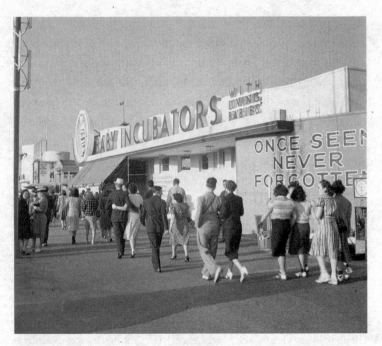

The baby incubator show at Coney Island, which was very much part of the midway, provided a high quality of care to premature infants; the "living babies" in their incubators astonished visitors by their small size—and perhaps reinforced for the public the idea that medicine had made a commitment to save even the smallest, weakest newborns. *Wurts Bros. (New York, NY) Museum of the City of New York. X2010.7.1.14272.*

Cruelty to Children tried unsuccessfully to close down the Coney Island exhibit, and some doctors dismissed incubators altogether because they were somehow tainted by the midway. But the doctors who tended these exhibitions included legitimate pioneers of neonatology, from Couney to Zahorsky to Dr. Julius Hess in Chicago, one of the most important academic neonatologists in America, who worked with Couney to set up the incubator show at the Chicago Century of Progress International Exposition in 1933. And generally in his day, Silverman noted, Dr. Couney "enjoyed a fine reputation among the obstetricians in the New York area; they sent infants to his exhibit confident that the babies would receive skilled care."[19] In their heyday, the shows were celebrations of a new and gleaming technology, but what made the technology so interesting were the freakishly tiny inhabitants, premature babies who by implication would otherwise be dead, growing and thriving in a brave new world of medical infancy. Even now, in the newborn intensive care unit, the same juxtaposition makes visitors gasp; the technology is ever more complex and impressive, and the babies tinier than ever, so that anyone unaccustomed to the scene can easily find it futuristic, terrifying, and profoundly moving all at once. In some ways, neonatology has never completely lost its sideshow atmosphere; those unbelievably tiny infants who can now be saved from those pushed-back borderlines still represent clear visual displays of the power of medical technology, the nearness of medical miracles.

In January 1945, a baby girl was born in a Bronx hospital four and a half months before her due date. She weighed only six hundred grams, less than a pound and a half. As Dr. Silverman told the story, decades later, the obstetrician who delivered her was surprised when she started to breathe spontaneously, and when he came back the next day, "he was even more amazed to find her alive."[20] So he sent her to Babies Hospital, in upper Manhattan, where she became the prize patient of one of the house officers—Dr. William Silverman, then at the beginning of his training.

Silverman told the story in a 1992 essay reflecting on the origins—and ethical dilemmas—of neonatology. Although no infant this small had ever survived at his hospital, Dr. Silverman diligently tended the baby for more than three months, treating her with continuous oxygen, putting food directly into her stomach with a tube, and even transfusing her every day with tiny doses of his own blood. "The baby was presented at grand rounds as a triumph of mechanism-guided treatment, and I was made to feel like a hero," the doctor wrote.[21] The baby's parents, he remarked, were less enthusiastic about his medical prowess. They were both in their late forties, with grown children, and to the doctor's dismay, they kept asking about the long-term prognosis and the baby's future. "The longer the baby lived, the more angry the parents became at the thought that I—a young, childless house officer, with no personal experience in rearing a normal child (much less one who might be disabled)—now held in my hands an important determinant in the fate of this family."[22] The baby ultimately died at the age of three and a half months, and the parents, still resentful, refused permission for an autopsy. Silverman would go on to be one of the founding fathers of neonatology, and a voice of historical perspective and conscience. In his own professional practice, he reckoned with both the miracles of technology and the moral, ethical, and scientific questions that followed almost immediately when saving babies who would otherwise have died at or soon after birth.

As neonatology came into its own, the people attending births and caring for babies had to look at newborns very differently. Each tiny body was a patient to be battled for, assessed and measured in every possible function, and, when necessary, resuscitated under bright lights. The state of being at the very beginning of life, which had once been the rationale for holding back and letting a baby "declare itself," would become the zone of aggressive treatment, pushing back the borders of viability.

When I was training in pediatrics, the most often cited neonatology benchmark—cited to show us how far neonatal medicine had come in the previous two decades—was a much bigger and less premature preemie than Dr. Silverman's six-hundred-gram girl. In 1963 the thirty-four-year-old first lady, Jacqueline Kennedy, had gone into labor five and a half weeks early. It was August, and she was on Cape Cod, vacationing with her other two children; she was taken by helicopter to a nearby air force base, where the baby was born, by cesarean section, and he was then transferred by ambulance to Children's Hospital in Boston, because he had developed trouble breathing. He weighed four pounds, ten and a half ounces, and he was the first—and only—baby to be born in the twentieth century to a sitting president and first lady.

But there was no way, almost twenty years after Silverman's efforts, to ventilate a newborn who was having trouble breathing, no matter who his father happened to be. Patrick Bouvier Kennedy lived for only thirty-nine hours. By the time I began my residency in those same Boston hospitals, in 1986, a baby of that gestational age and weight—thirty-four-plus weeks, almost five pounds—seemed to us a very mature, very big preemie. Our newborn intensive care unit, or NICU, was full of "twenty-eight weekers," babies who weighed only a little over two pounds, and even twenty-six and twenty-seven weekers (full term would be forty weeks). And though they were complicated and fragile, we had the capacity to ventilate even those tiny infants, as well as the drugs to help their stiff premature lungs soften and breathe better.

The very first night of my internship, I found myself in the NICU at the Brigham and Women's Hospital in Boston. Women who were known to be carrying babies with serious fetal anomalies came to the Brigham to deliver their babies, so that pediatric heart surgeons could be standing by, or pediatric kidney specialists, or neurosurgeons. Fascinated and terrified, I watched two more advanced residents rehearsing, working from the ultrasound showing how a pair of twins was conjoined so that they would be ready to resuscitate both babies at once.

It was a scary place to be starting an internship. The babies in the NICU, most of them so much more premature than a thirty-four-week infant, looked impossibly, ridiculously tiny, on their warming tables, and they all had so many tubes going in and out of them (breathing tubes for oxygen, IV lines through their umbilical arteries, more IVs in their arms and legs, nasogastric tubes to put food down into their stomachs), and they were connected to so many monitors, for temperature, heart rate, respiration, blood pressure, oxygen, and the alarms kept going off. The nurses, supremely competent and deeply invested in the well-being of their fragile patients, were by tradition fairly harsh with the newly minted doctors who arrived every July to be nominally in charge. Most of us were deeply grateful for their skill; we depended on them to keep us from doing any damage or, frankly, killing any babies, but we knew we were being measured and assessed, and generally found wanting.

By the mid-1980s, neonatology had come a long way. We were already worrying about the ethics of resuscitating "borderline" babies, those at about twenty-six weeks of gestation. Today, we would probably push that borderline of viability back to twenty-four weeks, but in either case, we are talking about very premature infants, babies at high risk for premature lung disease, or respiratory distress syndrome, or bleeds into the brain, or necrotizing enterocolitis, a scary syndrome in which the immature gut can get infected and destroyed. These are the babies who can weigh between one and two pounds, whose eyes are still fused closed, whose very thin skin we describe as "gelatinous." Their GI tracts are not always mature enough to absorb food; their immune systems are not mature enough to fight off infection. The great and comparatively rapid twentieth-century achievement of neonatology, over the course of twenty years or so, was to find technologies that made it even thinkable—though still fraught with danger and difficulty—to keep many, and then most, of those babies alive. The further trajectory, over the past few decades, has been to make those babies safer and to reduce the devastation of those dangers, though none of this is safe or easy, even now.

The obstetrical history of almost every woman up through the early decades of the twentieth century included at least one or two infants who had died at birth. Jacqueline Kennedy, for example, was actually on her fifth pregnancy when she gave birth to that premature baby; she had already endured two pregnancy losses, back in the 1950s: one a miscarriage, the other a stillbirth.

When a woman died during or soon after childbirth, history, in some sense, took notice. The status of those who survived her was changed—her husband was left a widower; her baby, if it survived, and her other children, if she had any, were left motherless. Her death was noted by her religious community, marked with funeral rites— so her name will turn up, for example, in a parish register. But when a baby was born apparently already dead, or born too premature to survive, or even born frail or with obvious congenital anomalies, it was rare for anyone, from doctors to clergymen to demographers, to keep rigorous track. Well into the twentieth century, the lines between miscarriage and stillbirth, and between stillbirth and delivery room death, were often allowed to blur.

In 1945 at Babies Hospital in New York, Dr. Silverman wrote, all newborns who weighed less than a kilogram were considered "pre-viable," too young to survive. If the little girl from the Bronx had been born at his own hospital, she would never have made it out of the delivery room: "'Pre-viable' and severely malformed newborns were placed in a cold corner of the delivery room and allowed to die. The decision was made by the obstetrician, who knew the family, knew the parents' circumstances, and often knew the parents' wishes. There was little or no discussion of the dark drama. . . . Everyone tried to ignore the gasping respirations—death never came quickly enough to relieve their acute, but silent, discomfort. The outcome of the delivery was reported as 'stillborn.'"[23]

Many of the deaths that take place soon after birth are linked to prematurity; that was true in 1945, when Dr. Silverman described those tiny babies gasping in a cold corner, and it is true today. Prematurity and congenital anomalies are now the two major causes of death at birth or in the first month of life. We now worry much more than we used to about babies born only a few weeks early. Now that we are much better able to establish the exact dates of a pregnancy, babies have been reclassified, so that from thirty-four weeks up until thirty-seven weeks gestation is called "late preterm" and we recognize that even though these infants may be of normal birthweight, their systems are notably less mature than full-term infants' and they are at higher risk for a wide variety of problems.

When I was in training, I always wanted to tend the baby in the delivery room, rather than the mother. The badges of office were the delivery room beeper, which summoned a pediatric team to the delivery room, and the DeLee catheters we used to suck meconium out of the baby's airway. (In 1982, you sucked out meconium by putting one tube of a suction catheter into the baby's airway and then putting the other tube into your mouth; there was a little plastic trap in between where the meconium was supposed to go. The suction is now supplied by a machine.)

Carrying that delivery room beeper meant, as every intern knew, that you were only one beep away from a delivery room resuscitation. Because of the dramatic physiological transitions that take place at the moment of birth, every delivery brings with it that suspenseful moment so often dramatized in movies, where everyone waits for the baby to cry—and sometimes, the baby doesn't. Midwifery and obstetrics through the ages had recommended a variety of techniques for stimulating newborn babies who did not immediately breathe or cry, from giving forms of mouth-to-mouth breathing to putting a little wine in the baby's mouth to placing the baby in a lukewarm bath to more strenuous endeavors, including administering enemas, burning the baby's feet with a hot iron, and swinging the baby vigorously.[24]

Historically, a baby with a problem generally came as a surprise to the midwife or doctor attending the delivery, but in the twenty-first century we tend to have a good deal of information about babies before they are born. Tests done during pregnancy can include full genetic profiles and incredibly high quality ultrasounds. (As recently as thirty years ago, when I was going through my pregnancies, even "good" ultrasounds looked mostly like weather patterns to non-radiologists like me.) More immediately, as labor progresses, we have data about the fetal heart rate and how it reacts to contractions, and we can sample the fetus's blood (from the scalp as the head descends) to see whether there's any metabolic stress, which is reflected in the acid-base balance of the blood. To tell a complex story very briefly, when there is not enough oxygen, shifts in cellular metabolism can make the blood more acidic, producing a dangerous condition called acidosis.

For all of the sophistication of these forms of monitoring, as soon as the baby is out, we use a less technologically bound measure, the Apgar score, to assess a baby's well-being. On your first night covering a delivery room as a pediatric intern, you learn to make these assessments at one minute and five minutes after birth, though the scores are often assigned by delivery room nurses or, indeed, by obstetricians. The baby gets either a 0, a 1, or a 2 in each of five categories: color, heart rate, reflex irritability, muscle tone, and respiratory effort (or, since mnemonic devices are important in medicine, Appearance, Pulse, Grimace, Activity, and Respiration). For example, blue all over, including the lips, means a 0, blue hands and feet only means a 1 (by far the most common), and no blue tinge anywhere means a 2. Similarly, no heart rate is a 0, a heart rate less than 100 beats per minute is a 1, and a heart rate over 100, which is normal for a newborn, gets you a 2. Reflex irritability is a measure of the baby's reaction to stimulation—for example, to having its mouth suctioned out; no response is a 0, a grimace or motion is a 1, and full-blown crying is a 2.

These scores become almost second nature to anyone who spends time in a delivery room, and you can see how these qualities describe a healthy baby. Blue only on the soles of the feet (1 point), heart beating over 100 times a minute (2 points), moving actively (2 points for muscle tone), crying lustily (2 points for respiratory effort, 2 points for reflex irritability) means an Apgar of 9, which is as high as we usually go, since it's pretty normal to be a little blue around the hands and feet; an Apgar of 9 means the baby looks great. On the other hand, limp and blue with a low heart rate and some weak attempts at breathing but no response to stimulation would be an Apgar of 2, and that baby would get a full-court resuscitation.

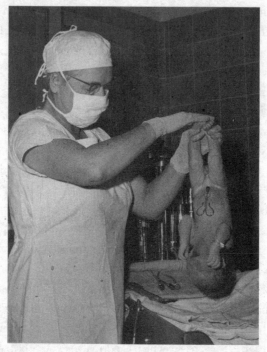

Dr. Virginia Apgar demonstrates assessing a newborn and awarding an Apgar score at Columbia Presbyterian Hospital. She is testing for reflex irritability, one of five criteria for the score, and is looking to see how the baby reacts to having his feet gently slapped. *Mount Holyoke College, Archives and Special Collections, L. Stanley James Papers (MS 0782). Used with permission from March of Dimes.*

The Apgar score was developed by the pioneering obstetrical anesthesiologist Virginia Apgar, and it's just a fortunate coincidence that her last name has five letters and those letters can be stretched to cover the five qualities she sketched out on a handy piece of paper in 1949 in the Columbia hospital cafeteria, when a medical student asked about how to evaluate newborn infants.[25] First published in 1953, the Apgar score continues to be used around the world. The opening lines of that 1953 article give a sense both of Dr. Apgar's voice and of the state of delivery room resuscitation at the time: "Resuscitation of infants at birth has been the subject of many articles. Seldom have there been such imaginative ideas, such enthu-siasms, and dislikes, and such unscientific observations and study about one clinical picture."[26]

Dr. L. Stanley James, a pediatrician who was a close colleague of Dr. Apgar's at Columbia and Babies Hospital, wrote after her death that the Apgar score "made people look at the baby immediately after birth."[27] Oddly, this was something new for doctors as a formal drill, looking at the baby. And it required medical students and physicians to assess several different qualities, rather than relying on any one sign. "It has been most gratifying to note the enthusiastic interest and competitive spirit displayed by the obstetric house staff who took great pride in a baby with a high score," Dr. Apgar wrote.[28]

Dr. James recounted that Virginia Apgar

carried a small bottle containing an 8-week-old fetus, as a teaching device, in her purse. The fetus had a failure of clo-sure of the neural tube and therefore had a visible defect which could clearly be seen at that early age. Producing this for the first time when we were flying to the West Coast, she showed it to the air hostesses. All service stopped for half an hour. The fetus was even named Billy, and at a recent dinner meeting of the Spina Bifida Association of America, where Virginia was the principal speaker, she produced Billy. He was handed round and examined by all the parents. No one was shocked. All were fascinated and intrigued.[29]

It was another era, no question, and perhaps not so far removed from the spectacle of the incubator shows.

———————— // ————————

In the novel *A Tree Grows in Brooklyn*, set in the early twentieth century, the protagonist's aunt Sissy endures one pregnancy after another; all go to term and all the children are stillborn, delivered at home by her relatives and a midwife. Finally Sissy announces, to the horror of her family, that she intends to have her baby in the hospital, though the poor immigrant community in which she lives is deeply fearful of hospitals, believing them to be places where people go to die. She also tells them that she plans to have a Jewish doctor. The baby is born in the hospital, and once again, he looks blue and limp; Sissy asks God, "Why couldn't You let me have one? Just one out of eleven?" Then she hears the doctor, Aaron Aaronstein, say "a word that she had never known. She heard the word 'oxygen.'" The baby is resuscitated: "She saw the dead blue change to living white. She saw an apparently lifeless child draw a breath. For the first time she heard the cry of a child she had borne." In gratitude, Sissy gives him the middle name Aaron.[30]

The ability to supply newborns with oxygen helped elucidate the benefits of enriched air—but it also meant controversy, continuing today, about the damage oxygen can do. This is another story of great goodness and joy and scientific advance, but it is also, again, a story that shows how good intentions do not always lead to good medicine, and how when you play at the boundaries of life, you inevitably come up against unintended effects and deeply complicated questions without simple answers.

As far back as 1783, only a decade after the gas was discovered, oxygen was administered to infants who didn't immediately start breathing on their own at birth. It was given in a variety of ways, including into the nostrils with bellows, intravenously into the umbilical cord, and into the stomach.[31]

So at the beginning of the twentieth century, oxygen was being used in hospitals, as it had been for over one hundred years, to "jump-start" babies who failed to start breathing independently— and it was being delivered by inhalation. In 1942, researchers found that the "regularly irregular" periodic breathing that was typical of premature babies would often correct itself if the baby was exposed to higher concentrations of oxygen. And then a new concern arose:

in 1951, a British doctor, Mary Crosse, raised the question of whether a strange new eye pathology that was being seen all over the world might possibly be related to these high oxygen levels.

The story of retrolental fibroplasia, later called retinopathy of prematurity (or ROP) went on to become one of the cautionary tales of modern medicine, taught to medical students and residents to keep them humble, to remind them that even miraculous new therapies may come with unexpected costs to the patients they are meant to benefit. There is always an obligation to study the long-term effects of even the most appealing—and the most apparently benign—breakthroughs. Dr. Silverman called supplemental oxygen "the albatross of neonatal medicine."[32] It turns out that highly concentrated oxygen can stimulate the growth of additional blood vessels in the eyes of premature babies, and those abnormally overgrowing blood vessels can damage the baby's vision, even causing blindness. Lower oxygen concentrations might protect their eyes, but what if the breathing got worse, what if the babies were more likely to die? The only way to determine the safest course was a clinical trial in which some babies were assigned to one kind of treatment and some to another. The first such trial, in 1952, Dr. Silverman wrote, was sabotaged by nurses who "surreptitiously" dialed up the oxygen on those babies who had been assigned to receive lower concentrations "because they were convinced restriction was threatening the lives of their patients."[33]

The study was published in 1954; it showed that limiting oxygen did not increase mortality but did cut down on the eye disease by two-thirds; oxygen concentrations over 40 percent were dangerous, and those under 40 percent were safe. "American juries began to award millions of dollars in judgments of malpractice if the hospital record indicated that concentration of oxygen in an incubator had been, even momentarily, >40%," Silverman reported.[34] But it turned out that there were problems with that original study. One analyst suggested that for each baby whose sight was saved, sixteen might have died from the lower oxygen concentrations. And then the issue of brain damage was raised—maybe the lower oxygen concentrations were preserving babies' vision but hurting their brains?

The second half of the twentieth century also saw the development of the essential technology for delivering oxygen directly into the lungs of babies who couldn't breathe for themselves, rather than putting the baby into an oxygen chamber or introducing oxygen into the stomach. Alexander Graham Bell himself had designed a "respirator" for newborns as early as 1889, but it was never used on human infants, though he tried it out on a baby lamb. The first scientific studies on respirators for newborns were published in the 1950s, using a machine called the "puffer," which worked through a mask on the baby's face. There were also attempts to adopt the "iron lung" technology that was used on polio patients for newborns. These tank-style machines work by negative pressure—the pressure around the chest is decreased until the chest expands in an inhalation. They were tried on newborns with some success, along with respirators, often manually operated, that could pump positive pressure into the lungs.

Dr. Mildred Stahlman, who graduated from the Vanderbilt University School of Medicine in 1946, founded the first modern newborn intensive care unit in the country there in 1961. All through the 1960s, newborn nurseries got better at monitoring their tiny patients. "We frequently measured blood gas values and pH with modern electrodes, sampling from indwelling arterial catheters; monitored heart and respiratory rates and did ECG studies . . . and administered mechanical ventilation in infants with respiratory failure, sometimes successfully," Dr. Stahlman wrote.[35] And then, around 1971, a technique was developed for delivering continuous positive pressure into the newborn's lungs through an endotracheal tube inserted into the baby's airway, keeping the stiff lungs from collapsing even at the end of expiration. Ventilator technology has continued to develop, with more sophisticated machines making it much less common to use the punishing high pressures that can damage a baby's lungs for life.

The oxygen saga continued, but it didn't get any easier—not for academic medicine, and not for parents. Oxygen, that invisible life-saving delivery room miracle, that substance Dr. Silverman called "the most frequently prescribed 'drug' in the care of small neonates," had turned out to be, like so many drugs, a mixed blessing, capable of harming as well as helping. Neonatology was saving babies—thousands of babies—and they were all getting oxygen, but it was not clear how much to give to any individual baby or for how long, in order to do as much helping and as little damage as possible. Different NICUs in different hospitals were following different guidelines. More clinical trials were conducted, using the newer technology of pulse oximetry, in which a sensor on the baby's skin reads the oxygen saturation in the baby's blood; the Supplemental Therapeutic Oxygen for Prethreshold Retinopathy of Prematurity (STOP-ROP) and the Benefits of Oxygen Saturation Targeting (BOOST) trials seemed to suggest that higher oxygen concentrations were not helping the babies.[36]

The SUPPORT (Surfactant, Positive Pressure, and Oxygenation Randomized Trial) study, which ran from 2005 to 2009, also involved surfactant, a therapy that helps keep premature lungs working well. The infants in the study were randomized to receive enough oxygen to keep them either 85–89 percent saturated or 91–95 percent saturated, both within the range of standard medical care at the time. The point of the study was to see whether tightening the controls and deliberately keeping infants at the lower end of that supposedly safe range could reduce damage to the retina. The consent form the parents signed promised that all the infants in the study—and, indeed, this applied to all infants not in the study—would be given enough oxygen to keep them in this standard range of 85–95 percent and stated that "the benefit of higher versus lower oxygen levels of oxygenation in infants, especially for premature infants, is not known."[37]

To the surprise of the doctors who had designed the SUPPORT study, more of the infants who got lower concentrations of oxygen died. Subsequently, parents and public interest groups protested that the parents had not been told that their babies might be exposed to a therapy that could cause brain damage and death. In 2013, the federal Office for Human Research Protections investigated; it ruled that the study had violated the rules of informed consent.[38]

Dr. John Lantos, a pediatrician and bioethicist, reviewed the studies and the criticism. He concluded that the study had been ethically designed; that the information provided to the parents had been consonant with the information available to the researchers, as well as with their beliefs; and that, in fact, the babies in the study—in both the high-oxygen arm and the low-oxygen arm—had done better than equivalent premature infants who were not enrolled in the study. Even so, the government censure, the public outcry, and the anger of parents did lasting damage to what was already a very complicated and often unpalatable cause in medicine—the need for randomized trials. "It is difficult to convey the need for randomized trials to any patient, but perhaps particularly to parents of critically ill children," Dr. Lantos wrote. "Perhaps for this reason, there have been very few prospective randomized trials in neonatology. As a result, many therapies in neonatology have not been validated and may be dangerous."[39]

Babies now receive higher concentrations of oxygen than they used to, building on the hard-won knowledge from the SUPPORT trial, while eye damage remains a major concern. Working in the NICU teaches you to be a little afraid of your own medications and interventions (never a bad lesson for doctors). We used to give antibiotics to tiny babies, knowing that certain drugs might damage their kidneys or their hearing but also understanding that we were treating what might be fatal infections. We used to dial up the pressure on ventilators to try to force air into stiff premature lungs, aware that the high pressures might blow holes in those lungs. Technological fixes for these problems have been developed since my training days—less toxic antibiotics, gentler higher-tech ventilators—but the babies remain vulnerable and the stakes remain high.

"Baby shows are no novelty now and certainly not the source of amusement," Dr. Zahorsky wrote in 1949 in his autobiography. "Visit any large hospital, find some excuse to be admitted to the obstetrical department, and you can see a baby show; some tiny ones are in incubators (or brooders)."[40] Thirty years later, William Silverman ended his article reconstructing the story of the incubator-baby shows this way:

> I find it hard to ignore the resemblance between the theatrics of the side-show exhibits and the dramatic actions in present-day neonatal intensive care units. In both cases, I find a disturbing detachment from reality. . . . The feeble infant is plucked up and deposited in a theater-like setting in which superb technical experts make all-out efforts to support life. And when this has been accomplished successfully the infant graduates. But no comparable effort is mounted to deal with the enormous problems which face the graduate at home and in the community.[41]

A few years later, Dr. Stahlman, who had started the first NICU in the country, published an article titled "Newborn Intensive Care: Success or Failure?" She reflected, "Spectacular gains have been made . . . and costs, both tangible and intangible, have been equally spectacular."[42]

Dr. Mary Ellen Avery, one of the senior neonatologists at Boston Children's Hospital when I was doing my residency, played a key role in researching the pathophysiology of respiratory distress syndrome, the disease of stiff premature lungs that killed Patrick Kennedy. In her lab, and in other labs around the world, researchers identified a particular molecule missing in premature lungs—a surfactant that keeps air sacs supple and allows oxygen exchange to take place. They developed artificial surfactants, which could be administered through the endotracheal tube into a baby's lungs, and these have dramatically improved survival in premature infants. "I hate to be a prophet," Dr. Avery said in a 1998 oral history interview, "because I remember hearing myself say 30 years ago that I didn't think any babies under 1500 grams should be resuscitated, because the chances of their survival were so poor. So having been so wrong in the past, I'm a bit humble." Babies well below that weight were routinely being resuscitated by 1998, and many of them were doing well, in part thanks to the artificial surfactant work that Dr. Avery and her colleagues had carried out. But she went on to caution, "I'm afraid that I still think it's very risky to go below 24 weeks with the present state of knowledge."[43]

By the 1960s, and even more so in the decades that followed, every full-term pregnancy was supposed to yield a viable child; as the mother's survival had reflected on the skills of the birth atten- dant, now the infant's survival was emblematic of the skill of the pediatrician. And the fact that survival rather than loss had become the norm meant new attention to deaths, which seemed more and more tragic as they became more rare. The first medical article to take note of the phenomenon that parents might grieve after stillbirths or deaths in the delivery room appeared in the medical literature in 1959: "The Management of Grief Situations in Obstetrics." Twenty years later, Emanuel Lewis, from the department of child and family psychiatry at Charing Cross Hospital, contributed a "Personal Prac- tice" column to the *Archives of Disease in Childhood*. In "Mourning by the Family after a Stillbirth or Neonatal Death," he spoke about how parents who lost children in this way were surrounded by a kind of conspiracy of silence. He argued for letting parents spend time with the dead infants, for photographs and mourning and funerals, and for acknowledging the loss and the sadness. "It is my impression that if a stillbirth has been a real experience for the family in the ways that I have described, mourning will have been facilitated," he wrote. "This leads to fewer psychological problems for the mother and her family."[44]

————— // —————

Birth and the days that follow it remain a liminal zone, in spite of everything that has been done to make it safer. The border may be pushed back and back, but it remains a borderland, one where some dreams die and others come true in complex and sometimes less-than-happy ways. The modern specialty of neonatology has brought about so many joyous outcomes—just look at the bulletin board outside any NICU or ask among your friends, and you will find people right at hand whose families owe everything to this most high-tech care. I remember talking to a fellow resident who was bound for neonatology as a specialty, and in addition to citing all the happy endings, she told me contentedly that taking care of a preemie was like flying a plane—when you had mastered all the variables and all the instruments, when you had a baby fully "plugged in" and hooked up, you could be truly in control, and use all your skills to bring that baby through to safety. Yet there will be decisions to be made; the perinatal period is an edge, an inflection point, a place where doing good can do harm—or at least, where the two can be mixed, as you might, for example, face the possibility that by giving babies enough oxygen to maximize their chances of survival, you may also be clouding their vision, reducing their chances to see the world in which they will—miraculously enough, by all the standards of human history—live to grow up.

CHAPTER 9

"Something Children Always Have"

Measles and Chicken Pox

When I was a resident, if a child came in with an unusual rash, and measles was suspected, we would sometimes call in older attending physicians, trusting more in their memory than in our textbook pictures of a rash that most of us had never seen. Inevitably, the attending would tell us, *Your grandmother could diagnose measles from across the room—she probably wouldn't even have bothered to ask the pediatrician.* Our grandmothers would have known it as a disease you wanted to get young but not too young—dangerous to babies but usually pretty routine in schoolchildren—and extremely contagious. When I was learning medicine in the 1980s, we were taught as a vaccination rule that if people were born before 1957, you could assume they were immune to measles without testing them, because *everyone* born in the pre-vaccine era got the disease. Jerome K. Jerome, the English writer and humorist, wrote in an 1886 essay, "Love is like the measles; we all have to go through it."[1]

Measles spreads rapidly and efficiently by small droplets of fluid from the nose and throat that are coughed or sneezed from one person to another, or the virus may hang in the air as an aerosol to be breathed in, or get onto someone's hand and then be inoculated into the eyes, nose or mouth. Most people who are exposed, unless they are immune, will get sick within seven to fourteen days. The illness can at first look very much like a cold, with fever, a runny nose, and a harsh cough. Our teachers told us over and over that children with measles were likely to seem particularly miserable; if a child seemed more irritable than the symptoms of a bad cold would warrant, they said, think about measles. In fact, the extreme "irritability" may be evidence of some inflammation of the central nervous system, which is one of the places the measles virus likes to go. The cold symptoms get worse, especially the fever and the runny nose. The throat gets red, and little bright red spots with tiny blue-white centers may appear on the inside of the mouth. These are Koplik's spots, which we were always trained to check for when there was any suspicion of measles, named for their discoverer, Dr. Henry Koplik (1858–1927), who was on the pediatrics faculty at Bellevue Hospital.

Because Koplik's spots allow you to make the diagnosis of measles a few days before the rash appears, recognizing them can stop a sick patient from exposing even more people. After two or three days of this sick but hard-to-identify stage, the rash appears, first as red spots at the hairline, then on the face, and then spreading down over the body. And it is quite a rash: red and blotchy and "confluent," with the patches of rash running together until all the skin is covered. Subsequently, in uncomplicated cases, the fever goes away, the rash fades, and the patients recover. Except when they don't.

In 1885, Ella O'Neill left her two little sons, James Jr. and Edmund, with her mother, Bridget Quinlan, to join her husband, the famous actor James O'Neill, on the road, because he was so jealous of her affections that he resented the children keeping her away from him. While his parents were touring, James Jr. developed measles, that standard and highly contagious disease of childhood. His younger brother, Edmund, who was just a year and a half old, caught it from him and died. In her distress and anger, Ella O'Neill promptly sent her surviving son away to boarding school. She did not intend to have more children, but three years later, she gave birth to another son, Eugene, who would grow up to tell his family's story in *Long Day's Journey into Night,* a play so personal that he did not want it produced and refused to publish it during his lifetime. "If I hadn't left him with my mother to join you on the road, because you wrote telling me you missed me and were so lonely, Jamie would never have been allowed, when he still had measles, to go in the baby's room," Ella O'Neill's dramatic counterpart, Mary Tyrone, says onstage to her husband. *Her face hardening,* according to the stage directions, she goes on: "I've always believed Jamie did it on purpose. He was jealous of the baby. He hated him."[2]

The play involves a somewhat unusual instance of measles playing a tragic literary role; more often, the disease turns up as an inevitability of childhood, sometimes faintly comic, with its dramatic red rash. In *Cheaper by the Dozen,* the 1948 book by Frank Gilbreth Jr. and his sister Ernestine Gilbreth Carey, about growing up in a family of a dozen children with two efficiency-expert parents, eleven of the children get measles at once: "Two big adjoining bedrooms upstairs were converted into hospital wards—one for the boys and the other for the girls. We suffered together for two or three miserable, feverish, itchy days, while Mother applied cocoa butter and ice packs." The general tone is humorous, and the doctor is highly reassuring: "Dr. Burton, who had delivered most of us, said there was nothing to worry about."[3] Although *Cheaper by the Dozen* and its sequel, *Belles on Their Toes,* as well as a host of movie versions, make much of the even dozen Gilbreth children, six boys and six girls, there were really only eleven of them alive for most of the story. Mary Elizabeth Gilbreth, the second of the six daughters, actually died of diphtheria in 1912 at the age of five; several of the children got sick, but the others recovered (this is mentioned in a footnote in *Belles*). This death hit the parents very hard, their son wrote in another memoir, saying his father "was so overcome with grief that he simply couldn't cope with things, and went into a shell," and that "for years thereafter, if one of the younger children asked Mother about Mary, she'd do her best to answer calmly, and then retire hastily to her room, with her shoulders shaking in sobs."[4] But even with this history—the death of a sibling following after a group illness—the idea of everyone coming down with measles is presented largely as comedy; later in the chapter, the father anoints himself with red ink and fakes an attack of measles himself, fooling no one.

In *Our Hearts Were Young and Gay,* the 1942 memoir by Cornelia Otis Skinner and Emily Kimbrough about a Grand Tour of Europe in the early 1920s, Cornelia gets sick on the boat crossing the Atlantic and her friends have to sneak her past the health authorities, so that she won't be quarantined. Their main worry is that Cornelia may develop her measles rash, which has not yet emerged, because when it does, it will make her illness unmistakable. But even without the rash, her face is flushed and swollen, and sneaking her into France turns into a bit of a caper, with thick stage makeup on her face and a bright red hat with a feather. "I topped off my startling appearance with a flowing white veil which, I pointed out, would make me less conspicuous. I guess I'd gotten a little delirious by then." She does make it past the health inspector, "who merely shuddered and passed me as rapidly as possible."[5]

And yet, even in its distinctly comic identity, fictional measles could be lethal to fictional characters. In *Gone with the Wind,* Scarlett O'Hara's first husband, the besotted Charles Hamilton (whom she married only to make Ashley Wilkes feel bad), "died ignominiously and swiftly of pneumonia, following measles, without ever having gotten any closer to the Yankees than the [Confederate training] camp in South Carolina."[6] This was historically accurate: measles was a major killer of the boys and young men conscripted into the army for the Civil War; like all soldiers, they lived in close confinement, ideal conditions for the spread of infections. For the Confederates, one surgeon wrote, "The disease consequent to and traceable to measles cost the Confederate Army the lives of more men and a greater amount of invalidism than all other causes combined."[7]

In the early part of the nineteenth century, there were six thousand or so deaths a year from measles in the United States, and the death rate for the disease was highest of all among children in orphanages.[8] By the late nineteenth century, those responsible for children in institutions knew that measles posed a particularly serious threat to their charges—and, again, the danger of the disease in hospital settings may have been partially due to that weakened or vulnerable population. In 1892, a measles epidemic in the Nursery and Child's Hospital in New York City killed 33 percent of the infants under a year of age and 50 percent of those between one and two. (The younger infants probably still had some protective maternal antibodies, especially if they had been breastfed.) In 1897, an outbreak in the Municipal Hospital of Philadelphia killed 39 percent of those infected, and 48 percent of children from one to five.[9]

Measles can be particularly devastating to malnourished children and to children with a vitamin A deficiency—this is still evident in the developing world today—and so, with improved nutrition in the twentieth century, the general population of children in the United States became better able to survive the infection. In 1926, 6,771 children under five died of measles in the United States. In 1937, less than a third as many perished, probably reflecting better nutrition. By 1945, the number had dropped to 214, probably because the new sulfa drugs offered the first effective option for treating the pneumonia that often followed, usually caused by bacteria infecting the weakened child after a bout of measles.

In 1946, with World War II over, and with no vaccine for measles on the horizon, Dr. Spock took the disease seriously in his *Common Sense Book of Baby and Child Care*, that bible of midcentury parenting. He urged parents not to fret too much about polio, since most children wouldn't catch it, but he knew that everyone would get measles, and he advised parents to worry if the fever stayed high for too many days after the rash appeared, and to call the doctor or bring the child to a hospital. "The complications are dangerous," he warned, especially in younger children.[10]

Inoculation against measles had been considered back in 1758, in Edinburgh, when Francis Home (1710–1801), a Scottish professor of medicine, tried to do for measles what others had done for smallpox: he scarified areas on the arms of people who had never had the disease and rubbed in blood from people sick with measles, blood he had taken from the areas of most intense rash. He explained his rationale: "Considering how many die . . . considering how it hurts the lungs and eyes; I thought I should do no small service to mankind, if I could render this disease more mild and safe, in the same way as the Turks have taught us to mitigate the small-pox."[11] In ten of the twelve children on whom he experimented, a mild case of measles developed, and he was able to conclude that, indeed, "the blood of a measly patient . . . contains a sufficient quantity of the morbific matter, to produce, by some fermentative power natural to it, the measles."[12] However, other doctors were not able to replicate his results, and the idea of battling measles by inoculation never attained the popularity—or the urgency—of smallpox inoculation.

Dr. Home, of course, had no way of knowing what the "morbific matter" was that he was transferring from child to child. John Enders and T. C. Peebles identified the cause of measles as a virus two hundred years later, in 1954, in the same lab in Boston that would be recognized with a Nobel Prize that same year for the discovery, by Enders and two colleagues, of how to grow the polio virus in culture. As a virus that infects only humans, measles, like smallpox, could be targeted for eradication: in theory, if we could immunize everyone, we could wipe out the disease. It cannot do what influenza can do— hide out in animals—and the virus cannot survive for long periods away from a living human host.

"When I got to the Enders lab, polio was still going on," recalled Samuel Katz, a prominent pediatric infectious diseases specialist who became Dr. Enders's research fellow in 1956. Speaking in an oral history project interview, Katz said, "But Dr. Enders had always been much more interested in measles than in polio. It had been his first love among the virus infections."[13] Enders did not treat patients himself, but Katz suggests that he was extremely aware of the amount of sickness and death the measles virus caused every year. Also, Katz said, Enders was not satisfied with the way the polio virus that he had so painstakingly cultured had been adapted into vaccines by Salk and Sabin. "I think in the back of his mind," Katz speculated, "he decided he could do a better job, and he was going to do a better job with measles. Not looking for glory or anything of that sort, but just the fulfillment of what he felt was a logical scientific approach."[14]

Enders, whom Katz described as a "Connecticut Yankee," was legendarily parsimonious as a researcher and a lab director. He had an eye out for human tissues that were likely to be discarded and could be collected and used to get cells for cell culture.[15] "Foreskins abounded," Dr. Katz remembered, so foreskins were collected after circumcisions and used to make those initial cell cultures. Then there were kidneys, because for a while there was a popular operation for treating hydrocephalus that involved taking out the child's kidney— so they used those cells to grow the measles virus. Later, they were able to grow measles in cells taken from placentas that were being discarded across the street at the Boston Lying-In Hospital, but ultimately, they wanted to move the virus, which only infects humans, into chick embryo cells, in hopes of making it less dangerous.

Like the oral polio vaccine, measles would be a live-virus vaccine, made less dangerous by being passed through a series of non-human cells. Using a particular strain of the virus that was isolated from a thirteen-year-old boy named David Edmonston during an outbreak in Boston, Enders and his fellows set to work to develop a modified viral strain that, when they tested it on monkeys, could be used to produce immunity without producing disease. It took three years of work, passing the virus twenty-four times through human kidney cells, twenty-eight times through human amniotic cells taken from placentas, six times through fertilized hen's eggs, and finally thirteen times through chick embryo cell cultures, to develop a live but sufficiently attenuated strain of measles virus. For testing, they took it to a local institution that provided residential treatment for severely handicapped children, the Walter E. Fernald State School, near the town of Waltham. "You parked your youngster there and they lived there forever after," as Dr. Katz put it.[16]

Testing anything new—a vaccine, a drug—on institutionalized patients is ethically problematic, even if they have the capacity to give consent. Institutional power can be an unspoken factor. The children at Fernald did not have the capacity to consent, and the school had previously been the site of a notorious set of experiments on children's nutrition in which, without telling parents or family members what they were doing, researchers had fed cereal coated with radioactive marker substances to the children. Yet testing the measles vaccine in this population had a certain logic: measles outbreaks were still terrible in institutionalized children, and the Fernald State School was no exception. "We knew, from pediatricians who worked there, that they had severe outbreaks of measles every year, in which there was a significant morbidity and indeed mortality among these youngsters," Katz said. "So we went to the officials who ran the school and proposed to them that we thought we had a product that would protect their children."[17]

The scientists met with the parents of all the children who had come to the school since the previous measles outbreak, because those children would not have been exposed, would not be immune, and would be vulnerable if measles broke out again. They laid out all the potential benefits of the vaccine, telling the parents that they believed it was safe. (In accordance with all the traditions of vaccine history, they had already given it to themselves, of course.)[18] They also, Katz added, "explain[ed] honestly that these would be the first children to whom this product would have been administered."[19] All the parents agreed to let their children be vaccinated, Katz recalled. Children at the institution for whom there were no parents available weren't included in the study. The researchers made this process of parental "informed consent" very explicit in their eventual article announcing the success of the vaccine. As it turned out, many of the Fernald children did run fevers after they were vaccinated, and some developed mild rashes, which went away. None encountered serious problems. The children at Fernald also developed antibodies, suggesting that the vaccine would be effective in producing immunity. The researchers extended their trial, involving pediatricians at a number of different medical centers, working with children in the general population as well as with institutionalized children. They announced their results in a special issue of the *New England Journal of Medicine*, in 1960.

The researchers were essentially making up the ethics of this trial as they went along. Dr. David Morley, a colleague working in Nigeria, contacted them when he heard about a possible measles vaccine. Among his patients, many of whom were undernourished, the mortality rate from measles was 10 percent or higher, with many dying of measles pneumonia or lung disease. Dr. Morley was eager to see if he could protect them with the vaccine, but, Katz recalled, "Dr. Enders and I agreed that we would not go to Nigeria until the vaccine was approved in the United States. . . . We were very concerned we could be thought of as using these poor black kids as 'guinea pigs.'"[20]

It's easy to imagine the tension between the doctor in Africa who is taking care of the children, and wants them to stop dying as soon as possible, and the researchers in Boston, worried about how the experiment will be viewed. It's also interesting that the researchers didn't have the same concerns about testing the vaccine at the Fernald State School, and, in fact, their procedures there with the parents were regarded as open and forward-thinking. After the vaccine was licensed, Katz and his team did go to Nigeria, with support from the Office of the Surgeon General, the armed forces, and the Health

Research Council of the City of New York, to study the immune response in a population of children at high risk, a population in which many of the children had malaria—but the vaccine continued to work.[21]

The measles vaccine was introduced in the United States for general use in 1963. At the time, though there were hundreds of thousands of cases and hundreds of deaths every year, many people did not think of a measles vaccine as important precisely because they saw measles as a routine childhood illness, and not a particularly frightening one. Everyone, it seemed, had had measles and recovered, so what was the big deal? That, together with the cartoonish quality of those red spots made the disease a non-threatening, non-scary illness, with perhaps a certain Dr. Seuss quality to the rash. Measles gave you spots, mumps gave you puffed chipmunk cheeks, chicken pox made you scratch. Everybody got sick, and almost everybody got well.

Smallpox, the other rash to which measles has historically been compared, was a much scarier disease, starting out with red spots but progressing to pustules, killing many of its victims and leaving others scarred for life. Polio, though much rarer, was a more terrifying specter because it paralyzed and killed a greater proportion of the children who did get sick. So the smallpox vaccine and the polio vaccine seemed like logical and even lifesaving heroic science, but measles was different. The head of the Centers for Disease Control called measles a disease "of only mild severity," although he acknowledged the "infrequent complications."[22]

Yet when scientists looked more closely, they found that those infrequent complications, spread across the enormous numbers of children who got measles, added up to a substantial number of children seriously harmed. During the first few years the measles vaccine was available, although many children were vaccinated, physicians and public health authorities were frustrated that there was not wider demand among parents.

The measles virus itself can attack the lungs, causing respiratory symptoms that can be serious, especially in young children, but more commonly, the measles infection may be followed closely by bacterial pneumonia. This sequence, bacterial pneumonia complicating the viral infection of measles, was responsible for many of the deaths in measles epidemics, perhaps especially in institutions. Children who recovered from the infection were sometimes left blind or with their vision badly damaged. Pediatric authorities advised that patients with measles should be kept in darkened rooms. In *The Five Little Peppers and How They Grew*, Margaret Sidney's 1881 novel of New England family life, the poor but plucky Pepper family is devastated by a bout of measles, which strikes down four of the five Pepper children. Their mother explains that measles is "something children always have," adding, "but I'm sure I hoped it wouldn't come just yet."[23] One brother gets so sick that he comes close to dying, and the eyes of eleven-year-old Polly Pepper, the heroine of the book, are threatened by the disease, so that her mother fears she will go "stone-blind." Thus poor Polly's eyes are bandaged to keep out the light, and she endures an interminable convalescence of darkness and inactivity: "Not to *do* anything! The very idea at any time would have filled her active, wide-awake little body with horror; and now, here she was!"[24] Since we now know that malnutrition and vitamin A deficiency add to the risk that measles will lead to blindness, you might wonder whether the rather restricted diet of the impoverished Pepper family (mush for breakfast, potatoes for dinner) contributes to Polly's risk. But Polly's eyes are eventually unbandaged, the measles vanquished, and the family restored to health.

The virus can also attack the gastrointestinal system, causing vomiting and diarrhea, and one in every five hundred children will develop encephalopathy, or brain damage, after the infection is over. But the scariest are the later neurologic complications, most importantly subacute sclerosing panencephalitis, or SSPE, an untreatable degenerative neurologic disease that comes on five to ten years after the initial infection, leaving the children who survive (nearly 50 percent don't) neurologically damaged.

In an editorial in December 1965, the *Journal of the American Medical Association* (*JAMA*) compared the mortality from measles with that from polio, pointing out that "means are at hand to prevent measles and poliomyelitis." In 1964, the editorial said, polio had caused seven deaths in the United States, while measles had caused about four hundred, mostly among preschool children. The editorial emphasized the serious complications of measles: "It is a disquieting thought that brain damage may result from what might appear to the clinician to be straightforward and uncomplicated measles." But though the writers had started by warning that "many parents regard it as an unwelcome but inevitable minor ailment of childhood," by the end of the editorial, they were worried that doctors also weren't taking the disease seriously: "Physicians . . . who do not consider measles to be serious enough to warrant immunization, would do well to ponder these facts."[25]

In 1965, Ann Landers answered a question from a reader about intentionally exposing children to infectious diseases:

> Dear Ann Landers: My kookie sister makes me mad. Her
> four children are always sick with something. When her
> eldest got the measles she intentionally exposed the other
> kids. Last weekend she came to my house and brought her
> children. The 5-year-old looked as if he had the mumps. I
> took his temperature and it was 103. I said. "Beatrice, I think
> Percy has the mumps." She said, "So do I." I told her she had
> a lot of nerve to bring a sick child to my house. "It is best for
> kids if they get everything early," she replied. Is she right or
> wrong?—MAD

The sister was not alone—some parents did deliberately expose their children. There were reports of measles parties as late as the early 1960s.[26] With a disease that all children were bound to catch sooner or later, parents could consider trying to control when it happened. Once a child was out of the most dangerous early years, they could look at measles as something to be scheduled at a convenient moment. The advice columnist, however, did not hesitate to take sides and, in particular, to offer a warning that measles, especially, could be very dangerous:

> Dear Mad: She is wrong. Every normal precaution should be taken to protect children against all diseases (particularly measles, which can be crippling or fatal). Most children get enough illnesses without inviting more.[27]

Ann Landers wasn't actually recommending the vaccine yet—though she would play a role later on in the campaign to get all children vaccinated—but she certainly wasn't treating measles as a joke.

The anti-vaccine movement has circulated a carefully assembled eight-minute online video called *Measles, Back in the Days Before the Marketing of the Vaccine,* which splices clips from a number of sitcoms in which measles is a fun and funny disease. On a 1959 episode from *The Donna Reed Show,* a visiting teen idol comes down with measles; on *The Flintstones* in 1961, it's Betty and Wilma with cartoon speckles all over their faces just before they're supposed to leave for a bake-off (Barney and Fred decide to go instead); and on *The Brady Bunch* from 1969, in the spirit of *Cheaper by the Dozen,* well, you can just imagine: one child gets sick, and soon all six are down. The clip helpfully emphasizes the various remarks characters make about how trivial and unserious the disease is. Thus, Barney Rubble: "Aw, don't worry, Fred. Measles don't hurt." Or Marcia Brady, as the Brady Bunch children, home from school in their pajamas and bathrobes, happily play Monopoly: "If you have to get sick, sure can't beat the measles." Leaving aside the dubious value of getting your health information from *The Brady Bunch* (let alone from *The Flintstones*), it's perfectly fair to say that families did not live in terror of the measles. Historian Elena Conis has argued that as a disease becomes rarer, thanks to vaccination, more attention is paid to the less common and more dangerous complications, and the deaths, than to the many more routine cases of an illness that used to be part of daily life (and sitcom plots).[28]

Measles immunization programs were nowhere near universal in the United States all through the 1960s and into the 1970s. Targeting measles with a vaccine represented a change in medical and public health thinking: a disease that had been a standard part of childhood was redefined as a potential menace. As childhood death became increasingly rare—and therefore increasingly unthinkable—in the decades after the war, campaigns would be launched to prevent even a relatively small number of deaths, or perhaps lasting injuries. Furthermore, in a world in which all children were routinely vaccinated, it was evident that vaccines not only saved lives but, on a much more mundane level, prevented lost schooldays for sick children and lost work days for their caretaking parents.

Would modern parents react calmly to the idea of a child coming down with an infection that is usually benign but still fatal in hundreds of cases and able to cause permanent neurological damage? It's hard to imagine, as a pediatrician, telling a parent to relax, that their child will almost certainly be fine, though hundreds die every year from what he's got. On the other hand, in 2019 the United States experienced a surprising and resurgent measles epidemic because many parents have avoided having their children vaccinated, believing what they have been told by the anti-vaccine movement—that the disease is benign and the complications too rare to worry about.

Dr. William Huffman Stewart, who became surgeon general in 1965, was a pediatrician (and the son of a pediatrician) and an epidemiologist. On November 1, 1966, he called for the eradication of measles in 1967, laying out four major goals. All children should be immunized at the age of one; of the older, unimmunized children, susceptible kindergarteners and first and second graders who had not yet had the measles should be immunized; better reporting systems should be developed; and epidemics should be addressed with crash immunization programs. The *Morbidity and Mortality Weekly Report* (MMWR), the statistically oriented publication of the CDC, sounded unusually excited when it initiated a special supplement, *Measles Eradication 1967*, and described the campaign: "The *Morbidity and Mortality Weekly Report* has enlarged its regular coverage of measles to present an up-to-date appraisal of what is clearly an unprecedented period in preventive medicine. Never before has the eradication of an important communicable disease been readily within reach."[29] The special supplement went on to quote a number of professional groups, from the American Medical Association and the American Academy of Pediatrics to the American School Health Association, all calling for the elimination of measles from the United States. The resolution passed by the American School Health Association emphasized the seriousness of the disease: "In the past measles has killed hundreds of children each year and left many others with handicapping conditions. Now there is no longer any reason for any child to die or suffer disability from measles."[30]

On March 6, 1967, President Lyndon B. Johnson put out a presidential announcement: "Our goal is to eliminate measles from the United States in 1967. The Surgeon General's target for this year is the vaccination of between 8 and 10 million children—all susceptible children between the ages of one and seven."[31] The national campaign stressed the idea that measles could be serious, enlisting everyone from the surgeon general to Ann Landers and aiming particularly at mothers.

"Many parents who survived childhood measles themselves without mishap may wonder what's so bad about having a case of measles," wrote Joy Miller, the Associated Press women's editor, in a 1967 column that went out to a number of newspapers.[32] (Miller's own cause was to make the so-called women's pages more substantive.) The column ran under such headlines as "Measles . . . A Crippler," "Measles Can Make a Child Retarded," and "Beware of the Danger!"

Miller cited statistics about measles encephalitis from the National Association for Retarded Children's 1966 report, ending the passage with "And that brings us to little Kim Fisher." Kim was the 1966–67 Poster Child for the National Association for Retarded Children (NARC). According to that same report, Kim was a ten-year-old from Fort Wayne, Indiana, "a normal baby, a bright child," who had developed measles encephalitis at the age of two, leaving her "mentally retarded, hard of hearing, unable to walk, talk, or hold up her head." She was attending "classes for the trainable," the report explained. "Gradually her handicaps are being counteracted. But measles robbed Kim of a normal life. It need not happen to others."[33]

This national campaign used many of the same techniques as the successful campaign to wipe out polio in the United States, from nonprofit advocacy groups to poster children. The 1966 report by NARC gave the statistics: 4 million cases of measles a year, 500 deaths, 4,000 cases of measles encephalitis, 1,600 of whom ended up intellectually disabled. Measles vaccines had been available for three years, the report said, but many children were not immunized. "In cooperation with the Public Health Service, NARC in 1966 joined the nationwide attack to wipe out this disease. Each of the 1,100 State and Local Associations was given a kit of information on measles and the measles vaccine, together with the steps that may be taken to assist health departments in initiating and conducting immunization programs."[34] The illustration for this passage is a pile of newspaper clippings with headlines like "Measles Is a Child Killer" and "Measles Vaccination Urged for Milford Area Children."

On another front, the *MMWR* supplement celebrated a series of *Peanuts* cartoons that took on the issue of the measles vaccine; the editors credited Dr. Mary Jean Trudeau, immunization project leader of the California State Department of Public Health, with getting Charles M. Schulz interested in the subject. In one comic strip, Linus complains to his older sister, Lucy, that his arm "hates to get shots," and she hands him a piece of paper to read. "Measles is the most

Target: measles

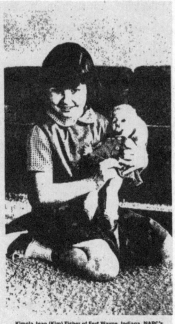

To lead the way . . .

Ten-year-old Kim Fisher was selected by NARC to spearhead the drive on prevention as the 1966-67 Poster Child.

Kim was a normal baby, a bright child, but at two, measles struck and measles encephalitis followed. This inflammation of the brain left her mentally retarded, hard of hearing, unable to walk, talk, or hold up her head.

Today Kim attends classes for the trainable mentally retarded at the Johnny Appleseed School and Training Center in Fort Wayne. Gradually her handicaps are being counteracted.

But measles robbed Kim of a normal life. It need not happen to others.

Kimela Jean (Kim) Fisher of Fort Wayne, Indiana, NARC's Poster Child, a victim of measles encephalitis.

Ten-year-old Kim Fisher, the official 1966–67 poster child for the National Association for Retarded Children, holds her doll and smiles. Here, Kim is the face of a campaign against measles led by the NARC, which hoped to mobilize parents to vaccinate. *Image provided courtesy of The Arc New York Historic Archives.*

common and serious 'childhood disease,'" he reads. "Complications are middle-ear infections, pneumonia and even brain damage." He holds up his arm and says to it, with a smile, "Did you hear that, arm? It's going to be worth it!"[35]

As measles vaccination was adopted, the number of cases dropped dramatically.[36] In 1978, the CDC again set a goal of eliminating measles from the United States, this time by 1982, and universal vaccination of young children brought measles rates down dramatically. But it turned out that a single dose of vaccine—which was what the campaign was based on—didn't protect everyone. In 1989, there was an outbreak among children who had gotten that single dose, and the recommendation had to change to include a second shot.[37] In 1971, the U.S. Public Health Service recommended that routine immunization against smallpox should be ended in this country, where the disease had not occurred in more than twenty years. But the national anti-measles campaign never got there; in 2000, the CDC declared another kind of victory, announcing that there had been no continuous transmission for over twelve months. Measles had essentially been eliminated as an endemic disease—that is, there were only sporadic outbreaks. Still, the goal of eradication remained elusive, and certainly no one was suggesting that it would be safe to stop vaccinating, since measles remained endemic in many countries around the world, and small measles outbreaks continued (and continue) to occur in the States, often started by cases imported from abroad and then spread to people who were either unimmunized or not completely protected by their immunizations.

Increasingly, what we now call "vaccine refusal" is to blame for those unprotected people. In 2013, an imported case sparked the largest outbreak New York City had seen since 1992, with 58 cases of measles. The median age of the patients was three, and 45 of them were old enough to be vaccinated but had not been, "owing to parental refusal or intentional delay." There were also 3,351 exposed contacts, who had to be tracked down and notified—and protected when possible—by the city health department; the total direct costs were estimated at $394,448.[38]

The much larger measles epidemic of 2019 involved more than a thousand cases reported in twenty-eight states in the first half of the year, the worst numbers, by far, since 1992. In New York in particular, the epidemic was centered in the Orthodox Jewish community, which had been targeted by a very specific anti-vaccine campaign by a group called Parents Educating and Advocating for Children's Health, or PEACH. PEACH had produced the glossy *Vaccine Safety Handbook*, which contained false information that emphasized the dangers of vaccination and compared government vaccination programs to Nazi Germany. In addition, they spread rumors claiming that the MMR vaccine contained monkey, rat, and pig DNA and was therefore forbidden to anyone following Jewish dietary laws. The booklet also falsely reassured parents that measles is not a dangerous disease.[39]

The anti-vaccine movement views measles as a normal, unalarming childhood disease that has been transformed into a terrifying bogeyman by the profit-oriented pharmaceutical companies and vaccine-mongering doctors. The vaccine developed in the Enders laboratory, based on the Edmonston strain of measles, became the basis for later vaccines, in which the virus had been weakened even more. That vaccine was eventually incorporated, in 1971, along with vaccines against mumps and rubella, into the MMR vaccine, which we now give to all children at ages one and five. Some parents who felt that measles was just not a serious disease continued to refuse the vaccine. (Ironically, David Edmonston himself decided not to vaccinate his son for this reason.) In Great Britain in the 1980s, a version of the MMR vaccine was withdrawn when it turned out that the particular strain of mumps that had been used had caused some cases of mumps meningitis. A safer version of the vaccine was made available, but many British parents continued to refuse the vaccine, arguing that measles was not particularly dangerous, especially in modern times.

In truth, deaths from measles had begun to drop well before the introduction of the vaccine, especially when antibiotics provided a way to cure the bacterial pneumonia that accounted for so much of measles mortality. Yet the rarer measles pneumonitis, in which the measles virus itself attacks the lungs, and the still rarer but devastating measles encephalitis both remained untreatable. It was measles encephalitis that killed Olivia Dahl, the seven-year-old daughter of the writer Roald Dahl and the actress Patricia Neal, in 1962. Her father wrote an essay about it in 1986, during the British vaccine controversies: "As the disease took its usual course I can remember reading to her often in bed and not feeling particularly alarmed about it. Then one morning, when she was well on the road to recovery, I was sitting on her bed showing her how to fashion little animals out of coloured pipe-cleaners, and when it came to her turn to make one herself, I noticed that her fingers and her mind were not working together and she couldn't do anything." He asked her if she was feeling all right, and she told him she felt sleepy. "In an hour, she was unconscious," he recalled. "In twelve hours she was dead."[40] He went on to explain that measles encephalitis was still untreatable twenty-four years later, but that parents in 1986 had the option that he had not had, because the vaccine was now available. "It is not yet generally accepted that measles can be a dangerous illness. Believe me, it is," he wrote. His children's book *The BFG* is dedicated "For Olivia, 20 April 1955–17 November 1962."

That double identity of measles—the not-scary disease that everyone gets and the relatively rare agent of death and devastation—echoes back to before the vaccine was developed. It complicated the eradication campaigns of the 1960s and 1970s, and it was still getting in the way of immunizing the children of Great Britain in the 1980s, as Roald Dahl offered his daughter's story in an attempt to convince parents that the disease was dangerous. (In his essay of appeal, Dahl cited the United States as a paragon for making measles vaccine compulsory and almost doing away with the disease.) The biggest and arguably most destructive vaccine controversy of them all was the MMR debate that started with the 1998 publication in the British journal the *Lancet* of a controversial "research" article by a doctor named Andrew Wakefield who claimed to have found traces of the altered measles virus used in the vaccine in the intestinal tracts of children who had developmental disorders. He suggested that the MMR vaccine might be implicated as a cause of autism.

Promoted as a way to fight intellectual disability and the brain damage that could come from encephalitis, the measles vaccine now stood accused of damaging the developing brain. The science and research in Wakefield's article have been thoroughly debunked, as have his ethics (he had an alternate vaccine of his own that he wanted to market, which he did not declare when he published the article). The journal retracted the whole article in 2010, with the editor calling it "utterly false." Wakefield himself was struck off the register of Britain's General Medical Council; he moved to Texas, where he continues to work against vaccines and is hailed as a hero in the anti-vaccine movement. Extensive epidemiologic studies have repeatedly failed to show any links between the MMR vaccine and the development of autism in children, but the claim comes up again and again, playing on the fears of parents.

The story of Wakefield and his claims—and of the journalist, Brian Deer, who exposed much of his scientific wrongdoing—is a long and complex saga of science and pseudoscience. I've been involved in teaching journalism students about science writing, and we often use it as a case study of the dangers of false equivalency (that is, if all the respectable doctors and scientists say that unbelievably extensive research has failed to show any link between the MMR vaccine and autism—which they do—and you are writing about the controversy, you are not journalistically obliged to go find some dubious "expert" who disagrees, just for the sake of "balance"). But it is also a sad case study in how hard it is to change people's minds. If you believe in your heart that there is a link between the MMR vaccine and autism, I am probably not going to be able to convince you otherwise with my long list of large-scale, painstaking, expensive epidemiologic studies.

There is no medicine that we can be sure will take out the measles virus once a child is infected. We can treat some of the complications, like the bacterial pneumonia that can follow measles, but we can't treat measles, and we can't protect the central nervous system from the attacks by the virus, either encephalitis right after the measles infection or, in the case of SSPE, years down the line. (For that matter, we can't protect an unimmunized child against mumps meningitis, either.) The fatality rates among malnourished children continue to be higher than anything seen in the developed world, and children in the developing world also have tended to contract measles at younger ages, when it is more dangerous. As we learned again in 2019, it is still a disease capable of causing epidemics close to home, especially in areas where what we now call "vaccine hesitancy" and "vaccine refusal" are common among parents. Because measles is so contagious, it is one of the diseases frequently cited by physicians who do not want to include such families in their practice, evoking the nightmare scenario of a deliberately unvaccinated child in the waiting room infecting an infant too young to be immunized, and the subsequent severe illness (and perhaps the subsequent lawsuit).

The measles campaigns of the 1960s and 1970s reminded parents—and physicians—of rare complications and unpreventable deaths, which showed far more starkly against a background of decreased child mortality. But the anti-vaccine controversy turned that inside out, with measles, as an almost-forgotten disease, less frightening to many parents than the idea of autism, which seemed as inexplicable and as scary as infectious diseases used to be.

So we didn't see measles when I was in training—but we certainly saw chicken pox, which we thought of as the remaining wildly infectious classic rash of childhood, a recognizable and non-threatening entity where the goal was often to keep children out of the office—pediatricians would diagnose it over the phone when they could, and thereby prevent infected children from lingering in the waiting room. When the varicella vaccine was first licensed in the United States, in 1995, I was a pediatrician in practice with three children of my own, and I wasn't particularly enthusiastic about it. Chicken pox represents a step beyond measles, immunizing against an equally universal disease with even rarer complications. Surely, I thought, it was a kind of overkill to vaccinate every child in America against this familiar disease, an inconvenient itch rather than a serious danger.

I have come around, however, as a doctor, to agree completely with the medical point of view that the chicken pox vaccine is a good idea—not just because it prevents routine suffering, loss of school, and loss of workdays but also because it prevents the vulnerable, including children undergoing chemotherapy and children with immune problems, from being exposed. And vaccination protects all children from very rare but serious and even fatal complications; there are periodic tabloid headlines about so-called flesh-eating bacteria, which cause a rare but devastating and often unstoppable skin infection, necrotizing fasciitis, in previously healthy, immunologically normal children. That can happen when a scratched and irritated chicken pox lesion is invaded by particularly virulent skin bacteria.

Cows get cowpox, a viral disease that has played a not inglorious part in the history of vaccination (cowpox was the virus that protected the dairy maids, and that Edward Jenner made into a smallpox vaccine in 1796), but chickens have nothing to do with chicken pox (they have their own related virus, fowl pox). Chicken pox is not, in most cases, a killer or even a crippler of children. There were millions and millions of cases over the years before the vaccine, billions and billions of itchy little skin lesions, so it's a virus that in some sense truly did pepper our collective history—but the words "chicken pox" probably don't chill your blood, and with rare exceptions, they never left parents praying that their children might be spared. Everyone got chicken pox, and pretty much everyone ended up okay.

It wasn't a disease to be afraid of. In Ray Bradbury's classic work of science fiction *The Martian Chronicles*, he uses the familiar not-scary character of chicken pox to ironic effect. The first human expeditions to Mars bring the virus, and it wipes out the indigenous Martian population, a clear reference (one of many in the stories) to the colonization of the New World, when highly developed native civilizations suffered massive fatalities from the new diseases brought over from Europe. The story called "—And the Moon Be Still as Bright," first published in 1948 in *Thrilling Wonder Stories,* is set in a beautiful abandoned Martian city; Hathaway, the "physician geologist" on the mission, tells the captain what he has discovered among the Martian corpses: "I made tests. Chicken pox. It did things to the Martians it never did to Earth Men. Their metabolism reacted differently, I suppose." And the captain, staring into the fire, reflects, "Chicken pox, God, chicken pox, think of it! A race builds itself for a million years, refines itself, erects cities like those out there, does everything it can to give itself respect and beauty, and then it dies. . . . In the name of all that's holy, it has to be chicken pox, a child's disease, a disease that doesn't even kill *children* on Earth! It's not right and it's not fair. It's like saying the Greeks died of mumps, or the proud Romans died on their beautiful hills of athlete's foot! . . . It can't be a dirty, silly thing like chicken pox. It doesn't fit the architecture; it doesn't fit this entire world!"[41]

The chicken pox virus, technically known as the varicella zoster virus (often abbreviated in medical language as VZV), is very catching, almost as easily transmitted as measles. Chicken pox starts out with fever and headache, and then the pox blisters appear, filled with little clear drops of fluid, each one sitting on its own bright red patch of skin. Generally, they first appear centrally, on the face and the trunk, and then spread out to the extremities. In dermatologic jargon, each spot is a vesicle on a red base—or, in one of those famous medical similes you never forget, a dewdrop on a rose petal. The rash doesn't look anything like the flatter rashes of measles or rubella or scarlet fever, and it doesn't look like pustules, either. That's why we used to take people's word—or their parents' word—that they had had chicken pox; if you had the rash, you had the disease. The clinical hallmark of chicken pox is that those dewdrops on rose petals don't happen all at once; they keep erupting. Each one starts as a red mark, evolves into a full-blown vesicle on its red base, and then, over the course of a couple of days, dries up and crusts over. Children with chicken pox have spots at all those different stages because new ones keep appearing. The severity of the infection is directly related to the number of pox vesicles, and back in the old days, researchers who studied the disease employed assistants (often medical students) as spot counters. That's why I can tell you that the average number of vesicles per person is three hundred, but the range goes all the way from ten up to fifteen hundred.

Dr. Moses Grossman, who had put in time on the polio ward in San Francisco in the 1940s, noted that polio had disappeared, and so had measles, to the point where the young doctors couldn't make the diagnosis. Speaking in 1996, he went on to say, "Rubella followed; mumps followed. There is hardly a young pediatrician now who knows what mumps look like. And then as time went on, chickenpox, which is still the one disease that everybody sees on a regular basis, will disappear, because chickenpox vaccine has been introduced just recently."[42] Before the vaccine, there were maybe a hundred deaths a year from chicken pox in the United States, half of them children. Since 2010, no U.S. resident under twenty has died of it.[43]

Those who were already suspicious of vaccines and vaccine manufacturers objected strenuously to vaccinating against chicken pox, arguing that it was a disease that everyone got, a familiar and non-frightening infection with a funny name. Anti-vaccine polemics argued that the complications of chicken pox were rare, and not something parents needed to worry about, the same kinds of false reassurances that helped set off the 2019 measles epidemic. On the other hand, and this is generally true of anti-vaccine rhetoric, the specter of very rare vaccine-related complications was used to induce tremendous parental anxiety. The most famous and newsworthy anti-vaccine response to the varicella vaccine was the idea of chicken pox parties. In Britain and the United States, there were lots of stories in the media about parents choosing to expose their children deliberately. The crunchy granola magazine *Mothering* (slogan: "The home for natural family living") recommended in 2004 that parents encourage "pox parties," with whistles passed around to make sure that infectious saliva got from child to child. The authors emphasized all the research they had done before deciding that "we at the party were doing what we felt was safest, after weeding through the propaganda and rhetoric about America's latest 'Red Scare': the deadly scourge of chickenpox panic."[44] The article is full of somewhat nonsensical rhetoric, and it suffers from many of the usual anti-vaccine logical lacunae: the authors expressed intense anxiety over a possible serious side effect from the vaccine, but they were not at all worried that chicken pox could—and did—kill children with leukemia.

It's not clear how many parents actually went so far as to organize or attend chicken pox parties, though certainly they continued—and, even now, continue—as something between an urban legend and a shadowy Internet presence.[45] Nowadays, when a child with chicken pox comes into the clinic, we call all the residents and medical students in to see—and, of course, they have all had to provide evidence of their own immunity, either from a vaccine or from a natural infection. (As time goes by, it becomes more likely that the medical students were vaccinated.) Chicken pox has become exotic, like measles, a rash they have learned about from books, and may need to identify on a test, but not an everyday rash of childhood, easily remembered from your own past.

By the 1980s and 1990s, infectious diseases were no longer killing children in large numbers in the United States and other developed countries. There was an increasing conviction that all infectious disease mortality should be preventable, at least in normal, healthy children, and that the possibility of rare complications was reason enough to vaccinate every child. Instead of being seen as a stage of life when we are particularly vulnerable to infections, instead of thinking in terms of "routine" diseases, childhood had become a zone deserving absolute protection. The chicken pox vaccine, like the shift from the oral live-virus polio vaccine to the injected killed-virus polio vaccine, meant taking a step toward zero tolerance.

I used to lie awake nights as a resident, worrying about comparatively rare but extremely serious bacterial infections, about *Hae-*

mophilus influenzae type b, Streptococcus pneumoniae, and Neisseria meningitidis. These bacteria haunted my training years in the 1980s; they were capable of causing fierce invasive infections, sepsis, meningitis, and pneumonia, and we had all seen children die of these infections in the ICU, or survive them with devastating damage done. Nowadays we vaccinate every child against these bacteria, and to the residents today, these diseases seem almost as remote as diphtheria and polio. Doctors in training study them, memorize facts about the damage they do, answer questions about them on tests, but don't really ever expect to see them. The cases of bacterial meningitis and bacterial sepsis which turned up regularly—and tragically—when I was training have now been almost eliminated, along with the rare but deadly manifestations like epiglottitis (Haemophilus influenzae type b can infect the epiglottis in young children, cutting off the airway). These three bacteria, Haemophilus influenzae type b, Streptococcus pneumoniae, and Neisseria meningitidis, were the targets of a new round of vaccine development, made possible by very new scientific technology, and also by the conviction that it would be worth immunizing every child to deliver this new level of assurance: your child is safe from even the rarer dangerous infections, the ones you probably haven't even heard of. After all, parents, unless they had bitter experience, did not lie awake worrying about these infections. They were not asking themselves the questions that haunted us as pediatric residents: Is this particular feverish baby's ear infection possibly Haemophilus influenzae type b? Could that especially cranky toddler's fever be Streptococcus pneumoniae or Neisseria meningitidis? But in the emergency room, for fear of them, we drew blood and did spinal taps on baby after baby after toddler after toddler.

It's much rarer now to see that scary news story that used to come around every year, about an outbreak of meningitis in a college dormitory killing healthy, normal college students, who had been totally fine a week earlier, or leaving them without fingers, toes, even limbs, because they went into shock from the overwhelming infection and lost the ability to pump blood properly throughout their bodies. All adolescents now get vaccinated against *Neisseria meningitidis*, also known as meningococcus.

Many of the diseases I have described in this book are outside my own medical experience; I first learned the details of their pathophysiology in medical school, memorizing them out of books, and went through my training and my time in pediatric practice without ever getting the chance to recognize the symptoms in a real live patient. Smallpox and polio, diphtheria and neonatal tetanus, even TB meningitis and measles—you could see some of these diseases if you traveled to other parts of the world, but in Boston, in the United States, they had largely faded from medical memory. The coronavirus pandemic in 2020 harshly reminded us all of the fear and uncertainty that a new and untreatable infectious threat can bring, and also, by driving down immunization rates around the world, raised the specter of resurgent infections, from measles and chicken pox to *Haemophilus influenza* type b and meningitis. For contemporary medical trainees, who will mark their medical era by the coronavirus, the invasive bacterial infections that so terrified us as recently as the 1980s—the cases of bacterial sepsis and meningitis, the specter of epiglottitis—have moved further from experience and memory. For doctors my age, who remember the fears of our own training years, working with smart and knowledgeable young doctors who feel no immediate sense of dread and doom at the idea of *Haemophilus influenzae* type b or meningococcal disease is a daily reminder of how quickly frightening infectious diseases can fade from the collective memory, even the educated medical memory. And I understand better why some of our teachers, back in the 1980s, looked at us students and shook their heads, remembering the polio wards and wondering why we weren't grateful every day of our medical lives that we would never have to worry about that diagnosis, never have to try to save those children.

CHAPTER 10

"Safe to Sleep"

Postwar Parents, Postwar Pediatricians

D r. Benjamin Spock was a wartime navy doctor who used his spare time to write a book that would become the child-rearing bible of the 1940s and beyond. He had been born in Connecticut, the child of a mother who was partial to some of the faddier turn-of-the-century child-rearing practices; he was sent to an experimental progressive school that met outside to take advantage of the fresh air. He would grow up to believe in the precepts of Freud, to explore his own relationship with his parents through psychoanalysis, to train both in pediatrics and in psychiatry and work as a psychiatrist in military hospitals, and to bring those ideas to his discussion of child-rearing. His first book was published in 1946: *The Common Sense Book of Baby and Child Care,* reprinted in paperback the next month as *The Pocket Book of Baby and Child Care.* It would go on to sell so many copies that it was regularly compared to the Bible, not just because it became the book families lived by but because only the Bible, supposedly, had sold more copies. Spock's book began with a famous first sentence of reassurance to parents: "You know more than you think you do." He went on, in that first passage, to tell parents, "Don't take too seriously all that the neighbors say. Don't be overawed by what the experts say. . . . Bringing up your child won't

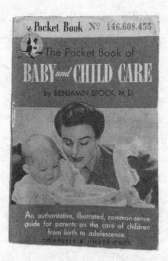

This 1946 paperback, priced at thirty-five cents, brought Dr. Spock's advice into thousands—and eventually millions—of homes, and encouraged parents to trust their own judgment. *Dr. Spock's Baby and Child Care by Benjamin Spock, MD (New York: Scribner, 1945). Reprinted with the permission of Scribner, a division of Simon and Schuster, Inc. All rights reserved.*

be a complicated job if you take it easy, trust your own instincts, and follow the directions that your doctor gives you."[1] So at the same time he was telling parents to take the experts lightly—at least in the abstract—he was recommending the individual physician as a specific source of instructions.[2]

He was writing for families who would have access to those individual physicians, as well as to clean water, pasteurized milk, refrigerators, and the other modern conveniences of postwar suburban America. The first edition of his book offers a snapshot of expert advice at a moment when midcentury medical advances were imminent but not yet available, when infant and child mortality was half what it had been at the turn of the century and parents were turning their attention—and anxiety—to child development and behavior, areas he clearly defined as pediatric territory. And yet, Dr. Spock, that avatar of reassurance, grappled with a long list of frightening childhood infections, still untreatable after the war. By 1946, sulfa drugs (the first antibiotics) were in use, and penicillin was very newly available, but Dr. Spock was concerned that parents might dose small children on their own initiative, risking serious side effects. Though scarlet fever, diphtheria, and polio were still dangerous, and occupied a full section in the first editions of the book, Dr. Spock reassured parents that each disease was either not so scary or not so likely.

"Nowadays scarlet fever is not apt to be as severe as it used to be," he wrote, making nonspecific references to "modern drugs and serums," though he warned parents about the lasting damage of rheumatic heart disease, another unpreventable and untreatable danger. Diphtheria, on the other hand, was "a serious but completely unnecessary disease"—children should get the series of four vaccinations so they would not be at risk. For polio, or infantile paralysis, he acknowledged, "As yet, there is no known way to prevent the disease, or to stop the infection in a case after it has started." Still, he was mostly concerned with allaying parental anxiety: a child who got a fever or a headache in the summer probably didn't have polio; most children who did get polio did not end up paralyzed. And, above all, parents should consult the medical expert: "Your doctor who knows local conditions can advise you best."[3]

In that first 1946 edition, Dr. Spock matter-of-factly mentioned both tuberculosis and polio, along with rickets, as diseases that might affect a child's posture, but he went on, in the next paragraph— and at greater length—to discuss children who "slouch because of lack of self-confidence."[4] Writing at about the same moment that Dr. Edith Lincoln was first trying out new drugs on the children in the Bellevue Chest Clinic, Dr. Spock recommended that any household member with a chronic cough should of course get a chest X-ray, and he warned in particular about the danger that a child might be exposed to an infected servant: "If you are hiring a maid or nurse, she should be examined and have a chest X-ray before becoming a member of the household where there is a baby or child." This echoes

Abraham Jacobi's concerns about diphtheria, from sixty years earlier, and the persistent idea that diseases associated with poverty might be brought into upper-class nurseries by servants. As of 1946, right before the disease was medically "solved," all Dr. Spock could offer by way of treatment and reassurance was this: "If there is any suspicion of *active* tuberculosis, the doctor may limit the child's activity to a greater or lesser degree, even put him to bed for a prolonged period."[5]

The tone of the book, that mix of reassurance, trust-yourself support, and medical expertise, was predicated on a certain faith in science to round out the common sense and the instincts of the dedicated loving parent. Most of *The Common Sense Book of Baby and Child Care,* after all, was about healthy children, about understanding behavior, and about nurturing the child's development, all strongly based in child psychiatry. In this way, his emphasis predicted the shifting focus of postwar pediatrics.

That was the information parents wanted, as pediatricians found themselves increasingly involved in questions of child development and child behavior, education, and social policy, many of which would have been too subtle to claim pediatric attention in an era focused on epidemics and untreatable infections. And there were plenty of parents looking for advice in the United States in the middle of the twentieth century, as the baby boom began. The Second World War ended, and the soldiers and sailors and airmen came home, married, or rejoined their families. As their children were born, parents expected more room, more technology, more modern comfort, from cars to washing machines to packaged convenience foods. And in that domesticity, they wanted the most modern scientific medical care for their babies, and pediatricians changed and evolved along with the new demographics.

In the early decades of the twentieth century, pediatricians had not provided what we now think of as well-child care or seen children with "routine" illnesses; rather, they stepped in when children were catastrophically ill to provide specialty care. General practitioners took care of most children and adults. That is still the model followed in many countries, but in the United States, the field evolved differently. In the 1920s and 1930s, pediatrics became, increasingly, about the care of well children in addition to sick children. When pediatricians tell this story, we tend to see it as strongly positive for children; we portray ourselves as advocates and point to a long list of projects and causes taken on to improve outcomes for children: as childhood deaths became more rare, pediatricians began to look more and more at the behavioral, psychological, developmental, and social issues that were worrying parents. It has also been characterized, however, as a story of professional expansion, and medical sociologists have addressed this history in a different light, looking at what they call "medicalization," in which professional forces (boundary battles, financial incentives) play a strong role in "the extension of medical forms of social control to a broadening range of social behaviors."[6]

Everyday pediatrics became more and more about preventing childhood infectious diseases with vaccines, treating infections with antibiotics, and then looking more closely, for the first time, at preventing the problems and accidents that were still killing children; though these occurred in smaller numbers, they became much more visible as the infections disappeared. The people who were having those baby boom children grew to be less and less afraid in terms of infectious disease. But in other ways, the postwar years, in particular the 1950s, are remembered as a time of political and social anxiety. Two of the top best-selling nonfiction books of 1948 were *How to Stop Worrying and Start Living,* by Dale Carnegie, and *Peace of Mind,* by Joshua L. Liebman, guidance from a salesmanship guru and a psychoanalytically oriented rabbi, respectively; they were at Nos. 3 and 4 for the year, sandwiched between a memoir of the war by Dwight D. Eisenhower and Kinsey's *Sexual Behavior in the Human Male.* Parents had objectively less to worry about than their own parents in the 1920s and 1930s had had, but they were generally characterized as an anxious and self-critical group, concerned not only about their children's physical safety but also about their own responsibility, as parents, to bring up their children according to modern best practices, and to shape them into physically and psychologically healthy adults.

Like many of the children born in the postwar years, I was of course brought up on Spock, and I have my parents' battered copy. My mother, hoping to get pregnant for the first time, brought Spock with her to Trinidad when she and my father went there in the late 1950s so he could do his anthropological fieldwork. My mother told the story in her memoir of the year in Trinidad, describing how the women around her in the small East Indian village where my parents lived were immensely entertained by the idea of any mother needing a book to tell her what to do with a baby. Trinidadian women often lived in multigenerational households, so they had plenty of older female relatives around to advise them. Most dramatically, my mother said, they were shocked by Dr. Spock's rule that the baby should never be taken into the parents' bed, or even laid down upon it, and they regarded the idea of putting a baby to sleep in a separate bed in a separate room as somewhere between cruel and crazy.

Today we avoid bed sharing to prevent SIDS, but for Dr. Spock, and for my parents and their contemporaries, the baby in the parents' bed posed behavioral hazards—a baby might become habituated to sleeping there and refuse to be moved to an appropriate crib in an appropriate second bedroom—and also suggested the psychosexual complexities of a more Freudian view of childhood. Parents like mine who had grown up poor and made it into the middle class may have felt there was something that smacked of tenement life about a bed where the whole family slept together, something very far from the baby boomer ideal of a comfortable suburban home with parents in the master bedroom and children down the hall.[7]

The women my mother knew in Trinidad in 1958, living with their extended families, also presumably believed in raising their children as they themselves had been raised, under the eyes of the older women in their households. But my parents, children of immigrants who had grown up in poverty in New York City in the 1920s and 1930s, were determined to bring up their own children differently. I doubt they would have said "scientifically," but certainly, as liberal academic parents in the 1960s and 1970s, they were heavily invested in understanding child psychology, in avoiding corporal punishment, in bringing up their children with lots of educational toys and intellectual stimulation, and in providing frank and clear answers to childish questions about human reproduction—all hallmarks of liberal postwar parenting.

Dr. T. Berry Brazelton, the pediatrician who was most often regarded as Dr. Spock's successor, argued for supporting, not blaming, parents and for appreciating the profound temperamental differences between one baby and another. He said of Spock, whom he knew well (and whose grandchildren were his pediatric patients), that he "changed the model of parenting to a much more child-oriented approach, much more sensitive to what parents brought with them, their strengths. I think he changed life for everybody in the 40's."[8]

In *Raising America: Experts, Parents, and a Century of Advice About Children*, Ann Hulbert conjures the materially prosperous but insecure and socially isolated suburban parents of the baby boom, whose children would be brought up according to Dr. Spock and would learn to read from Dr. Seuss:

Dr. Spock was the confiding companion whom suburbanizing mothers yearned for, living as they did miles away from their parents and a well-manicured lawn away from everyone else. . . . Meanwhile, the other Dr. S was conjuring up a thrilling (and terrifying) babysitter who swept in when Mom slipped out for a moment. The Cat in the Hat, hardly your

ordinary nanny, defied adults and joined Spock in introducing us—and our parents—to our libidinal urges.[9]

The anarchic, let's-break-all-the-rules character who came in off the
street into that neat suburban house was perhaps a harbinger of other
disruptions to come in the lives of those baby boom children, who
would grow up to be the generation of the 1960s.

It's kind of amazing to remember now how famous a figure Benjamin Spock was in the 1960s and 1970s. For years, he wrote a
column, which ran with a photo—and that, of course, made him
particularly recognizable in those years before social media. I had
dinner with him one night in the 1980s at Legal Sea Foods in Cambridge; he was pleased that I had named my first child Benjamin and
wanted to talk about some of the writing I was doing about pediatric
issues. Both my husband and I were more than a little overwhelmed
to find ourselves in his presence, but I don't think we were completely prepared for the experience of the evening, in which dinner
was interrupted, every few minutes, by someone who recognized Dr.
Spock and wanted to say, *I was brought up on your book—my mother
always trusted everything you said.* Toward the end of the meal, the
owner of the restaurant appeared; the staff had called him and told
him that Dr. Spock was having dinner there, so he'd driven over to
ask if he could take a photo. It was the closest I have ever come to
having dinner with a rock star, and since I was starting out myself
in pediatrics at the time, it left me with a strong sense of the connection that parents form with the people who help them navigate the
complexities of taking care of their children.

Dr. Spock's single most famous recommendation, the one that
most assertively upended the pediatric wisdom that had come before,
was what came to be called "demand feeding," the idea that babies
should be fed—preferably breastfed—when they were hungry, and
not according to the kind of rigid schedule pediatricians had been
advocating as necessary for both physical health and also proper

character formation. Demand feeding would come, over time, to stand in for a whole host of more "permissive" parenting strategies, as the social ideal of good parenting moved away from spanking and discipline and closer to the more individualistic nurturing of a child's character and personality. The whole "demand feeding" controversy was dictated by the extremism of the pediatric recommendations from the first half of the twentieth century. In making infant feeding their business, pediatricians had become deeply embroiled in the questions of breastfeeding, concerns about women with inadequate milk supplies, and how to ensure healthy alternatives to breast milk. They had worried endlessly about how to mix formulas with the correct proportions for infant nutrition, and they had been involved in the campaigns to purify the cow's milk on which such formulas were based.

Dr. Spock himself clearly understood that it might be an uphill battle to get women to nurse their babies in 1946, and he started out his chapter on breastfeeding by confronting the "disadvantages." He acknowledged that bottle-feeding had become "safe and easy," and he discussed a variety of maternal fears, everything from not being able to see how much milk the baby was getting to sagging breasts (he recommended "a good brassiere" and limited weight gain). He conceded that women who really didn't like the idea of nursing to the point of "revulsion" shouldn't do it, but then he came down strongly in favor of breastfeeding for pretty much everyone else: "On general principle, it's safer to do things the natural way. . . . Breast feeding has definite advantages that we know of, and it may have others that we aren't smart enough to see."[10]

By 1955, breastfeeding had decreased dramatically in the United States; only 29 percent of one-week-old infants in the country were being breastfed, either exclusively or in combination with bottle-feeding. (In contrast, 77 percent of the babies born between 1936 and 1940 were breastfed.)[11] There was no longer any worry about contamination or infection; the formulas were safe, and the principles of hygiene and sterilization were part of the modern appeal of bottle feeding. Marketing by infant formula companies became more sophisticated and more intense, targeting mothers with advertisements that emphasized the convenience, scientific excellence, and hygiene of the available formulas, while also lavishing obstetricians and pediatricians with attention. Hospitals were stocked with formula samples and branded swag, while doctors were courted by the formula manufacturers, invited to meetings and dinners, and even offered trips to exciting destinations (with an occasional commercial thrown in).

Since childbirth in the United States, over the course of the twentieth century, had moved almost completely from the home into the hospital, and since hospital stays after childbirth lasted for a week or longer in those days, women who wanted to breastfeed had to get started in the hospital. Between nursery schedules, easy formula availability, and the effects of obstetrical anesthesia on both mothers and babies, those hospital maternity wards were not necessarily set up for breastfeeding. Mary McCarthy's best-selling 1963 novel, *The Group,* features an unforgettable episode on a maternity ward, back in the 1930s, in which Priss, a young upper-class woman married to a pediatrician, attempts, following his instructions, to breastfeed her baby; but she must do it in the most medically approved and scientific way, with nurses swabbing her breasts with alcohol and the baby brought to her only following the prescribed rigid schedule. Poor Priss feels terrible guilt when her hungry newborn son cries loudly and long for off-schedule feedings, and she is not fully comforted by the regular weight gain that makes her pediatrician husband so proud; what she feels, guiltily, hearing her son's voice screaming down the hall, is that "it was making a natural request, in this day and age; it was asking for a bottle."[12]

Priss's breastfeeding was also a sensation in her circle. (The chapter begins, "Priss Hartshorn Crockett was nursing her baby. That was the big news."[13]) She indignantly rejects the idea of writing about it for *Reader's Digest,* and she clearly feels that there is something freakish and unnatural about what she is doing. By the middle of the century, bottle-feeding had become a social norm for many women; to decide to breastfeed in many American social circles was to do something a little ostentatious. It might look old-fashioned or lower-class to your own family and friends, and it also, in the first decade of *Playboy* magazine (its debut cover in 1953 featured Marilyn Monroe), drew attention to a part of the female body that was increasingly regarded as sexual, to be featured in push-up bras and pinups. Breasts were not maternal and nurturing but private and prurient.

The turn away from breastfeeding served mothers who wanted to be freed from the constraints of breastfeeding, those who had no choice because they needed to work, and those who felt they were unable to nourish their babies sufficiently. Yet even with all the barriers in hospitals and even with the social marginalization of breastfeeding mothers, some women wanted to nurse their infants. In 1956, seven women who had done it and wanted to help others do it formed a group in a suburb of Chicago. The mothers' group grew into the La Leche League, a grassroots organization of support groups that numbered 430 by 1966 and 3,000 by 1976.[14] They were supported by pediatricians, and they pushed mothers to vet pediatricians thoroughly for their attitudes toward breastfeeding, and to avoid any doctor who didn't seem knowledgeable and supportive.

Today, the recommendation of the American Academy of Pediatrics (AAP) is that mothers should breastfeed exclusively for the first six months of life (that is, no formula at all) and continue breastfeeding for the whole first year, which is when we recommend starting cow's milk. I believe deeply in breastfeeding, and I nursed all three of my own children. With the youngest, given the official advice that I was by then handing out in my practice, I felt obliged to follow the most recent AAP recommendations. I nursed him exclusively for six months, pumping and freezing and schlepping the breast milk to day care once I was back at work, and I kept up the pumping and the nursing till he was a full year old, not so much because I believed that it would make a big difference but because I would have felt like such a hypocrite if I hadn't. I was an experienced mother who had breastfed before, and a well-paid and well-supported physician—and it was still quite a project.

I am the product of a loving mother who did *not* breastfeed her children. She wanted to, she said, as she wanted to have a "natural childbirth"; she was, after all, a writer who had spent the 1950s in Greenwich Village. But like many women of the time, she was told that she would not be able to. I have to remember, when I talk with mothers about what they want to do, that my own perfectly satisfactory life and robust good health are built on a foundation of formula feeding, as are those of pretty much all my contemporaries. I would have been deeply distressed to hear anyone make my mother feel she had done something irreparable to harm her children. She did her best, and we turned out fine, and that should be the luxury of having finally achieved a safe way to feed infants who for one reason or another don't get nursed. Yet developing that safe way to feed infants and removing the high infant mortality rate that used to accompany impure milk has not made the breastfeeding debate any kinder, gentler, or easier. The "DON'T KILL YOUR BABY!" poster that was used to frighten women into breastfeeding in 1910 is a thing of the past, but the message to mothers now is actually strong enough that you can search the Internet and come up with "How to Let Go of the Breastfeeding Guilt" (on The Bump), "Diary of a Reluctant Breastfeeder" (Mumfidential), and "7 Reasons to Forgive Yourself for Not Breastfeeding" (Scary Mommy)—or, on the other hand, "I Didn't Breastfeed, and It Took Years to Get Over My Shame and Guilt" (Scary Mommy).

Breastfeeding is linked to lower rates of SIDS, and breastfeeding advocates also point to an array of scientific research supporting the neurocognitive and medical benefits of nursing. So a lot of mothers at a very vulnerable moment end up feeling inadequate, unnatural, and, above all, guilty if they don't breastfeed. It's a great achievement to have made formula feeding pretty safe after all those centuries when anything other than breastfeeding was likely to be deadly, and it's a step forward to have science and medicine recognize and honor breastfeeding as important and protective—but somehow, all this progress can still end up making mothers feel anxious and guilty.

With the successful battles against the major child killers, diarrhea and infectious diseases, largely won by the end of the 1950s, other dangers to children's lives began to figure more prominently. Children's deaths in car accidents, for example, became dramatically "visible," as they came to be seen as deaths that could be—and then should be—prevented as a medical imperative. Dr. Spock's 1946 book made no mention of car seats or car safety. A plastic surgeon in Detroit, Dr. Claire Straith, noted in the 1930s that he was doing reconstructive operations on a lot of people, especially women and children, who had been injured in car crashes while sitting in what he called the "death seat," beside the driver. He fitted out his own car with seat belts and crash pads, then talked Chrysler into adopting some of his ideas for its 1937 cars. In a photo of the crash pad he invented—and patented—his smiling small granddaughter, Grace, perches in the front seat beside the driver (Dr. Straith's daughter), leaning her curly head against the pad on the dashboard.[15] The photo looks so disturbingly wrong to us now—the smiling child in her pretty dress, in the front seat, where no small child should be, unrestrained (because, in fact, there were no seat belts), trustingly, smilingly, pillowing her head on the dashboard crash pad. But, in fact, it looks wrong precisely because Dr. Straith was so right—and so ahead of his time. It was the first step toward passenger protection.

In 1965, Ralph Nader published his best-selling exposé, *Unsafe at Any Speed: The Designed-in Dangers of the American Automobile*, in which he accused car manufacturers of deliberately failing to build in safety features that were well within reach. A new small organization, Physicians for Automotive Safety, formed in 1965 by a doctor named Seymour Charles, got off to a dramatic start by picketing the New

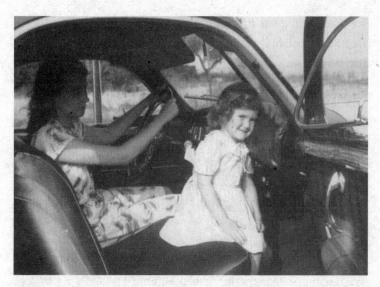

The daughter and granddaughter of Dr. Claire Straith, who was the chief of plastic surgery at Harper Hospital in Detroit during the 1920s and '30s, demonstrate his car safety innovations, with little Grace Jeffries leaning against the dashboard pad. *Used with permission of Grace Quitzow.*

York Auto Show. The doctors were part of a more general awakening, and with legislators pushed into action, in 1966 the National Traffic and Motor Vehicle Safety Act set some safety standards and created a federal agency, the National Highway Traffic Safety Administration, with oversight to enforce them. Among other things, the new bill required seat belts in every new car. The first car seats were developed in the late 1960s, and in 1971 the relatively new federal agency established its first car seat standards. But car seats were not mandatory (the first laws requiring them were passed in the late 1970s), and there wasn't much standardization in terms of what designs were truly effective; in 1972, *Consumer Reports* published an article showing that car seats that met the new federal standards were not actually able to stand up to the forces of car crashes.

In 1978, the NHTSA, that relatively new federal agency, held the first national child passenger safety conference in Nashville. Tennessee then became the first state to pass a law requiring car seats.[16] A local pediatrician, Dr. Robert Sanders, played a major role in passing that law, but six years later, in an article titled "Bless the Seats and the Children: The Physician and the Legislative Process," he pointed out that "more than 90% of children ride unprotected in automobiles." He urged doctors to join the battle—and to think about extending protection to older children as well.[17] By 1982, twenty states had passed laws about infant seats, and by 1985, every state had one. Because of wide publicity about the importance of car seats—and, even more than that, because of the new state laws—the market expanded enormously, and car seat testing brought about new safety standards. The technology got better and better.

In the 1990s, attention turned to safety seats for older children. A Washington State journalist named Autumn Alexander Skeen, who had advocated for car seats for infants, lost her own four-year-old son, Anton, in 1996, when he was riding beside her in the front seat and the car rolled over. Her son had been excited to sit next to Mom, she recalled, and for herself, "I was going by the law," she explained. "I told myself someone must have tested this."[18] But no one had tested it, and the seat belt did not hold Anton, who weighed only forty-five pounds; he was thrown from the car and killed. His mother launched a campaign to require booster seats for kids aged four to six and from forty to sixty pounds; Washington did pass such a law—"Anton's Law"—in 2001, and so did other states. And today that image of a four-year-old riding in the front seat with an adult safety belt (or, indeed, at all) seems as scary and what's-wrong-with-this-picture as the image of little Grace demonstrating her grandfather's crash pad.

When my children were young, in the 1980s and 1990s, my own parents made it clear that they considered car seats a lot of fuss about nothing. They loved their grandchildren dearly, of course, but they had loved their children as well, and we had always been just fine in the car. The safest place for a baby in a car, really, they assured me, was in its mother's arms, and they were not particularly interested to know that a medical study had shown that a parent's arms were pretty useless for protection in a crash. They were willing to indulge us, since car seats were evidently important to us, but they couldn't repress a little smile as they watched us struggle with the complex catches and straps and buckles of those relatively early and idiosyncratic contraptions.

Parents in the eighteenth century wrote poems to their dead children or had statues carved, if they had the means. Parents and grandparents in the nineteenth and early twentieth centuries sometimes founded colleges (Vassar, Stanford) or arts colonies (Yaddo) or scientific institutions (Rockefeller). But Autumn Skeen told *People* magazine that she had vowed that "death would not have the last word," and as a memorial for her son, she wanted laws that would make sure that children his age were required to be safely buckled into booster seats.[19] The idea that a fitting memorial to a child's death was legislation to make the world safer for other children, that you could give the child's death meaning by eliminating the hazard, was a powerful postwar twentieth-century idea, and it reflected a commitment—and an expectation—that the world could truly be made safe for children, if adults only took the time and the trouble.

Strapping a baby into a car seat was a reassuringly concrete way of making the world safer. The mysterious entity of "crib death" posed a different terror: infants who were laid down to sleep apparently healthy and then never woke up. Probably everyone who trains in pediatrics remembers, as I do, a first case of sudden infant death syndrome, or SIDS (the term was first used in 1969): a perfect, "previously healthy" baby brought into the emergency room by EMTs who were trying to keep a resuscitation going, an all-out effort in the trauma room to start a heart that had stopped, and then finally the necessity of breaking the news to the frantic, shocked, disbelieving parents, who had put a vigorous infant down for a nap on what seemed to be an unremarkable day, and now found themselves holding on to each other as the recognition of a tragedy unfurled around them. I remember the repetition of some of the formulas doctors use at times like this, especially the idea that we did everything, that the resuscitation had been as complete and thorough and extreme as possible. Were we reassuring the parents or reassuring ourselves? Everyone in the emergency room was left shaken and devastated. Even back in the 1980s, when we knew so much less about SIDS, and had so much less ability to prevent it, it felt wrong, shocking, and outrageous that such a thing should happen.

The definition of SIDS we still use (though we now call it SUID, for sudden unexpected infant death), "the sudden death of an infant younger than 1 year of age, which remains unexplained after a thorough case investigation, including performance of a complete autopsy, examination of the death scene, and review of the clinical history," was developed in 1989 by the National Institutes of Health. What that means is that if you find another explanation—the baby had an undiagnosed congenital heart problem, or there was an infection that no one suspected—we don't call it SIDS. When all is said and done, and after years of research, we are left with a kind of negative definition of these heartbreaking events. The current medical explanation involves the intersection of three different kinds of risks: First of all, the baby has some intrinsic risk factor but one we cannot yet diagnose, such as a propensity to cardiac arrhythmia or an abnormality in the brainstem that controls the respiratory drive. Second, there is a critical period of vulnerability in the first six months of life when the baby does not yet have full neuromuscular control. And the third component involves the dangers in the environment, from sleeping position to bed-sharing to overheated rooms.

SIDS was starting to be discussed and treated as a major menace at the end of the 1960s and the beginning of the 1970s. Congress passed legislation in 1974 calling for increased research. In the late 1980s and early 1990s, studies from both Europe and Australia showed the link between babies sleeping on their stomachs and the risk of SIDS, and the American Academy of Pediatrics recommended that babies be laid down to sleep on their backs or sides. In 1994, the Back to Sleep campaign was launched by the National Institute of Child Health and Development, working with the AAP and the largest SIDS advocacy groups. With increasing evidence that sleeping on the back was the safest position of all, the recommendations were strengthened in 1996, and they began to include language about avoiding soft bedding. Tipper Gore, the wife of the vice president, became a national spokesperson, and the message was put out to the public on Gerber rice cereal boxes, mailed to parents (this was just before e-mail), and reinforced by Pampers and Johnson & Johnson.

The campaign went on to target African American parents in particular, since evidence was accumulating that African American mothers were less likely to be laying their children down on their backs. The surgeon general, David Satcher, himself African American, made special efforts to put out messages to reach minority parents, partnering with African American organizations, from sororities to Women in the NAACP, the National Coalition of 100 Black Women, and the National Medical Association. The campaign would go on to include public service announcements on radio stations with large African American audiences, a call for faith leaders to raise awareness in churches on designated "SIDS Sundays," and ads on buses in African American neighborhoods.[20] There was also an effort with the Indian Health Service and American Indian and Alaska Native organizations to get the word out to their populations.

And it worked. The rate of SIDS in 1990 was 130.3 deaths for every 100,000 live births; in 2016, it was 38 deaths for every 100,000 live births. In 2016, only 1,500 infants in the entire country died from SIDS.[21]

Meanwhile, the safe-sleep guidelines continued to evolve, ever stricter and more stringent. If the initial advice (1992) had included laying babies down on their sides (which had spawned a small cottage industry in prop pillows), newer iterations specified the back (1996) and then later warned specifically against the dangers of placing babies on their sides (2000) and against bed-sharing. The blanket was supposed to be tucked in firmly at the bottom of the mattress (1999) and reach no higher up than the baby's chest; then there were to be no blankets or any other loose bedding (2005). As of 2016, safe-sleep recommendations had expanded to include keeping the baby in the parents' bedroom (though emphatically not in the parents' bed) for the first year of life, and a certain amount of pushback was coming from parents who found that hard to do. Still, the Back to Sleep campaign is often cited as an example of a successful public awareness and education movement.

The campaign has now evolved into Safe to Sleep, with a logo showing a brown-skinned infant peacefully asleep on his or her back, no bedding in sight, wearing a stretchy pajama suit that, presumably, is warm enough to replace a blanket, without making the child so warm that there is any risk of overheating. The illustration looks perfectly normal and healthy to me; I have to remind myself that when my third child was born, and the first recommendations had been issued for putting babies on their backs, it looked completely implausible and even scary to me to lay him down in that position. When my second child was born, in 1989, we were still telling parents to put babies on their stomachs, confident that this was the right thing to protect them against the dangers of SIDS. Now I had to put my baby down in exactly the opposite position. I didn't really believe he would be able to sleep that way—but, of course, he could and he did.

When the shadows cast by constant infectious illnesses and frequent newborn deaths lessened enough to let us see the landscape more clearly, pediatricians developed new ways of thinking about children's lives, instead of just concentrating on saving them. The term "the new morbidity" was coined in the 1970s by Dr. Robert Haggerty, referencing the increasing importance of behavioral, developmental, psychosocial, and emotional problems in pediatric practice. The hospital-based training pediatricians received did not necessarily prepare us to deal with such issues. In his career at the

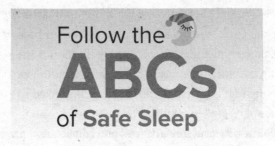

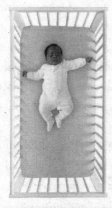

Baby should sleep
Alone

On their
Back

In a safe
Crib

In a
Smoke-free home

Make sure everyone caring for your baby follows these tips!

health.ny.gov/safesleep

NEW YORK STATE | Department of Health | Office of Children and Family Services

One of the many posters developed as part of the campaign to inform parents about the ABCs of safe sleep—that a baby should sleep Alone, on its Back, in a Crib— which now extend to specific recommendations against stuffed animals, blankets, crib bumpers, and anything else that could possibly obstruct the baby's breathing. *New York State Department of Health.*

University of Rochester School of Medicine, Dr. Haggerty championed the field of "community pediatrics," emphasizing the idea that taking care of children meant taking care of the whole family and thinking about the context of the community in which that family was living.[22] Along with spotlighting behavioral issues, school problems, and developmental delays that kept children from thriving, the wider focus on the family and the community drew attention to larger social issues that might be holding children back or putting them in danger, like gun violence today. Pediatrics was, from the beginning, a somewhat socially minded field, and there was never any denying that children's health was much affected by the socioeconomic status of their families.

In 1982, a statement from the AAP proclaimed, "As a primary care physician and consultant, the pediatrician is increasingly expected to be concerned with the prevention, early detection, and management of psychosocial problems pertinent to optimal child and family health and development."[23] The statement listed the need to advise and support families in crisis, whether from the birth of a premature infant or a parental divorce, and it also staked out pediatric territory in "the evaluation and treatment of common behavior disorders such as temper tantrums, breath-holding spells, or sleep problems." And there was more: identifying abuse (both physical and sexual) and neglect, dealing with school problems—all were pediatric duties. In 2001, at the beginning of the new millennium, the AAP said in a published statement that "the behavioral needs of our patients are now recognized as core elements of pediatric care."[24] Some of these were problems that might have been handled by other professions in the past, perhaps by teachers, perhaps by the clergy, but others were issues that were newly being formulated as real problems, the kind for which parents might seek expert help—and be willing to pay for it.

Sydney Halpern, a medical sociologist, argues that the decline in childhood disease and death led community pediatricians, in order to stay in business, to start diagnosing children once seen as healthy with conditions that need pediatric care. This analysis implies that only the pediatrician's agenda matters in the pediatric visit, which feels a little strange to anyone who regularly sees patients. Parents consistently—and persistently—bring up behavioral issues at primary care visits. And in any case, there is no money in psychosocial pediatrics. Even Halpern concludes that "the treatment of behavioral and developmental problems is time-consuming and poorly compensated when compared to other types of services that pediatricians deliver."[25]

T. Berry Brazelton told the story differently. Going into primary care practice in Cambridge, Massachusetts, after the war, he said, "I could see that these problems were really what needed documentation, like crying at the end of the day, or toilet training, or thumb sucking. And those were the things that really intrigued me, the sort of normal events that went on during a parent's day. I thought if I could document what was normal and what was out of range, that pediatricians would have more idea about what to do about them, and patients really led me into that kind of research."[26]

Babies and children see their primary care provider—whether a pediatrician, family physician, or nurse-practitioner—regularly during their early years of life, most frequently during the first two years, and then later at least annually. There is no other system to reach all children in the first five years of life, reinforced by the medical forms that children need in order to qualify for government assistance with food or, later, to attend preschool or day care or Head Start or summer camp. If psychosocial issues are important—and they are—and if screening is important—and it is—then building it into or onto the primary care system as it exists is faster, cheaper, and much more effective than trying to construct an alternative system. And when those babies and children come to see their primary care providers, behavioral and psychosocial issues are going to come up, even if the providers don't go looking for them. We worry now about "missing" early signs of autism spectrum disorder, as we worry about missing other diagnoses, precisely because we believe that early diagnosis and therapy can mitigate the course of the disorder.

As the postwar babies grew up and became parents themselves, they expected a safer world than their own parents had known, a world in which, if the experts gave the right advice, if the regulations

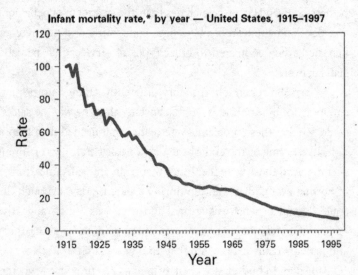

Infant mortality rate,* by year — United States, 1915–1997

*Per 1000 live births.

This simple graph from the CDC illustrates the remarkable progress over the course of the twentieth century as infant mortality in the United States was reliably tracked and steadily brought down, leading to a huge relief of loss, pain, grief, and suffering for families. It should remind us of how far we have come, and of what it is possible to do for all families and children. *Centers for Disease Control and Prevention / Dr. Demetri Vacalis.*

were sufficiently strict, not only diseases but also accidents could be prevented. Parents and pediatricians together now demand more security than their own parents and grandparents and their professional predecessors ever did.

When I chose pediatrics, in the mid-1980s, I was choosing the medical territory where you could hope and expect *not* to have to preside over patients at the end of life. I trained in a children's hospital where we did a lot of highly specialized care for children with rare syndromes, but we also took care of plenty of what we called "bread-and-butter pediatrics" cases: high fevers in small children (all those blood draws and spinal taps), asthma exacerbations, diarrhea and dehydration. Every single one of the children with every single one of those common diagnoses was supposed to walk—or crawl— out of the hospital. Not one single child at Boston Children's Hospital in the 1980s was supposed to die of asthma or diarrhea or any other common childhood disease. When something went wrong, when a child actually died of asthma or croup or gastroenteritis, it would be a "sentinel event," the subject of M&M (morbidity and mortality) conferences to figure out what had gone wrong.

But children did die at children's hospitals in the 1980s, as they still do now. In fact, we would talk sometimes about the irony that we had chosen pediatrics because we enjoyed being around children, we took pleasure in their resilience and their recuperative powers— but in order to train, we were spending our lives in a building full of children who were suffering, often from rare and incurable diseases or chronic conditions that doomed them to lives of pain and repeated medical procedures. Children died—and still die—on the pediatric cardiology ward after heroic surgeries to repair malformed hearts. Children died—and still die—on the oncology ward when every experimental chemotherapy regimen had failed, or in the bone marrow transplant unit when infections overwhelmed their heavily suppressed immune systems. Children with cystic fibrosis died on the adolescent ward because the vicious bacteria in their lungs had grown resistant to every antibiotic we could administer (and also, though we didn't know it at the time, because we were making things much worse by hospitalizing all the kids with cystic fibrosis together when they came in for their antibiotic "clean-outs," thereby letting them exchange those resistant bacteria back and forth on the ward). Children died in the ICU from rare but exceptionally virulent bacterial infections, especially sepsis and meningitis. Babies died in the NICU because they were just too premature to resuscitate or because we had resuscitated them but then the rigors of ventilation blew holes in their lungs or they developed terrible infections, often because of the many tubes and lines going into their tiny bodies. And, of course, children died in the emergency room because of terrible accidents and apparently random events, from SIDS and poisonings and car crashes and gunshot wounds and beatings.

But those were the unforeseen tragedies of the emergency room; I think I remember every one of the ER deaths that happened on one of my watches, and I would be willing to bet that most of the people I trained with remember them, too. Even in the NICU, even on the oncology ward, where everyone knew that deaths would happen, where the nurses had protocols worked out for comforting families, death was relatively rare.

That training was intense and life-altering, and it left me with, I think, a permanent sense of my identity as a pediatrician, and my place in the ongoing chain of medical training. Pronouncing—even rarely—a child dead, filling out those death certificates, left all of us connected to the great enterprise of keeping children alive. We had signed up for a field that was not about dying children but that offered a great deal of hope to the majority of patients—even on the oncology ward—and looked ahead to better and better numbers, the individual victories of watching even the sickest patients live to grow up. It used to be relatively unusual for kids with congenital heart disease or cystic fibrosis to grow up into internal medicine patients; now adult cardiologists and adult pulmonologists see these patients all the time (though sometimes these adult patients yearn for the tiny needles and the bright murals of the pediatric treatment centers that helped them through childhood).

Back in the early days of postwar pediatrics, at the beginning of his 1946 book, Benjamin Spock wrote, "I want to urge you not to worry or decide that you've made a mistake with your child on the basis of anything that you read in this book (or anywhere else, for that matter)."[27] But the tone of parenting—and, often, the tone of pediatrics—would increasingly include a sense that parents must monitor the remaining rare dangers lurking in a supposedly safe world, whether in a common and ostensibly mild disease, like measles or chicken pox, or in rare but terrifying infections, or, even, in the vaccines themselves. Dr. Spock had told parents to follow the directions from their child's doctor, but many parents would come to feel that listening to expert advice was not enough, that their responsibility extended to evaluating and questioning all such advice, and many, nowadays, feel an imperative to search out information on the Internet, where they often find a sea of conflicting information and opinions that leaves them anxious about any decisions they may make.

The world of the 1940s and 1950s and 1960s in which the baby boomers were growing up was clearly safer for children than the world in which their own parents had grown up; the world in which the children of the baby boomers grew up—the 1970s and 1980s and 1990s—was objectively safer still. But the climate of parental responsibility was very different, and parents were not necessarily more likely to trust themselves—or their pediatricians.

The Promise of Safety

Beating back infant and child mortality was no single story. Our babies and children live to grow up now because of so many different changes in how we live and how we feed them and care for them and how we handle sanitation and how we respond to illness. As parents—and also as pediatricians—it can be terrifying, even at a historical distance, to contemplate that time, not so long ago, when so many newborns never breathed, when so many babies died in the summer of mysterious intractable diarrhea, when some number of sore throats in older children signaled the onset of untreatable and devastating infections. It was a grand and not necessarily coordinated effort, by scientists and social reformers, nurses and nutritionists, parents and physicians, that collectively, gradually, over time, has given us a world of such privileged parenting and doctoring that we can expect our children to live and thrive. As we have looked to modern-day epidemiologists and scientists to help us understand and mitigate a modern-day pandemic, we can surely appreciate the ambition and the sweeping grandeur of this past project, which harnessed so many kinds of human ingenuity, understanding, and activism to the noble overarching goal of reducing suffering and unnecessary death. Protecting our children has been one of our most remarkable human achievements, transforming what seemed for centuries to be a sad inevitability of the human condition.

But as we get closer to the present day, and the child deaths diminish, we see in sharper relief the illnesses we still can't treat, and especially the deaths we can't—or don't—prevent. They stand as challenges to medical science, which has failed to keep a promise, or as reproaches, evidence that safety nets were not sufficient. When I was training in the 1980s, children were no longer supposed to die. We had immunizations, we had generations of ever-more-sophisticated antibiotics, we had high-tech ICUs and a gleaming, buzzing NICU, where we were engaged in saving "micropreemies" at the very edge of human viability. When a full-term newborn was sick enough to spend time in the NICU, that seven- or eight-pound baby would look impossibly big and robust and vigorous next to the tiny preemies, who weighed in at one and a half or two pounds. You would look at the full-term infant and wonder how anything could possibly go wrong with a baby so big and strong.

In the years since my training, the technology of ventilating premature newborns has improved tremendously, and most of the remaining bacterial "bad actors" we worried about in healthy children who came in sick with fever have been eliminated by vaccination. And there are many other important stories to be told about applying science and public health and parental activism to the diseases that threaten children, from the triumphs of pediatric oncology to the progress in repairing congenital heart disease to the complex science of helping children with rare metabolic syndromes to the developments that have extended life expectancy and improved quality of life for children with the most common genetic syndromes, sickle-cell disease and cystic fibrosis.

We are, no question, the luckiest parents—and pediatricians—in history. However much we may whine and cry (and we do) about the hazards and problems of parenting in the here and now, none of us, I suspect, would trade any of our first-world issues, from screen time and social media to cyber bullying and the pressure of college applications, for a supposedly simpler world that doubled the chance of losing a child. A century ago, that chance was much more than double, and a century or so before that, even greater. All other parental and pediatric woes have to pale a little in the face of that larger miracle.

So why are we so anxious, and why don't we feel safer, either as parents or on behalf of our lucky children? We have reached the stage, in the United States, where we can worry about protecting our children against even relatively rare accidents. As I was writing an early part of this book, I got a bulletin from the American Academy of Pediatrics about the danger of children being injured and even dying as a result of strangulation on window blind cords; 271 children had died between 1990 and 2015.[1] The AAP advocated legislation in 2018 to ban the cords entirely. Parent advocacy—often in the wake of a tragedy—has been important in working to draw attention to the risk that a baby might strangle on the cord of a baby monitor and to promote guidelines to make drawstrings safe (if, for example, there are two separate strings at the front of a sweatshirt's hood, rather than one that goes all the way around, they are much less likely to be a problem).[2] We are able to look at each childhood death now as a death that should have been prevented or should be preventable in the future.

Sometimes I wonder how I ever lived to grow up, and other times I feel that my own children's survival through infancy and childhood was a minor miracle. There I was, rattling around in the back seat with no car seats or seat belts, riding my bike in the street with no helmet, growing up in the era before childproof caps on dangerous medicines, in homes with window blind cords, with walls painted before the rules on lead paint reduction. No vaccines against meningitis, pneumonia, or even chicken pox. I'm absolutely grateful for each of the hard-won measures that have collectively made all our children so much safer. But when you look at all of them together, is it possible that all these campaigns and perhaps even all these protections, which have made children safer, may have made some parents, if anything, more anxious?

Certainly, modern parents are acutely aware of their own responsibility to create safe environments for their children, and this responsibility plays out many times every day. "The most important safety feature to keep in mind, though, is proper use," warned the *New York Times* in a March 2018 article on car seats.[3] This is perfectly true—to work, car seats have to be the right size, have to be correctly installed, and have to be used whenever the baby or child is in the car. But what about the dangerous drivers out on the roads with you, the safety features that were or weren't built into the car, the speed limits and whether people around you do or don't respect them? What about the vigor with which alcohol-related driving offenses are prosecuted, or even the controls on emissions and their effects on air quality? Too often, the life-and-death responsibility lands squarely on the parent.

Parents and pediatricians alike have come to believe that we have the power to keep children safe, if we make the right choices and take the right precautions. When a baby or a child dies, our response now is to ask why, what was not done that could have stopped the death. When I hear a story about a death with a pediatric practice element—like a baby sent home from the emergency room who died the next day—I ask first about possible errors: Did they do the right blood test? Did anybody record the vital signs, and was the pulse actually elevated? I am always looking for something in the story that I can at least tell myself I would have done differently.

This response is not only about blaming the parents—or the pediatrician—though that is certainly partly how we hear it. Parents who lose a baby to SIDS often undergo the further distress of being suspected of having murdered the child (since one of the alternative explanations to rule out in making the diagnosis of SIDS is inflicted injury). Parents whose only crime was letting the baby sleep on an "inappropriate sleep surface," such as a sofa, may one day stand trial for criminal negligence, if not homicide. Criminal prosecution has already been brought against parents who failed to put their baby in the car seat, as it has for parents who, without realizing it, left an infant to die in a hot car. And pediatricians do, of course, face lawsuits for missing diagnoses and failing to do tests that might have made all the difference.

Convincing ourselves that the bereaved parents are somehow at fault may help us tell ourselves that we are different from those parents, and therefore our own children are safe. I want to believe that I am different from the pediatrician who sent the dangerously sick child home. We need to believe fervently that the same scenario would never apply to our own child, our own patients, that there is a thick, dark line between the child who dies and the child we care for.

I don't ever want to see the head injuries that were so common before bike helmets, or the car crash disasters before car seats, let alone the resurgence of the vaccine-preventable diseases. But I think that there was probably some comfort for parents in the acceptance that do what you might, the world was not completely safe, and life and death were more than a little bit beyond your control. You could buy the best advice books and follow that advice (or, for that matter, not follow it), you could write to the government or to a women's magazine, you could (and mostly did) pray to your God or resort to lucky charms and spells, but even so, everyone knew that sometimes luck turned bad. That understanding did not make parents' grief any less real or severe. Mary Todd Lincoln, Varina Davis, Ralph Waldo Emerson, Charles Dickens, Charles Darwin, Gustav Mahler, W. E. B. Du Bois, Harriet Beecher Stowe—all of them felt the losses of their children every bit as acutely as parents would today. But perhaps the higher child mortality all around them helped them, at least in some cases, understand that it was not their fault, that they were not negligent parents, just terribly, tragically unlucky parents of unlucky children. What we may have lost is a sense that some children don't make it, that accidents happen, that tragedies can strike.

Generations of parents (and theatergoers) wept at the death of Little Eva in *Uncle Tom's Cabin*. If the scene reads to us now as far-fetched in its extreme mix of religiosity and sentimentalism, we can perhaps understand how desperately parents craved the narrative of a perfect child, too good for life on this earth, ascending to a welcoming heaven.

In most ways, parenthood today can be more joyful, less shadowed. Many fewer parents live with the grief of a child's loss; in fact, losing a child begins to be seen as the kind of black hole in a life that admits of no recovery. The kind of intense mourning that Mary Todd Lincoln was once criticized for comes to seem a rational and even expected response. In plays and movies and novels, the memory of a child's death becomes reason for madness, depression, the kind of explanatory trauma that is at the root of a ruined life, a family destroyed. Those parents who have lost a child often find themselves feeling marginalized and isolated.

And yet, this promise of safety, this assurance that you can look at your baby and expect to see the toddler turn into the child turn into the adolescent—and then outlive you—also connects to a new and pervasive anxiety. The security that parents came to know in the second half of the twentieth century also carries with it an anxious corollary: if all children can live to grow up, then it becomes the parent's fault if something goes wrong. And so parents are haunted by the fear of making a wrong decision, forgetting a precaution, or exposing a child to the risks that continue to haunt parental nightmares.

To have made the world—our world—as safe for children as possible places us under an obligation to extend that safety. The racial inequalities that still exist in the United States in infant mortality and in maternal mortality stand out sharply, as beyond that, do the global inequalities. There was a time when even great wealth, to the tune of Rockefeller millions (John D. was the first billionaire), could not buy a young child's safety. Now that moderate wealth and privilege can keep most children safer than any nineteenth-century millionaire could have imagined, there is no excuse not to look outside our own protected neighborhoods and think about extending that safety to children everywhere. We need to protect children as they grow, not only from car crashes but also from medical inequalities, from epidemic gun violence, from pollution and environmental toxins. Having kept our children medically safe, we have a moral obligation to find ways to protect all children around the world. Children's vulnerability once reached across populations and social classes; our triumphant goal should be to create a world in which child health and safety does the same.

Parenthood leaves us all vulnerable, no matter how carefully we care for our children. The world has become safer for children, but it is not completely safe. Bad things do happen, sometimes. Growing up is still—and will always be—about taking some chances, exploring, establishing independence, walking to school, crossing streets, learning to drive. The microbes that live around us and on us and in us can still surprise us, sometimes in terrifying ways. As we have watched the Covid-19 pandemic sweep the world, we have learned again the hard lesson that this new virus, like old infections, does more damage among the poor, among minorities, among immigrants and refugees, among people who are kept on the margins. Plagues and dangers can remind us of our common humanity and our common vulnerability, but they can also underscore the inequities which make even relative safety a privilege. Keeping our children safe matters tremendously— but what they will do with that safety is thrive and grow and go out into the not perfectly safe world, where they will have to find their way. Remembering that lost world where children used to die, I believe, should make us feel connected to the historical parents who loved and tended their children in more dangerous times, and to the parents nowadays who love and tend their children in more difficult and dangerous circumstances. Appreciating our good fortune—and our children—should help open us to the wider world. Understanding how far we have collectively come should encourage us to continue the project—by staying alert for hazards close to home but also by recognizing that making the world safer has to remain a collective human endeavor. We should be able to cherish and appreciate our luck, and to understand it as the product of effort and achievement, struggle and science, and we should look to extend it to all possible children and all possible parents.

You have to give them credit, the mothers and fathers of the not so very distant past. They risked their hearts, and they carried with them all their lives the memories of children loved and lost, of possibilities snuffed out and promises unfulfilled. In 1902, Mary Putnam Jacobi, that indomitable American woman who awed the academic doctors of Paris and championed women's health in the United States, gave a speech at the annual alumnae breakfast of her own public high school, "dedicated to the interests of better education for girls."[4] She took as her topic the birth of a first child to her own one surviving child, her daughter. "There are those among you who can remember a fearful day," she told her audience, "day above all days when Life and Death came to wrestle together under your roof. For a time, perhaps, you look almost reproachfully on the tiny brown creature—a mere scrap of life, infinitesimal in comparison with the life that has been risked for her. . . . But what marvellous days follow fast upon one another's heels, as the miraculous creature begins to unfold its hidden capacities, one by one!" And she went on, experienced mother and physician and observer that she was, to describe the dawning of consciousness in the new grandchild's eyes:

> To watch from day to day the progress towards conscious thought and volition; on such a day a smile, on another a gurgling laugh; then daily periods of cooing laughter as the baby begins every morning to greet a new epoch of felicity coming so opportunely after its bath of sleep. And how radiantly it emerges from that sleep! How rapidly it learns to test the validity of its fingers, their continuity with the rest of its body, even to the mouth—their prehensile capacity—the joy of grasping things when at last this is known to be possible!

She also looked back at the difficulties of the lives that she and the other women in the audience had lived: "So many dangers barely escaped, so many others unescapable; one may well ask whether it is worth while to launch another sentient being upon such a difficult and dangerous course, one whose misfortunes, moreover, will wring our heart strings, and seem to us more intolerable than our own. Fortunate the decision is not left to our timid forethought, but that the Force of Life sweeps away forebodings and brings us the grandchild whether we will or no. If you must take the bitter with the sweet it is also permitted to take the sweet with the bitter."[5]

Mary Putnam Jacobi died four years later, in 1906, the year George Newman published *Infant Mortality: A Social Problem*. She died on June 10, 1906, the anniversary of her son Ernst's death from diphtheria twenty-three years before. That child—like so many children of the past—would certainly not die today, and that represents a great collective medical and social achievement. It's a shift that has substantially changed the human balance, as well as the practice of parenting and pediatrics for all of us: a triumph of the sweet over the bitter.

Epilogue to the Paperback Edition

In July 2021, Dr. Rochelle Walensky, the director of the CDC, testified before a senate committee. In response to a question from a senator about whether children should eventually get Covid vaccines, Dr. Walensky said, "One thing I just want to note with the children is: I think we fall into this flawed thinking of saying that only 400 of these 600,000 deaths from Covid-19 have been in children. Children are not supposed to die, and so 400 is a huge amount. . . ."

The assorted victories that have allowed us, in the late twentieth and early twenty-first centuries, to feel that it should be possible to keep our children safe drew on science, medicine, and public health, on parent advocacy and public policy, on sanitation and vaccination. During the pandemic, we have watched all those same forces at work in this new context. Many respiratory diseases are harder on young children than on adults; Covid-19 has been different. It has caused much more severe disease, hospitalization, and death among adults than among children and infants. But lots of children have gotten sick; and some have needed intensive care, and hundreds have died. In addition, there are persistent uncertainties about the possible long-term effects of Covid in at least some percentage of the children who become infected. We have a new danger in the world, a new set of imperatives for parents, a new target for science and safety.

Children are not supposed to die. This book, under the title *A Good Time to Be Born*, was initially published in the fall of 2020, that difficult pandemic year. But most of the book was researched and written before the world had ever heard of Covid-19, and certainly before so many aspects of our lives had been touched and changed by humanity's encounter with a new virus. We are now living in a world that feels much less safe; we have been through lockdowns and isolation; we have grown accustomed to wearing masks and seeing our children masked; we have learned to worry in ways that most of us never had to before. I had written (before the pandemic) that we are the luckiest parents—and pediatricians—in history. And even while the current moment does not feel like a lucky time in any way to most of us, we still expect our children to grow up. All of them. Along with the director of the CDC, we even demand it. *Children are not supposed to die.* We are able to start from the assumption that every pediatric death should be preventable only because of the protection, the privilege, and yes, the luck, conferred upon us by medicine and public health over the course of the twentieth century. That is why, as Dr. Walensky said, 400 deaths is a "huge" number, an intolerable number.

I remember looking down at my own first baby when he was put into my arms after a rather protracted labor and feeling both the rush of relief and the rush of responsibility. Here he was, safe (if a little smeared with blood and vernix), and it was my job to take care of him and keep him safe. When his father and I looked down at him, there was love and joy (here he was!) and also certainly anxiety (he was so small and helpless! we were so inexperienced!). Did I look over at my mother—who had talked her way onto a sold-out budget flight from New Jersey to Boston when my labor began by explaining to everyone that her first grandchild was being born, and had stayed with us all through that long night of labor—and wonder what *she* had felt when I was first put into her arms, in 1958, or even, back beyond that, what *her* mother had felt, back in 1927? Did it occur to me that my grandmother, looking down at her baby, faced very different odds and very different dangers?

We need to recognize and celebrate the remarkable decline in infant and child mortality over the last centuries, culminating in the changes since the early twentieth century, between my grand-mother's era and our current moment. Yet even before the pandemic, the twenty-first century was being described as an era of anxious parenting. People who wrote about parents and children were worry-ing over terms like helicopter parenting, snowplow parenting, lawn-mower parenting, attachment parenting, and free-range parenting, along with older words like permissive, authoritarian, and authori-tative, not to mention "tiger parenting" and its opposite number, "ele-phant parenting." Whenever I wrote about parenting issues, readers commented with heavy disapproval about all the mistakes they had observed other parents making, whether by being too indulgent or by being too distracted, whether by pressuring children with heavy expectations or by coddling them and giving everyone a trophy. It seemed pretty clear that many parents were receiving a consistent message that everything they did was wrong and potentially damag-ing. Parents have come to feel, as greater pressure mounts, that each small decision may put a child's happiness, or health, or future suc-cess at risk. This has become the new normal of parenting.

The pandemic has made us all—children, parents, health-care workers—much more anxious than before about children's health and well-being. With parents juggling questions about school and extracurricular activities and masks and exposures, with colleges instituting testing and tracing protocols, with the twenty-four-hour news cycle endlessly debating vaccine mandates, booster shot sched-ules, and antibody levels, nothing feels normal anymore. Pediatri-cians practiced remotely during the initial lockdowns, when parents were afraid to bring their children into the clinic or the office, and we worried that infants were missing their immunizations. I have colleagues who were giving shots in parking lots so that babies didn't have to come into the office, and going out into neighborhoods in a mobile van, trying to reach the families who would not come to the hospital clinic. During the lockdowns, at least, comparatively few children got sore throats and colds; when schools reopened, pediatric offices needed to deal with coughs and runny noses, common symptoms that we used to take for granted, but which now evoke anxiety and uncertainty. Pediatric offices are testing children for Covid—along with other viruses—and advising families about who can go back to school or daycare, who can visit grandma.

Pediatricians also worried, just as parents worried, about what was being lost to children when they spent months in isolation, about the drawbacks of remote education, the social deprivation, the increases in screen time. We worried about pandemic weight gain, which has been widespread in children (as in adults), sometimes connected to stress and emotional eating (and again, all that screen time, instead of outdoor time and exercise). We worried about the increase in anxiety among children and adolescents, about the increase in suicidal thoughts and the pressure building on already strained mental health services.

Living through a pandemic has reminded us all how vulnerable we are physically—but also how vulnerable our societies are. Covid showed us over and over where the inequities were—in our communities, in our country, and in our world. We've seen systemic racism play out in the high infection rates and the high mortality rates in Black, Hispanic, and Indigenous people in the United States. We've witnessed the increased vulnerability of low-salaried "essential workers" who had to show up in person every day, compared to the relative safety of those who could work from home, and we've seen the different kinds of medical care provided to the rich and to the poor. Each one of the pandemic impacts that I cite above has been harder on communities of color, harder on the poor. Black children and Hispanic children have disproportionately high rates of serious Covid infections and of multisystem inflammatory syndrome following the infection. When it comes to remote schooling, poor children and non-white children are more likely to live in areas where Internet access is unreliable or unaffordable. And in many parts of the United States, private schools were able to continue offering at least some in-class instruction, even while large urban school systems went completely remote.

But living through the pandemic has also reminded us of the possibilities of scientific progress, and of the absolute importance that scientific progress be guided by careful attention to public health. We've watched the experts learn in real time, and we've watched them struggle to explain their messages, not always successfully. We've watched high-speed science play out on social media with preprints and analyses on Twitter. And we've lived through the scientific miracle of astonishingly rapid and astonishingly effective vaccine development; through stumbling rollouts which have angered those who wanted vaccines and couldn't get them; through misinformation and the politicization of vaccines that prevented the high rates of vaccination which could protect the whole population. The "epidemic of the unvaccinated" stage has left many health-care workers in despair, as they have found themselves unable to convince patients they care for to get vaccinated, or as they have found themselves working in ERs and ICUs with sick and dying unvaccinated patients. The complex vaccine story of 2021 continues—and even illuminates— the long history of vaccines that I have touched on in this book, starting with the early victories over smallpox in the eighteenth century and continuing on to twentieth-century campaigns against diphtheria, polio, and many other diseases. One of the social media memes that circulated during the pandemic was a cartoon by the artist dawnymock in which a small child asks her mother about the mark on her arm and is told it's a smallpox vaccine scar. "Why don't I have one?" the child asks. "Because it worked," her mother replies.

What seemed clear all through 2021 was that until it was possible to vaccinate all children, the best way to protect them was to vaccinate all adults. Watching adults refuse the vaccine has been profoundly painful, in part because of all those unvaccinated children. Pandemic diseases teach us over and over again how connected we are to our communities and to our whole world; we can only keep ourselves safe by keeping others safe. Vaccinating the world should be everyone's urgent project. Within every country and every community, children who are too young to be vaccinated have had to rely on the adults and adolescents around them to keep Covid-19 rates and risks down—and in many cases, we failed to keep our children safe, just as we failed to protect other vulnerable groups.

The child pictured on the cover of this edition is Rebecca Ansah Asamoah, a little girl in Ghana who in 1969 received the twenty-five millionth dose of the smallpox vaccine in the campaign to eradicate the disease. She reminds us that vaccines can eliminate huge slices of human suffering. Smallpox had been killing and disfiguring children and adults for millennia, but humans found an answer: they used a related but milder virus to turn on the immune system, so that someone who had not actually had the disease could have the same protection as someone who had had a full-blown case of smallpox and recovered.

The scientific elegance of vaccines must be accompanied by the public health boots-on-the-ground hard work of vaccination campaigns. Vaccine equity across the world is as important now in the Covid-19 pandemic as it was when humans triumphantly eradicated the smallpox virus in the 1970s. Vaccines have helped so many children survive and thrive, and the Covid vaccines will also protect the parents and grandparents of the world. Protecting children means protecting families, acknowledging and undoing systemic inequities, and building communities where children can thrive in the safer and more just world that they deserve. Children are not supposed to die, and we should remember and celebrate the many triumphs across the twentieth century that averted and prevented childhood deaths. It's a worthy and inspirational human project, to be continued and extended into the twenty-first century: children are supposed to thrive and learn and live to grow up.

Acknowledgments

O ver the course of writing this book, I enjoyed the extraordinary hospitality of residencies at Yaddo, MacDowell, and Hedgebrook, and I was grateful for the protected time, the inspirational atmosphere of places where so much good work gets done, and the creative company of other writers and artists. I was mindful of the ways the heritage of Yaddo spoke directly to the subject of this book, in that the decision to make the estate into an arts residency was the result of the deaths of all four children born to the Trask family. The larger-than-life portraits of Spencer and Christina, the son and daughter who died of diphtheria in 1888, reminded me of the thread of childhood death and parental grief woven through all of human history and vividly illustrated the truth that great family wealth and all the medical care it could buy offered no protection to children at the turn of the century.

I have been profoundly aware, as I worked on this book, that it draws from a very broad subject area. I am neither a historian nor an expert in any one of the fields I have tried to cover, from neonatology to diphtheria to the literature of child mortality, and I am grateful to the colleagues, intellectual role models of mine and true experts in different areas, who were willing to read pieces of the manuscript and help guide me so that I got the details right and, even more, so that I was true to the larger story. Richard Meckel, professor of American Studies at Brown University, is the author of *Save the Babies: American Public Health Reform and the Prevention of Infant Mortality, 1850–1929,* which profoundly influenced my thinking and writing on the subject; I strongly recommend the book to anyone interested in the history of pediatrics, infant mortality, or social welfare in the United States. Professor Meckel very kindly read my chapters on the U.S. movement to bring down infant mortality, and I appreciate his advice, as well as everything I learned from his book. Dr. Jeffrey Baker, a fellow pediatrician who is professor of pediatrics and history at Duke University, where he directs the Trent Center for Bioethics, Humanities, and History of Medicine, read the manuscript and offered valuable comments and direction, and I similarly recommend his book *The Machine in the Nursery: Incubator Technology and the Origins of Newborn Intensive Care* to everyone interested in the very remarkable history of neonatology. It's a rare treat to hear from someone who is both a practicing pediatrician and a trained historian, and I was grateful for his guidance. I am also grateful for the careful reading and helpful comments and questions of Dr. Hughes Evans, a good friend since medical school days, and another pediatrician—now on the faculty at Emory—who is also a historian of science. Historian David Oshinsky, who is a professor of history at NYU and directs the Division of Medical Humanities at our medical school, is the author of two books from which I learned an enormous amount, *Polio: An American Story* and *Bellevue: Three Centuries of Medicine and Mayhem at America's Most Storied Hospital*; these were enormously helpful to me in thinking about medical history, and serve as models of integrating medical humanities and social history. He was good enough to read my chapter on polio and tuberculosis and provided me with very helpful direction. Dr. Adam Ratner, the division chief of pediatric infectious diseases at NYU, read an early version of the manuscript, corrected many of my errors, and talked through with me a variety of important issues in history, medicine, and bacteriology. Dr. Benard Dreyer, the director of pediatrics at Bellevue, read the manuscript and offered valuable perspectives on pediatrics, history, and the intersections of poverty and racism with children's health.

Needless to say, any errors or misconceptions that remain in this book are my responsibility and mine alone.

I am grateful to the chair of pediatrics at NYU, Dr. Catherine Manno, for supporting me in the department as I pursued my own particular mix of pediatrics and writing. My clinical colleagues at that "most storied hospital," Bellevue, with whom I have seen patients and precepted pediatric residents, have discussed many of the issues in the book with me over the years, and I want to acknowledge the "Wednesday afternoon group" in particular: Dr. Arthur Fierman, Dr. Herb Lazarus, Dr. Lori Legano, and Dr. Chris Bandera, to whom I have so often brought clinical, historical, and narrative conundrums for consideration and review. I have also been grateful for conversations with Dr. Mary Jo Messito, Dr. Bill Borkowsky, Dr. Andra Fertig, Dr. Julia Chang-Lin, Dr. Alan Mendelsohn, Dr. Cindy Osman, Dr. Suzy Tomopoulos, and Dr. Leo Trasande. I owe a special gratitude to my colleagues at the *Bellevue Literary Review,* especially Dr. Danielle Ofri, Dr. Jerome Lowenstein, and Dr. Ruth Oratz, for their commitment to combining medical practice with literary endeavor.

Other colleagues at NYU have helped tremendously as I attempted to understand cross-disciplinary questions and problems. I thank Professor Arthur Caplan, whose understanding of ethics and of the value of different kinds of narrative is without peer. I have found a wonderful professional second home at NYU Journalism, in the Arthur L. Carter Institute, and I want to thank Professor Brooke Kroeger, who initially welcomed me there, and my colleagues, especially Professors Charles Seife, Pamela Newkirk, Ted Conover, Dan Fagin, Meredith Broussard, and Steve Solomon. I have learned so much from them about high standards of reporting, and about the importance of narrative and making sure that essential stories get told and get told accurately.

Andrea Rosenberg at the Journalism Institute took on the job of locating and researching the photos and images for this book, and brought to the job a keen detail-oriented intelligence, a strong sense of design, and an appetite for tracking down historical truths—and myths. Her research uncovered many fascinating twists to the stories I was telling, and helped me see the ways that marginalized groups can easily be "erased" from the historical record, as she found, in particular, that images offered on the Internet of heroic African American women are often not really tied to those individuals—as if they were interchangeable. Andrea's hard work and enthusiastic sleuthing has enriched the whole project.

My wonderful editor at the *New York Times,* Roberta Zeff, has always encouraged me to look at issues in historical perspective and has helped me become a better writer, although I still get "that" and "which" wrong every time, by her standards (and I will never abandon the serial comma). Tara Parker-Pope has given me the opportunity to address a wide variety of pediatric issues in the setting of a wide-ranging and creative section, and Toby Bilanow has always improved the clarity and rigor of my writing. At the *New England Journal of Medicine,* Debbie Malina has encouraged me to think about the many stories that grow out of clinical medicine.

I am grateful to Professor Jill Lepore at Harvard for discussing this project with me early in its development and encouraging me. At Vanderbilt, Professor Jonathan Metzl and Professor Arleen Tuchman welcomed me and discussed medical history and medical humanities.

My agent, Jill Kneerim, strongly believed in this project, and helped me shape it and think it through. At Norton, I have benefited from the careful editing and the high standards of Alane Mason.

Eileen Costello and I met in our third year of pediatric residency, at Boston Children's Hospital, and practiced together for years at Dorchester House, seeing patients every Monday evening and talking over the clinical puzzles; we continue to call each other up when patient problems are worrying us or when there are amazing and unexpected outcomes. Eileen is one of the best clinicians I have ever known, and her consistent enthusiasm for the joys and rewards of taking care of children always helps remind me of what really matters; her perspective has been tremendously valuable as I have gone digging through pediatric—and parental—history. Mitch Katz and I met in our first year of medical school, when we were two of four students dissecting a cadaver (and proving to ourselves and each other, if it needed proving, that surgery was not our destiny). His own work, first in California and now in New York City, is connected to much of the social and medical history touched on in this book, and it reminds me, every time we talk, that medical advances and scientific miracles are no use unless patients and families have access to care. Martha Gershun and I met in our first year of college and have remained friends and (perhaps to our own surprise) colleagues in a number of enterprises across the past four decades; she has encouraged this project and listened patiently to my doubts and confusions, while showing me by her own example the value of bravely taking on new topics and intellectual adventures.

Dr. Gerald Hass was my preceptor—that is to say, my supervisor—back at Boston Children's Hospital in the 1980s, when I was learning how to do pediatric primary care. Because I thought he was the best of all possible pediatricians, I asked him to take care of my own child—and he was therefore also our pediatrician—and the best of all possible pediatricians. Over the years, Gerry has been a teacher, a mentor, and a friend; he has also been willing to discuss some of the most complex and personal issues in pediatrics and to give me the benefit of his wisdom and his experience.

I want to acknowledge my family—in particular, to start by saying that my daughter, Josephine, should get credit for making this book happen. She is a spectacular writer, a fast and true editor, and she knows me perhaps too well, as can happen with mothers and daughters. At several points along the way, when I was either overwhelmed by the scope of the project or just unsure how to proceed, she offered stimulating and galvanizing (and sometimes blistering) commentary, usually pointing out (fairly) that she was only saying to me what I would say to her in similar circumstances. She edited the manuscript with fierce intelligence and superb efficiency, and she also provided the kind of extraordinarily efficient technical assistance around revising and formatting that I would never ever be able to provide anyone in similar circumstances. Josephine and her brother Anatol also did me the enormous favor of working through my references, checking obscure sources, and formatting what I had messed up. They sacrificed a good deal of time to this over a holiday visit, and Anatol even managed to give me the impression that as a budding historian, he considered it an interesting challenge to be tracking down obscure newspaper clippings on the Internet Archive's Wayback Machine. He also read an early draft of the manuscript and offered useful structural comments. I am beyond grateful to both of them. Again, needless to say, any possible errors or lapses in sourcing are completely my own fault, and probably would not surprise my children one bit. My son Orlando, who was finishing his training as a psychiatrist as I was involved in this project, has discussed the nuances of grief and mourning with me—and the changing ways we formulate what is and is not normal grief—and helped me sort out some of the complexities of looking back at human behavior in earlier centuries from our modern perspective.

Larry Wolff has lived with me—and with this project—for quite a number of years now. The book probably has its origins in a course we first taught together in 2013 at NYU Shanghai, for which we began talking about how our professional interests intersect, in order to put together a course on children and childhood, including his perspective as a historian and mine as a pediatrician. Teaching the class together has been a joy, and has also helped me think about taking care of children from many new points of view; I am grateful to Larry, and also to the amazing students we have taught in Shanghai, year after year, coming from NYU Abu Dhabi for their January term, who have questioned us and pushed us on these topics. Larry has tried to help me understand how a historian looks back on the children of the past, and on the changing understanding of childhood, and he has always been open to my own pediatric perspective. (But what did the rash actually *look* like?) He has encouraged this project, read different drafts and corrected historical misconceptions, and helped me think about the parents of the past, as we have continued our own ongoing parental adventure.

Notes

Introduction: The Waning of Child Mortality
and the New Expectations of Parenthood

1. Molly Ladd-Taylor, *Raising a Baby the Government Way: Mothers' Letters to the Children's Bureau, 1915–1932* (New Brunswick, NJ: Rutgers University Press, 1986), 116–17.
2. Ladd-Taylor, *Raising a Baby,* 2.
3. Ladd-Taylor, *Raising a Baby,* 118.
4. Ladd-Taylor, *Raising a Baby,* 120.
5. Ladd-Taylor, *Raising a Baby,* 124.
6. Ladd-Taylor, *Raising a Baby,* 124.
7. Nancy Schrom Dye and Daniel Blake Smith, "Mother Love and Infant Death, 1750–1920." *Journal of American History* 73, no. 2 (1986): 329–53, 352.
8. Samuel H. Preston and Michael R. Haines, *Fatal Years: Child Mortality in Late Nineteenth-Century America* (Princeton: Princeton University Press, 1991), 188.
9. Melanie Rehak, *Girl Sleuth: Nancy Drew and the Women Who Created Her* (Orlando: Houghton Mifflin Harcourt, 2005), 48–49.
10. Charles Dickens, *The Selected Letters of Charles Dickens,* ed. Jenny Hartley (Oxford: Oxford University Press, 2012), 230–31.
11. Institute of Medicine, *When Children Die: Improving Palliative and End-of-Life Care for Children and Their Families* (Washington, DC: National Academies Press, 2003), 1.
12. Institute of Medicine, *When Children Die,* 20.
13. Linda Villarosa, "Why America's Black Mothers and Babies Are in a Life-or-Death Crisis," *New York Times Magazine,* April 11, 2018.
14. Maria Trent, Danielle G. Dooley, Jacqueline Dougé, Section on Ado-

lescent Health, Council on Community Pediatrics and Committee on Adolescence, "The Impact of Racism on Child and Adolescent Health," *Pediatrics* 144, no. 2 (2019), https://doi.org/10.1542/peds .2019-1765. In this first policy statement on racism by the American Academy of Pediatrics, issued in 2019, the authors review a large body of evidence on the intersection of racism and children's growth, health, and development, considering the additional stresses on children's lives that result from exposure to racism, but also the literature on the health effects of differential treatment by the health care system for a wide range of medical, developmental, and mental health conditions.

15. Historian Peter Stearns writes that in the twentieth century, parents were dealing with "the unprecedented unacceptability of death or serious illness among children. . . . Always before . . . the understanding that some children would die, despite the best efforts of parents and doctors, had provided some cold comfort. Now this prop was withdrawn. . . . This valuation of children meant, for those few parents actually confronted with death, an almost unbearable sense of sorrow and guilt." From his *Anxious Parents: A History of Modern Childrearing in America* (New York: New York University Press, 2003), 31.

Chapter 1: Postmortem Poetry and Comfort Books

1. Henry Wadsworth Longfellow, *Poems and Other Writings,* ed. J. D. McClatchy (New York: Library of America, 2000), 135. Longfellow also noted in his journal two months after her death, "I miss very much my dear little Fanny. An inappeasable longing to see her comes over me at times." His wife, also named Fanny, wrote, "Every room, every object recalls her, and the house is desolation." From: Sylvia D. Hoffert, "'A Very Peculiar Sorrow': Attitudes Toward Infant Death in the Urban Northeast, 1800–1860," *American Quarterly* 39, no. 4 (Winter 1987): 601–16.

2. George Newman, *Infant Mortality: A Social Problem* (London: Methuen, 1906), 2–3 (italics in original).

3. Newman, *Infant Mortality,* v.

4. Newman, *Infant Mortality,* 177.

5. All ages were susceptible to smallpox, which covered the body in a dra-

matic pustular rash, and killed at least 30 percent of its victims, with even higher death rates among babies. Many people who survived were left badly scarred, and often blind—but the survivors became immune to smallpox. That led to the early antecedent of immunization, the idea of directly inoculating people with the smallpox virus itself, the *Variola* virus, taken from pustules. That effective but dangerous technique seems to have developed in several places around the world; it had been practiced in Africa and Asia, and was imported to Europe in the eighteenth century from the Ottoman Empire. In America, it was first practiced by Cotton Mather, in 1721 in Boston, after he learned about the practice from enslaved Africans. At the end of the eighteenth century, the English physician Edward Jenner developed a new and much safer technique, built on the observation that dairy maids who caught cowpox from the cows they milked were immune to smallpox. The word vaccination comes from the Latin name for the cowpox virus, *Vaccinia*, the virus that Jenner injected into eight-year-old James Phipps in 1796, in the first act of deliberate vaccination. By the middle of the nineteenth century, many countries, including England and many states in the United States, had compulsory vaccination programs.

6. Philippe Ariès, *Centuries of Childhood: A Social History of Family Life* (New York: Vintage, 1965). For counterarguments and opposing views—specifically challenging the arguments that Ariès puts forward about the changes in parent-child connections—see (among others) Linda A. Pollock, *Forgotten Children: Parent-Child Relations from 1500 to 1900* (Cambridge: Cambridge University Press, 1983), and Stephen Orme, *Medieval Children* (New Haven: Yale University Press, 2001).

7. Laurence Lerner, *Angels and Absences: Child Deaths in the Nineteenth Century* (Nashville: Vanderbilt University Press, 1997).

8. I.C., *A Handkercher for Parents Wet Eyes Vpon the Death of Children: A Consolatory Letter to a Friend* (EEBO Editions, ProQuest, 2010), 8 (italics in original).

9. I.C., *A Handkercher for Parents*, 20.

10. I.C., *A Handkercher for Parents*, 34.

11. I.C., *A Handkercher for Parents*, 61.

12. Hannah Newton, *The Sick Child in Early Modern England, 1580–1720* (Oxford: Oxford University Press, 2012).

13. Viktor Aldrin, "Parental Grief and Prayer in the Middle Ages: Religious

Coping in Swedish Miracle Stories," in *Cultures of Death and Dying in Medieval and Early Modern Europe,* ed. Mia Korpiola and Anu Lahtinen (Helsinki: Helsinki Collegium for Advanced Studies, 2015).

14. Elizabeth Clarke, "'A Heart Terrifying Sorrow': The Deaths of Children in Seventeenth-Century Women's Manuscript Journals," in *Representations of Childhood Death,* ed. Gillian Avery and Kimberley Reynolds (London: Palgrave Macmillan, 2000), 73.

15. Charlotte Brontë, *Jane Eyre* (1847; repr., London: Penguin Classics, 1996), 94–95.

16. Charles Dickens, *The Adventures of Oliver Twist* (1839; repr., New York: Holt, Rinehart and Winston, 1962), 122–23.

17. Lerner, *Angels and Absences,* 82.

18. I was brought up on this story, which was particularly vivid in my father's imagination, as an example of the transatlantic power of a good yarn. In my father's telling, the people on the shore would call out to the sailors, who would of course have read the story on the way over, "What's become of Little Nell?" He told the story so often and so vividly that I think I came to believe that he had invented it, and I was actually surprised, later on, to find that slightly different versions of it turn up in all the Dickens biographies. Fred Kaplan, for example, mentions "the American readers who waited in anxious anticipation on the docks of Boston and New York to receive the installment of *The Old Curiosity Shop* that might break their hearts with the news of Little Nell's death" (*Dickens: A Biography,* p. 124). And the introduction, by Malcolm Andrews, to my Penguin Classics edition of the novel says that the public reception of the chapters in which Nell dies "is now almost as notorious as the death itself. Crowds gathered on the quayside in New York awaiting the news of Nell's fate" (p. 27). The *Victorian Calendar* blog will tell you that "when English ships reached American ports, people stood on the dock shouting, 'Is Little Nell dead?'"

19. Jenny Hartley, afterword to *Reading and the Victorians,* ed. Matthew Bradley and Juliet John (Burlington, VT: Ashgate, 2015), 160.

20. "The deaths of Nell and Paul have been so much admired, loved, hated, despised that the terrain may remind us of a muddy field trampled by crowds; even of a battlefield, where fine apprehensions of landscape are difficult," according to A.O.J. Cockshut, "Children's Death in Dickens: A Chapter in the History of Taste," in *Representa-*

tions of Childhood Death, ed. Gillian Avery and Kimberley Reynolds (London: Palgrave Macmillan, 2000), 137.

21. Charles Dickens, *Dombey and Son* (1848; repr., London: Penguin Classics, 1985), 149.

22. *The Letters of Charles Dickens,* ed. Graham Storey, Kathleen Tillotson, and Nina Burgis, vol. 6, *1850–1852* (Oxford: Clarendon Press, 1965), 353.

23. Laurence Lerner, in *Angels and Absences: Child Deaths in the Nineteenth Century* (Nashville: Vanderbilt University Press, 1997), writes: "Dickens was read, as all Victorian novelists were read, overwhelmingly by the middle classes; and in his pages, no aristocratic children die. . . . Nell is poor, but she has come down in the world; culturally she quite obviously belongs to the middle class. . . . When it comes to the death of proletarian children pathos may not be the only ingredient: it can be supplemented, even replaced, by indignation" (121).

24. Natalie Angier ("The Debilitating Malady Called Boyhood," *New York Times,* July 24, 1994) invoked Tom and Huck and the likelihood that they would be medicated in a piece on the "pathologization" of what had once been regarded as normal red-blooded American boyhood, with all its classic concomitants: getting into fights, feeling bored in school, running away to find adventure.

25. Mark Twain, *Adventures of Huckleberry Finn* (1884; repr., North Chelmsford, MA: Courier Corporation, 2012), 76–77.

26. Mark Twain, *My Autobiography: "Chapters" from the North American Review* (North Chelmsford, MA: Courier Corporation, 2012), 68.

27. Mark Twain, *The Writings of Mark Twain: The 30,000 Bequest and Other Stories* (New York: P. F. Collier & Son, 1917), 312.

28. Nicholas Parsons, *The Joy of Bad Verse* (London: Collins, 1988), 247–48.

29. Julia A. Moore, *Mortal Refrains: The Complete Collected Poetry, Prose, and Songs of Julia A. Moore, the Sweet Singer of Michigan* (Ann Arbor: Michigan State University Press, 1998), 34.

30. Moore, *Mortal Refrains,* 105.

31. Mark Twain knew her work and didn't like it; "bad grammar and slovenly English," he said. The president of Yale, Timothy Dwight, wrote a scathing attack on Sigourney and her poetry after her death, complaining about her "poetical obituaries." On the New England Historical Society's website, her page is titled "Mrs. Sigourney, Hart-

ford's High Priestess of Bad Poetry," and the text begins, "During the first half of the 19th century, Mrs. Sigourney wrote such bad poetry upon a person's death that she was said to add a new terror to dying." "Mrs. Sigourney, Hartford's High Priestess of Bad Poetry," *New England Historical Society* (blog), June 12, 2015, http://www .newenglandhistoricalsociety.com/mrs-sigourney-hartfords-high -priestess-of-bad-poetry/.

32. Lydia Huntley Sigourney, *Letters to Mothers* (Hartford: Hudson & Skinner, 1838), 208–9 (italics in original).

33. In *Centuries of Solace: Expressions of Maternal Grief in Popular Literature* (Philadelphia: Temple University Press, 1992), Wendy Simonds and Barbara Katz Rothman survey women's magazines from the nineteenth and twentieth centuries, collecting and discussing a range of forms of what they term "consolation literature," ranging from memorial poetry to confession magazines, and arguing persuasively for the continuity of powerful themes of maternal grief.

Chapter 2: "Ma'am, Have You Ever Lost a Child?"

1. Sarah Mapps Douglass (Zillah), "A Mother's Love," in *The Portable Nineteenth-Century African American Women Writers*, ed. Hollis Robbins and Henry Louis Gates Jr. (New York: Penguin Books, 2017), 39. Douglass spoke publicly about the way the abolitionist cause had come to seem much closer and more urgent to her with the new punitive legislation after the Nat Turner rebellion, laws that threatened black people's safety even in the non-slave states; she said in a public address: "One short year ago, how different were my feelings on the subject of slavery! It is true, the wail of the captive sometimes came to my ear in the midst of my happiness, and caused my heart to bleed for his wrongs; but, alas! The impression was as evanescent as the early cloud and morning dew." From Marie Lindhorst, "Politics in a Box: Sarah Mapps Douglass and the Female Literary Association, 1831–1833," *Pennsylvania History* 65, no. 3 (1998): 265.

2. Richard A. Steckel, "A Dreadful Childhood: The Excess Mortality of American Slaves," *Social Science History* 10, no. 4 (1986): 427–65, https://doi.org/10.2307/1171026.

3. Daina Ramey Berry, *The Price for Their Pound of Flesh: The Value of the*

Enslaved, from Womb to Grave, in the Building of a Nation (Boston: Beacon Press, 2017), 46.

4. Marie Jenkins Schwartz, *Born in Bondage: Growing Up Enslaved in the Antebellum South* (Cambridge: Harvard University Press, 2009), 27.

5. In 2018, New York City removed the statue of Dr. J. Marion Sims from Central Park. Sims had developed techniques for repairing vesicovaginal fistulas, a serious complication of childbirth in which urine leaks into the vagina because of internal tears. He experimented by operating repeatedly, without anesthesia, on enslaved women, who could not refuse the procedures. He named three—Anarcha, Betsey, and Lucy—in his records. See "City Orders Sims Statue Removed From Central Park," *New York Times*, April 16, 2018; Sara Spettel and Mark Donald White, "The Portrayal of J. Marion Sims' Controversial Surgical Legacy," *Journal of Urology* 185 (June 2011): 2424–27; Harriet A. Washington, *Medical Apartheid: The Dark History of Medical Experimentation on Black Americans from Colonial Times to the Present* (New York: Anchor Books, 2007).

6. Thomas Affleck, *Steward of the Land: Selected Writings of Nineteenth-Century Horticulturist Thomas Affleck*, ed. Lake Douglas (Baton Rouge: LSU Press, 2014), 206.

7. Todd L. Savitt, *Medicine and Slavery: The Diseases and Health Care of Blacks in Antebellum Virginia* (Champaign: University of Illinois Press, 2002), 20–22.

8. Stephen C. Kenny, "'I can do the child no good': Dr. Sims and the Enslaved Infants of Montgomery, Alabama," *Social History of Medicine* 20, no. 2 (2007): 223–41.

9. Affleck, *Steward of the Land,* 206. "Dirt-eating is frequent amongst young negroes, and it always kills them, if not cured," he went on. "Those under the best care are liable to it."

10. Savitt, *Medicine and Slavery*, 124.

11. Michael P. Johnson, "Smothered Slave Infants: Were Slave Mothers at Fault?," *Journal of Southern History* 47, no. 4 (1981): 493–520, doi:10.2307/2207400. The idea of an enslaved mother killing her child to save that child from living in slavery was important in Toni Morrison's 1987 novel, *Beloved,* which was inspired by the case of Margaret Garner, who in 1856 was escaping from slavery with her family

when they were found by federal marshalls; she killed her two-year-old daughter rather than allowing her to be recaptured.

12. Schwartz, *Born in Bondage*, 71.

13. Steckel, "Women, Work, and Health Under Plantation Slavery in the United States," in Gaspar and Hine, *More Than Chattel*, 48.

14. Sojourner Truth, *Narrative of Sojourner Truth* (1850; repr., New York: Penguin Classics, 1998), 56. Truth writes that her informant "had seen this brute of a man, when the child was curled up under a chair, innocently amusing itself with a few sticks, drag it thence, that he might have the pleasure of tormenting it." It's worth noting that in Truth's narrative, after the child died, the slaveholder himself became sick, and the enslaved mother had her revenge: "She was very strong, and was therefore selected to support her master, as he sat up in bed, by putting her arms around, while she stood behind him. It was then that she did her best to wreak her vengeance on him. She would clutch his feeble frame in her iron grasp, as in a vice; and, when her mistress did not see, would give him a squeeze, a shake, and lifting him up, set him down again, as *hard as possible*. If his breathing betrayed too tight a grasp, and her mistress said, 'Be careful, don't hurt him, Soan!' her ever-ready answer was, 'Oh no, Missus, no,' in her most pleasant tone—and then, as soon as Missus's eyes and ears were engaged away, another grasp—another shake—another bounce" (57).

15. William Wells Brown, *"Clotel" & Other Writings* (New York: Library of America, 2014), 40.

16. Truth, *Narrative of Sojourner Truth*, 25.

17. Thomas H. Jones, *The Experience of Thomas H. Jones: Who Was a Slave for Forty-Three Years* (New Bedford: E. Anthony & Sons, 1885), 5–6.

18. Josiah Henson, *The Life of Josiah Henson, Formerly a Slave, Now an Inhabitant of Canada, as Narrated by Himself* (Boston: Arthur D. Phelps, 1849), 4.

19. Margaret Burnham, "An Impossible Marriage: Slave Law and Family Law," *Law and Inequality* 5 (1987): 202.

20. Truth, *Narrative of Sojourner Truth*, 11.

21. Mary V. Cook, "Women's Place in the Work of the Denomination," in *The Portable Nineteenth-Century African American Women Writers,* ed. Hollis Robbins and Henry Louis Gates (New York: Penguin Classics, 2017), 475.

22. Harriet Beecher Stowe, *The Annotated Uncle Tom's Cabin,* ed. Henry Louis Gates Jr. and Hollis Robbins (New York: W. W. Norton, 2007), 67–68.

23. Stowe, *The Annotated Uncle Tom's Cabin,* 88.

24. Stowe, *The Annotated Uncle Tom's Cabin,* 86.

25. Charles Edward Stowe and Lyman Beecher Stowe, *Harriet Beecher Stowe: The Story of Her Life* (Boston: Houghton Mifflin, 1911), 139. In 1850, after the passage of the Fugitive Slave Act, Stowe received a series of letters from her sister-in-law Mrs. Edward Beecher about the evils of the new law. Years later, that sister-in-law took full credit for suggesting the book: "I remember distinctly saying in one of them, 'Now, Hattie, if I could use a pen as you can, I would write something that would make this whole nation feel what an accursed thing slavery is.'" Charles Stowe describes his mother's reaction to the letter, as recounted by another family member: "Mrs. Stowe rose up from her chair, crushing the letter in her hand, and with an expression on her face that stamped itself on the mind of her child, said: 'I will write something. I will if I live.'"

26. Stowe, *The Annotated Uncle Tom's Cabin,* 92.

27. Stowe, *The Annotated Uncle Tom's Cabin,* 92.

28. Stowe, *The Annotated Uncle Tom's Cabin,* 96.

29. Stowe, *The Annotated Uncle Tom's Cabin,* 96.

30. Harriet Beecher Stowe, "Letter to Delia Bacon, July 1849," in the Papers of Delia Salter Bacon, Folger Shakespeare Library, Washington, DC, MS Y.c.2599 (305), 2–3.

31. Charles Edward Stowe, *The Life of Harriet Beecher Stowe, Compiled from Her Letters and Journals* (1890; repr., Echo Library, 2006), 100.

32. Stowe, *The Life of Harriet Beecher Stowe,* 63.

33. Stowe, *The Annotated Uncle Tom's Cabin,* 289.

34. Stowe, *The Annotated Uncle Tom's Cabin,* 306.

35. "Eva's death owes a good deal to Nell's," wrote Laurence Lerner in *Angels and Absences.* "Both are etherealized, never disfigured by suffering, and both end up lying beautiful in their deathbeds, surrounded by emblems of innocence and regeneration. . . . Both are angels before their time and have a premonition of their end" (140).

36. Lydia Huntley Sigourney, *Letters to Mothers* (Hudson & Skinner, 1838), 206. It is worth noting that Sigourney was also a staunch abolitionist

and corresponded with Thomas Jefferson about the importance of ending the evils of slavery.

37. Stowe, *The Annotated Uncle Tom's Cabin*, 467.

38. Drew Gilpin Faust, *This Republic of Suffering: Death and the American Civil War* (New York: Vintage, 2009), xii–xiii.

39. Andrew Cliff, Peter Haggett, and Matthew Smallman-Raynor, *Measles: An Historical Geography of a Major Human Viral Disease from Global Expansion to Local Retreat, 1840–1990* (Oxford: Blackwell, 1993), 101.

40. The soldier's mother theme is certainly not unique to the Civil War; there are many songs with similar titles from the First World War as well, including "A Mother's Prayer for Her Soldier Boy" and "My Brown-Eyed Soldier Boy: A Mother Song." Still, the Civil War was taking place at the height of nineteenth-century reverence about the maternal bond, and the many sentimental songs provoked a certain amount of irony in response. Drew Gilpin Faust, in *This Republic of Suffering,* mentions a Civil War–era satirist who strung together the titles of many sentimental "mother songs" to create a parody, "Mother on the Brain," to be sung to the tune of "The Bonnie Blue Flag": " 'It was my Mother's customs,' 'My gentle Mother dear'; / 'I was my Mother's darling,' for, I loved my lager beer. / 'Kiss me goodnight, Mother,' and bring me a Bourbon plain— / 'Mother dear, I feel I'm dying,' with Mother on the brain" (p. 194).

41. Eleanor Cecilia Donnelly, *Out of Sweet Solitude* (Philadelphia: J. B. Lippincott, 1873), 49.

42. Jean H. Baker, *Mary Todd Lincoln: A Biography* (New York: W. W. Norton, 2008), 125.

43. Ruth Painter Randall, *Mary Lincoln: Biography of a Marriage* (Boston: Little, Brown, 1953), 141. Randall, who in this 1953 biography was focused on the Lincoln marriage—as the subtitle suggests—commented, "In the end it was doubtless the wife's response to her husband's need of her, and his response to her need of him, and the need of Bobbie for both, that enabled them to pull themselves together and take up normal life again" (141). Jean H. Baker in her 2008 biography uses the phrase "Mary Lincoln's difficult mournings" to characterize this pattern, and comments, "If her grief was such in 1850, then a pattern was already established" (126).

44. Mary Lincoln's party on February 5, 1862, was intended to showcase the power and magnificence of the presidency and the presidential mansion; an expensive caterer provided a sumptuous buffet dinner, with lavish sugar sculptures, including one of Fort Sumter and another of a warship. The party was widely criticized for extravagance at a moment of wartime suffering for so many. Eleanor Cecilia Donnelly wrote another of her Civil War poems, "The Lady President's Ball," which was printed in the newspaper four days before Willie's death. It tells the story of the party from the point of view of a wounded Union soldier:

> What matter that I, poor private,
> Lie here on my narrow bed,
> With the fever scorching my vitals
> And dazing my hapless head?
> What matter that nurses are callous,
> And rations meagre and small,
> So long as the beau monde revel
> At the Lady President's Ball?

Mary Lincoln herself always insisted that she had actually wanted to cancel the entertainment, worried about her sick sons, but had been persuaded not to; she would say to a visitor that those who had urged her to hold the ball were now ridiculing her, adding, "I have had evil counselors!"

45. Katherine Helm, *The True Story of Mary, Wife of Lincoln; Containing the Recollections of Mary Lincoln's Sister Emilie (Mrs. Ben Hardin Helm), Extracts from Her War-Time Diary, Numerous Letters and Other Documents* (New York: Harper & Brothers, 1928), 196–97.

46. Elizabeth Keckley, *Behind the Scenes in the Lincoln White House: Memoirs of an African-American Seamstress* (1868; repr., New York: Feather Trail Press, 2012), 36.

47. Harold Holzer, "Untold Civil War Stories: The Death of Willie Lincoln," *Washington Post,* October 7, 2011.

48. "The Train Accident That Broke a President, Estranged His Wife & Killed His Son," Carl Anthony Online, May 15, 2015, https://carlanthonyonline.com/2015/05/15/the-train-accident-that-broke-a

-president-estranged-his-wife-killed-his-son/. And "Frightful Accident on the Boston and Maine Railroad: Narrow Escape of Gen. Pierce and His Wife—His Son Killed," *Boston Journal,* January 6, 1853. Collected by historian Carl Sferrazza Anthony.

49. "Inaugural Address of Franklin Pierce," The Avalon Project: Documents in Law, History and Diplomacy, https://avalon.law.yale .edu/19th_century/pierce.asp.

50. Joan Cashin, *First Lady of the Confederacy: Varina Davis's Civil War* (Cambridge, MA: Harvard University Press, 2006), 68.

51. Cashin, *First Lady of the Confederacy,* 147.

52. Baker, *Mary Todd Lincoln,* 307

53. Randall, *Mary Lincoln,* 424–25.

54. Douglas C. Ewbank, "History of Black Mortality and Health before 1940," *Milbank Quarterly* 65 (1987): 100–128, doi:10.2307/3349953.

Chapter 3: "We Might Rather Wonder That Any Survive"

1. S. Josephine Baker, *Fighting for Life* (1939; repr., New York: NYRB Classics, 2013), 49.

2. Baker, *Fighting for Life,* 50.

3. Across generations and political persuasions, I am reminded of a joke Barbara Bush liked to tell in her speeches, about how if the three wise men in the Christmas story had been three wise women, "they would have asked for directions, arrived on time, they would have helped deliver the baby, cleaned the stable, made a casserole, and brought practical gifts." From Pamela Kilian, *Barbara Bush: Matriarch of a Dynasty* (New York: Thomas Dunne, 2002), 219.

4. Baker, *Fighting for Life,* 50.

5. "Achievements in Public Health, 1900–1999: Healthier Mothers and Babies," *Morbidity and Mortality Weekly Report* 48, no. 38 (October 1, 1999): 849–58.

6. "Achievements in Public Health, 1900–1999."

7. Abigail Zuger, "Josephine Baker's *Fighting for Life* Still Thought-Provoking Decades Later," *New York Times,* October 28, 2013.

8. David Meredith Reese, *Report on Infant Mortality in Large Cities, the Sources of Its Increase, and Means for Its Diminution* (Philadelphia: T. K. and P. G. Collins, 1857), 6–7.

9. Viviana A. Zelizer, *Pricing the Priceless Child: The Changing Social Value of Children* (New York: Basic Books, 1985), 27.

10. Richard A. Meckel, *Save the Babies: American Public Health Reform and the Prevention of Infant Mortality, 1850–1929* (1990; repr., Rochester, NY: University of Rochester Press, 2015).

11. Meckel, *Save the Babies,* 16.

12. Reese, *Report on Infant Mortality,* 12.

13. Baker, *Fighting for Life,* 26.

14. Most of these schools would be closed down in the early twentieth century as part of the consolidation and standardization of medical education, which did not make it any friendlier to women; many of the remaining medical schools, after this consolidation, were reluctant to accept many—or any—female students.

15. Baker, *Fighting for Life,* 42.

16. Baker, *Fighting for Life,* 42–43.

17. Thomas E. Cone, *History of American Pediatrics,* (Boston: Little, Brown, 1979), 112.

18. Meckel, *Save the Babies,* 35.

19. U. D. Parashar et al., "Global Illness and Deaths Caused by Rotavirus Disease in Children," *Emerging Infectious Diseases Journal* 9, no. 5 (May 2003): 565–72.

20. Cone, *History of American Pediatrics,* 49.

21. Cone, *History of American Pediatrics,* 44. Rush is a complex figure in the history of medicine; he was prominent as a physician, as a revolutionary patriot and signer of the Declaration of Independence, and also as an abolitionist and antislavery activist. Because he believed that Black people were immune to yellow fever, during the Philadelphia yellow fever epidemic of 1793, he asked Richard Allen and Absalom Jones, the founders of the Free African Society, to enlist the Black population of the city to stay and help during the epidemic, and many of them suffered and died.

22. Cone, *History of American Pediatrics,* 107.

23. Rebecca Crumpler, *A Book of Medical Discourses in Two Parts* (Boston: Cashman, Keating, 1883), 76.

24. Koch, who learned how to grow bacteria on agar gel in petri dishes (named for his assistant Julius Richard Petri), discovered the bacterium responsible for tuberculosis, and also the very different bacterium that causes cholera. He formulated a famous set of "Koch's Postulates," still

memorized and discussed by medical students, conditions he thought
needed to be satisfied in order to claim that a particular microorganism caused a particular disease: first, it must be found in all cases of
the disease but not in healthy animals; second, it must be isolated
from a diseased host and grown in a pure culture; third, samples from
the culture must cause the disease when inoculated into a healthy susceptible host; and fourth, the microorganism that is then isolated from
that inoculated healthy host must be the same as the organism isolated
from the original diseased host. (These conditions have not turned
out to be true in all cases, as we have learned more about microbiology; there are diseases with healthy carriers, as there are organisms
that cannot be cultured or are not infectious without passing through
an intermediate host. But at the time, Koch's postulates marked an
important step forward in systematic epidemiological thinking—and
Pasteur, naturally, refused to acknowledge or use them.)

25. Cone, *History of American Pediatrics,* 142.

26. Samuel H. Preston and Michael R. Haines, *Fatal Years: Child Mortality
in Late Nineteenth-Century America* (Princeton: Princeton University
Press, 1991), 16.

27. Hannah Newton, *The Sick Child in Early Modern England, 1580–1720*
(Oxford: Oxford University Press, 2012).

28. Russell Viner, "Abraham Jacobi and the Origins of Scientific Pediatrics
in America," in *Formative Years: Children's Health in the United States,
1880–2000,* ed. Alexandra Minna Stern and Howard Markel (Ann
Arbor: University of Michigan Press, 2002), 23. Dr. Jacobi's actual
title at New York Medical College was "professor of infantile pathology
and therapeutics," a designation he chose himself to emphasize his
focus on understanding and treating the diseases of childhood from
a strictly scientific point of view; Viner points out that Jacobi himself
was the first to use the term "paediatrics" in English (from the Greek
words for "child," *paed,* and "doctor," *iatros*).

29. Colin Phoon, "The Origins of Pediatrics as a Clinical and Academic
Specialty in the United States," *Hektoen International,* Winter 2018.

30. Meckel, *Save the Babies,* 82.

31. Jean-Jacques Rousseau, *Emile* (1762; repr., North Chelmsford, MA:
Courier Corporation, 2013), 161.

32. An American Matron [Mary Palmer Tyler], *The Maternal Physician: A*

Treatise on the Nurture and Management of Infants, from the Birth Until Two Years Old; Being the Result of Sixteen Years' Experience in the Nursery (New York: Isaac Riley, 1811), 10. The author warned against the dangers of wet nursing, again using Roscoe's translation of Tansillo's lines:

> Not half a mother she, whose pride denies
> The streaming beverage to her infant's cries,
> Admits another in her rights to share,
> Or trusts its nurture to a stranger's care.

33. An American Matron, *The Maternal Physician,* 11–12.
34. Crumpler, *A Book of Medical Discourses,* 43–45.
35. An American Matron, *The Maternal Physician,* 35.
36. Baker, *Fighting for Life,* 126.
37. Cone, *History of American Pediatrics,* 74.
38. Preston and Haines, *Fatal Years,* 21.
39. Preston and Haines, *Fatal Years,* 23.
40. Cone, *History of American Pediatrics,* 137.
41. Ann Hulbert, *Raising America: Experts, Parents, and a Century of Advice About Children* (New York: Vintage, 2004), 46.
42. Rima D. Apple, *Mothers and Medicine: A Social History of Infant Feeding, 1890–1950* (Madison: University of Wisconsin Press, 1987), 66. Apple describes arguments among the doctors about how to feed babies, though many approved of the laboratory milk: "At the same time, however, many more practitioners, both opponents and proponents of the percentage method, were very dissatisfied with the milk laboratories. Some praised milk laboratories for demonstrating that good, clean milk could be produced commercially but claimed that it was this milk, not the formula, that made laboratory-modified milk so efficacious. Other physicians claimed that infants fed laboratory milk over a long period of time were not as healthy as those brought up on home-modified milk."
43. Meckel, *Save the Babies,* 58.
44. Cone, *History of American Pediatrics,* 141.
45. Meckel, *Save the Babies,* 52.
46. L. Emmett Holt, *The Care and Feeding of Children: A Catechism for the Use of Mothers and Children's Nurses,* 8th ed. (1894; repr., New York: D. Appleton, 1916), 48.
47. Meckel, *Save the Babies,* 106–7.

48. Baker, *Fighting for Life,* 56.

49. Baker, *Fighting for Life,* 58.

50. Baker, *Fighting for Life,* 60–61.

51. Baker, *Fighting for Life,* 58.

52. Cone, *History of American Pediatrics,* 144.

53. Meckel, *Save the Babies,* 78–79.

54. Meckel, *Save the Babies,* 89.

55. Baker, *Fighting for Life,* 129.

Chapter 4: "Each Has a Right to Live"

1. S. Josephine Baker, *Fighting for Life* (1939; repr., New York: NYRB Classics, 2013), 85.

2. Alice Hamilton, *Exploring the Dangerous Trades: The Autobiography of Alice Hamilton, M.D.* (Boston: Little, Brown, 1943), 69. Alice Hamilton is another doctor who deserves much more recognition. She would go on to found the specialty of industrial medicine, doing research on the hazards of many different jobs; she would also be the first female faculty member at Harvard Medical School (where she was not treated particularly well by the rest of the faculty). Her appointment, in 1919, was marked by a *New York Tribune* headline: "A Woman on Harvard Faculty—The Last Citadel Has Fallen—The Sex Has Come Into Its Own."

3. Baker, *Fighting for Life,* 86–87.

4. Baker, *Fighting for Life,* 83.

5. Richard A. Meckel, *Save the Babies: American Public Health Reform and the Prevention of Infant Mortality, 1850–1929* (1990; repr., Rochester, NY: University of Rochester Press, 2015), 139.

6. Meckel, *Save the Babies,* 80.

7. Meckel, *Save the Babies,* 101.

8. George Newman, *Infant Mortality: A Social Problem* (London: Methuen, 1906), vi.

9. Meckel, *Save the Babies,* 100.

10. Sociologist Viviana A. Zelizer, in her landmark book *Pricing the Priceless Child: The Changing Social Value of Children* (New York: Basic Books, 1985), describes the growth of the child insurance business around the turn of the century: "The surge of concern with the

proper burial of poor children in the late nineteenth century, which became the main sales appeal of the insurance industry, suggests that working-class parents adopted the middle-class cult of child mourning. . . . Insurance sold primarily as a modern mourning device; it 'bought' a dignified death for children" (131–32).

11. U.S. National Library of Medicine, "Dr. Helen Cordelia Putnam," Changing the Face of Medicine, accessed July 8, 2018, https://cfmedicine.nlm.nih.gov/physicians/biography_350.html.

12. Newman, *Infant Mortality,* 257 (italics in original). Discussed in Meckel, *Save the Babies,* 100.

13. Samuel H. Preston and Michael R. Haines, *Fatal Years: Child Mortality in Late Nineteenth-Century America* (Princeton: Princeton University Press, 1991), 35.

14. Baker, *Fighting for Life,* 143.

15. Anne Baber Kennedy, "J. H. Mason Knox, Jr.," *American Journal of Public Health* 89, no. 3 (March 1, 1999): 409–11.

16. Jean-Jacques Rousseau, *Emile* (1762; repr., North Chelmsford, MA: Courier Corporation, 2013), 16.

17. Charles Richmond Henderson, *Introduction to the Study of the Dependent, Defective, and Delinquent Classes, and of Their Social Treatment* (1893; repr., Boston: D. C. Heath, 1901), 347.

18. Henderson, *Introduction to the Study,* 178

19. Henderson, *Introduction to the Study,* 179–81.

20. Henderson, *Introduction to the Study,* 196.

21. Henderson, *Introduction to the Study,* 198–99.

22. Newman, *Infant Mortality,* 63.

23. Meckel, *Save the Babies,* 117.

24. Meckel, *Save the Babies,* 117–18.

25. Similar involuntary sterilization laws were adopted by the Nazis when they came to power in Germany; these served as initial steps toward their own version of "racial hygiene" and the mass killing of "undesirables." The association with Nazi ideology, together with the general failure of eugenic "science," brought the whole field into marked disrepute in the United States by the 1940s, with organizations and periodicals renaming themselves to get rid of the word "eugenics" and respectable scientists disavowing it as "pseudoscience." Senator Edward Kennedy held Senate hearings in 1973, looking into the

extent of the forced sterilizations and advising state-by-state repeal of the laws that had allowed them.

26. Newman, *Infant Mortality,* 89.

27. Miriam Cohen, *Julia Lathrop: Social Service and Progressive Government* (Boulder, CO: Routledge, 2017), 102.

28. Thomas E. Cone, *History of American Pediatrics* (Boston: Little, Brown, 1979), 156.

29. Preston and Haines, *Fatal Years,* 27.

30. Ernst Christopher Meyer, *Infant Mortality in New York City: A Study of the Results Accomplished by Infant-Life Saving Agencies, 1885–1929* (New York: Rockefeller Foundation, International Health Board, 1921), 46.

31. Meyer, *Infant Mortality,* 59.

32. Jacqueline H. Wolf, *Don't Kill Your Baby: Public Health and the Decline of Breastfeeding in the Nineteenth and Twentieth Centuries* (Columbus: Ohio State University Press, 2001), 125.

33. Meckel, *Save the Babies,* 125–27.

34. Clare Coss, ed., *Lillian D. Wald: Progressive Activist* (1989; repr., New York: Feminist Press at CUNY, 1993), 43–44.

35. John Spargo, *The Bitter Cry of the Children* (London: Macmillan, 1906), 38.

36. Spargo, *Bitter Cry,* 233.

37. Baker, *Fighting for Life,* 133–36.

38. Preston and Haines, *Fatal Years,* 25.

39. Mrs. Max West, *Infant Care,* 1st ed. (Washington, DC: Government Printing Office, 1914), 63. The pamphlet is available at https://www.mchlibrary.org/collections/chbu/3121-1914.PDF and is well summarized in Dorothy Bradbury, "Children's Bureau: Part I," published by the Virginia Commonwealth University's Social Welfare History Project; available from https://socialwelfare.library.vcu.edu/programs/child-welfarechild-labor/childrens-bureau-part-i-2/.

40. Molly Ladd-Taylor, *Raising a Baby the Government Way: Mothers' Letters to the Children's Bureau, 1915–1932* (New Brunswick, NJ: Rutgers University Press, 1986), 72.

41. Ladd-Taylor, *Raising a Baby,* 85.

42. Ladd-Taylor, *Raising a Baby,* 104–5.

43. West, *Infant Care,* 73.

44. West, *Infant Care,* 59, 62–63. Mothers are also warned against kiss-

ing their infants on the mouth and against the dangers of any kind of rough or upsetting "playing" with a baby (which, it is suggested, fathers in particular may have a tendency to do). This was only in accordance with the best pediatric advice of the time; the eminent pediatrician L. Emmett Holt, in his contemporary (and popular) 1894 book, *The Care and Feeding of Children: A Catechism for the Use of Mothers and Children's Nurses* (1894; repr., New York: D. Appleton, 1916), said clearly that "babies under six months old should never be played with; and the less of it at any time the better for the infant. . . . They are made nervous and irritable, sleep badly, and suffer from indigestion and in many other respects" (171–72).

45. Molly Ladd-Taylor, " 'Why Does Congress Wish Women and Children to Die?': The Rise and Fall of Public Maternal and Infant Health Care in the United States, 1921–1929," in *Women and Children First: International Materna land Infant Welfare, 1870–1945,* ed. Valerie Fildes, Lara Marks, and Hilary Marland (1992; repr., New York: Routledge, 2013): 121–32.

46. Carolyn M. Moehling and Melissa A. Thomasson, "Saving Babies: The Contribution of Sheppard-Towner to the Decline in Infant Mortality in the 1920s," Working Paper (National Bureau of Economic Research, April 2012), https://doi.org/10.3386/w17996.

47. Institute of Medicine, Board on Health Sciences Policy, Committee on Understanding and Eliminating Racial and Ethnic Disparities in Health Care, *Unequal Treatment: Confronting Racial and Ethnic Disparities in Health Care* (Washington, DC: National Academies Press, 2009), 105. Abraham Flexner wrote: "The practice of the Negro doctor will be limited to his own race, which in turn will be cared for better by good Negro physicians than poor white ones. . . . A well-taught Negro sanitarian will be immensely useful; an essentially untrained Negro wearing an M.D. degree is dangerous" (106).

48. Baker, *Fighting for Life,* 119–22.

49. Deborah A. Frank et al., "Infants and Young Children in Orphanages: One View from Pediatrics and Child Psychiatry," *Pediatrics* 97, no. 4 (April 1, 1996): 569–78.

50. Baker, *Fighting for Life,* 169–70.

51. Baker, *Fighting for Life,* 171–72. The evolution of the German organization formed in 1909 to combat infant mortality, the German Union

for the Protection of Infants, later renamed the Deutsche Vereinigung für Säuglingsschutz und Kinderschutz, to include children as well as infants, reflected the troubled history of Germany as the Nazis came to power, as recounted by the Institute of Medicine, Board on Health Sciences Policy, Committee on Understanding and Eliminating Racial Disparities in Health Care, *Unequal Treatment: Confronting Racial and Ethnic Disparities in Health Care* (Washington, DC: National Academies Press, 2009): "Before 1933 nearly 50% of all pediatricians in Germany were Jewish and many of them were very active in this field. . . . They were all forced out of their practices and the scientific societies, and many of them were cruelly persecuted or even killed." In 1934, the organization was merged into a Nazi organization for mothers and children. "Many of these pediatricians had been more or less involved in the registration and examination of disabled children, some even in the killings," according to Volker Roelcke, Sascha Topp, Etienne Lepicard, eds., *Silence, Scapegoats, Self-Reflection: The Shadow of Nazi Medical Crimes on Medicine and Bioethics* (Göttingen: V&R Unipress, 2014), 341.

52. Friederike Kind-Kovács, "The Great War, the Child's Body and the American Red Cross," *European Review of History: Revue européenne d'histoire* 23 (2016): 1–2, 33–62, DOI: 10.1080/13507486.2015.1121971.

53. Baker, *Fighting for Life,* 171–72.

54. Cone, *History of American Pediatrics,* 202.

55. Douglas C. Ewbank, "History of Black Mortality and Health before 1940," *Milbank Quarterly* 65 (1987): 100–128, doi:10.2307/3349953.

56. Baker, *Fighting for Life,* 252–53. Baker was writing of social and scientific responsibility; it is worth noting that related language, adding in a strongly religious note, was later used in a very different way to justify the supposed "right to life" of the unborn fetus, and deny any authority of science or medicine: "Every human being, even the child in the womb, has the right to life *directly* from God and not from his parents, not from any society or human authority. Therefore, there is no man, no human authority, no science, no 'indication' at all—whether it be medical, eugenic, social, economic, or moral—that may offer or give a valid judicial title for a *direct* deliberate disposal of an innocent human life." From Pope Pius XII, "Address to Midwives on the Nature of Their Profession," October 29, 1951, Papal Encyclicals Online, https://www.papalencyclicals.net/pius12/p12midwives.htm.

Chapter 5: "The Plague Among Children"

1. Pierre Bretonneau (Fidèle) et al., *Memoirs on Diphtheria: From the Writings of Bretonneau, Guersant, Trousseau, Bouchut, Empis and Daviot*, selected and translated by Robert Hunter Semple (London: New Sydenham Society, 1859), 179.

2. Noah Webster, *A Brief History of Epidemic and Pestilential Diseases: With the Principal Phenomena of the Physical World, Which Precede and Accompany Them, and Observations Deduced from the Facts Stated* (London: G. G. and J. Robinson and G. Woodfall, 1800), 233.

3. Thomas E. Cone, *History of American Pediatrics* (Boston: Little, Brown, 1979), 108–9.

4. Gregory L. Kearns et al., "Developmental Pharmacology: Drug Disposition, Action, and Therapy in Infants and Children," *New England Journal of Medicine* 349, no. 12 (September 18, 2003): 1157–67, https://doi.org/10.1056/NEJMra035092.

5. When Jacobi arrived in New York City—and before he was made a professor—he found his mission and his vocation working among the tenement-bound poor on the Lower East Side. In 1857, he was one of the doctors who founded the German Dispensary at 132 Canal Street, where medical care was provided to the urban poor, especially the German immigrant population.

6. Mary Putnam's storytelling skills and sense of joy in medicine as a young woman make it a pleasure to read her letters home and provide a very immediate sense of how she got along with her fellow students, as is clear in this one, from Paris, May 1867:

> I encounter frequently along the rue de Rivoli whole families of English girls, all dressed alike, all wearing the same expression, all meek, subdued, conventional as a pack of sheep. In the anatomical class is a young Englishman who is the centre of amusement for the whole class, who get a great deal of fun out of him, without in the least infringing upon politeness. He seems a good innocent youth too, but so daisy-like, sandy and English. I always imagine him on his return to London seated at his father's substantial mahogany table, surrounded by his four well educated sisters, and relating his terrific adventures

in Paris,—and how finally he will say, as he tries to eye a glass of port with the air of a connoisseur, "Oh, by the way, there was a woman in our class—Yes there was, 'pon my honor, and by Jove she always answered just as well as us fellows." This is a modest statement, as it would be difficult not to know ten times as much anatomy as the youth in question. Then how Louisa and Emily will exclaim, and Amelia will say she was sure *she* never could do such a thing, and the Mama will observe sternly "I should think not, my dear, highly improper," and sniff with all the virtue of a solid British Matron. As I look at this student every day, and as every time I look at him this imaginary scene rises in my mind, it has become as distinct as possible,—I can tell the color of the curtains, and the difference in the noses of Emily and Louisa,—their chins are certainly identical, and retreating. (Mary Putnam Jacobi, *Life and Letters of Mary Putnam Jacobi* [New York: G. P. Putnam's Sons, 1925], 140)

7. Jacobi, *Life and Letters of Mary Putnam Jacobi*, 286.
8. Jacobi, *Life and Letters of Mary Putnam Jacobi*, 302.
9. Jacobi, *Life and Letters of Mary Putnam Jacobi*, 318.
10. Jacobi, *Life and Letters of Mary Putnam Jacobi*, 319.
11. A. [Abraham] Jacobi, *A Treatise on Diphtheria* (New York: William Wood, 1880), 27.
12. Jacobi, *A Treatise on Diphtheria*, iv.
13. Jacobi, *A Treatise on Diphtheria*, 223–24.
14. Abraham Jacobi, *Collectanea Jacobi in Eight Volumes* (New York: Critic and Guide Company, 1909), 444.
15. Carla Bittel, *Mary Putnam Jacobi and the Politics of Medicine in Nineteenth-Century America* (Chapel Hill: University of North Carolina Press, 2009), 172.
16. Evelynn Maxine Hammonds, *Childhood's Deadly Scourge: The Campaign to Control Diphtheria in New York City, 1880–1930* (Baltimore: Johns Hopkins University Press, 1999), 52.
17. Hammonds, *Childhood's Deadly Scourge*, 92.
18. Hammonds, *Childhood's Deadly Scourge*, 76. The *Medical Record* continued: "We shall watch the experiment with great interest."

19. Hammonds, *Childhood's Deadly Scourge*. The book examines in detail the complexities of the New York campaign to control diphtheria, looking at the ways publicity was part of the campaign and at the social complexities of public health. Hammonds points out that "while cholera had brought about the establishment of New York City's bacteriological laboratory, it was diphtheria that established its importance to public health and medical practice" (84). She also argues that "in a city with a multiethnic population of varying degrees of literacy, what is notable is the concerted attempts to reach all ethnic groups" and that "the ultimate success of the antidiphtheria programs was critically dependent on their being perceived by physicians and the public as classless rather than class-conscious interventions" (224–25).

20. Howard Markel, "Long Ago Against Diphtheria, the Heroes Were Horses," *New York Times,* July 10, 2007.

21. Canadian Social Hygiene Council, "Diphtheria: A Popular Health Article," *Public Health Journal* 18, no. 12 (1927): 572–76, 574.

22. William Carlos Williams, *The Doctor Stories* (New York: New Directions, 1984), 59–60.

23. Enid Nemy and William McDonald, "Bess Myerson, New Yorker of Beauty, Wit, Service and Scandal, Dies at 90," *New York Times*, January 5, 2015.

24. Denise Gellene, "Sherwin B. Nuland, Author of *How We Die,* Is Dead at 83," *New York Times*, March 4, 2014.

25. Michael T. Kaufman, "Peter W. Rodino Dies at 96; Led House Inquiry on Nixon," *New York Times*, May 8, 2005.

26. John Richardson, "Picasso's Broken Vow," *New York Review of Books*, June 25, 2015.

27. W. E. B. Du Bois, *The Souls of Black Folk: Essays and Sketches* (1903; repr., New York: New American Library, 2012), 210.

28. Alyn Brodsky, *Grover Cleveland: A Study in Character* (New York: Macmillan, 2000), 427. Ruth Cleveland achieved a mild immortality in that the Curtiss Candy Company, which renamed its Kandy Kake candy bar the Baby Ruth bar in 1921, claimed to be naming the bar for the president's daughter, rather than for the baseball player (probably in order to avoid having to pay royalties to Babe Ruth, while taking advantage of his celebrity).

29. The notion of a fatal "kiss of death" transmitting diphtheria between

mother and child was also invoked—in the other direction—in the death of Queen Victoria's third child, Princess Alice, from diphtheria in 1878. Alice's husband (the Grand Duke of Hesse-Darmstadt) and four of their seven children had the disease; the youngest child died, and the suggestion was that one of the children had passed it to their mother.

30. Their fourth and last child died soon after birth, and so they were left without heirs. Larger-than-life-size portraits of Christina and Spencer Jr. hang in the music room, and the children are among the many ghosts who are sometimes seen on the property.

Chapter 6: "Most Dreaded of All the Diseases"

1. You may remember that *Little Women* starts at Christmas: "Christmas won't be Christmas without any presents," Jo complains, reflecting on their poverty. On Christmas morning the girls, at Marmee's suggestion, take their celebratory Christmas breakfast to feed the starving Hummel children: "I want to say one word before we sit down. Not far away from here lies a poor woman with a little newborn baby. Six children are huddled into one bed to keep from freezing, for they have no fire. There is nothing to eat over there, and the oldest boy came to tell me they were suffering hunger and cold. My girls, will you give them your breakfast as a Christmas present?" The girls do, and the Hummel children call them "angel children": "Die Engel-kinder!"

2. Louisa May Alcott, *Little Women* (1868–69; repr., New York: Penguin Classics Deluxe Edition, 2012), 168. Within the Hummel family, scarlet fever is going to kill another one of those children with sore throats, by the way; but the only mention is slipped into a paragraph later in the book, when Beth gets sick, about how much everyone misses seeing her: "Everyone missed Beth. The milkman, baker, grocer, and butcher inquired how she did, poor Mrs. Hummel came to beg pardon for her thoughtlessness, and to get a shroud for Minna, the neighbors sent all sorts of comforts and good wishes, and even those who knew her best, were surprised to find how many friends shy little Beth had made" (Alcott, *Little Women,* 174). So poor Mrs. Hummel has lost not only her nameless baby but also little Minna to the disease; it was a disease well known for killing more than one child in a family.

3. The youngest Alcott sister, May (Amy in *Little Women*), died at thirty-nine, seven weeks after giving birth to a daughter; the cause of death is usually given as meningitis. Louisa May Alcott's own death has sometimes been attributed to complications from the dangerous anti-infection therapy of her time. During the Civil War, she worked as a nurse, and she came down with typhoid in 1863. She was treated for it with mercury, which was part of many standard medications, such as the calomel that Benjamin Rush had suggested almost a century earlier as a treatment for scarlet fever; antibiotic therapy had not come far in the intervening period. Alcott herself believed that the mercury had poisoned her, causing a range of symptoms for the rest of her life, including rashes, severe headaches, and vertigo. Some researchers have suggested that the mercury may have induced an autoimmune condition like lupus. (See Norbert Hirschhorn and Ian Greaves. "Louisa May Alcott: Her Mysterious Illness," *Perspectives in Biology and Medicine* 50, no. 2 [Spring 2007]: 243–59.) She died of a stroke at the age of fifty-five, within two days of her father, Bronson Alcott, who died at the age of eighty-eight. Of the original family, the parents and the four daughters, the last one alive was the oldest sister, Anna Alcott Pratt, the model for Meg; Anna married a local Concord gentleman, John Pratt, with whom she had two sons. So in addition to the historical microbiology of the novel, the real Alcott family offers another reminder of the ways life for children and for adults was shaped by infectious diseases. Two daughters died of infection—one from a childhood disease that had also killed the children of friends and neighbors, the other from an infection possibly connected to childbirth—and the third daughter was badly damaged by a treatment given to her for infection.

4. "Emerson's Hyacinthine Boy," *American Literary Blog,* January 27, 2010, http://americanliteraryblog.blogspot.com/2010/01/emersons-hyacinthine-boy.html.

5. Ralph Waldo Emerson, "Threnody," 1904, in *The Complete Works of Ralph Waldo Emerson: Poems* (Ann Arbor: University of Michigan Library, 2006).

6. William A. Altemeier, "A Pediatrician's View: A Brief History of Group A Beta Hemolytic Strep," *Pediatric Annals* 27, no. 5 (May 1998): 264, 266–67.

7. This statement was made by Dr. Charles Creighton, born in 1847, a

crucial figure in the development of epidemiology in England, who, paradoxically, did not believe in the germ theory of disease as it developed, and opposed vaccination. The changing virulence of scarlet fever is discussed in Stanford T. Shulman, "The History of Pediatric Infectious Diseases," *Pediatric Research* 55 (January 2004): 163–76.

8. Thomas E. Cone, *History of American Pediatrics* (Boston: Little, Brown, 1979), 111.

9. Cone, *History of American Pediatrics,* 126.

10. A. R. Katz and D. M. Morens, "Severe Streptococcal Infections in Historical Perspective," *Clinical Infectious Diseases: An Official Publication of the Infectious Diseases Society of America* 14, no. 1 (January 1992): 298–307.

11. Charles Darwin, "To Emma Darwin, 21 April 1851," accessed through Cambridge University's online Darwin Correspondence Project.

12. Chloride of lime was the disinfectant Dr. Ignaz Semmelweis had placed at the entrance to the obstetrical ward in Vienna in 1847 to make the medical residents clean the deadly contaminants off their hands when they came from the autopsy room.

13. For a full—book-length—consideration of the life of Annie Darwin, and the role her life and death played in her father's scientific thinking, see Randal Keynes, *Annie's Box: Charles Darwin, His Daughter and Human Evolution* (London: Fourth Estate, 2001). Keynes looks at the ways that Annie's short life—and her death—shaped and colored her father's thinking about religion and about human nature.

14. Charles Darwin, letter to W. D. Fox, July 2, 1858, Darwin Correspondence Project.

15. J. D. Hooker, letter to Charles Darwin, September 16, 1864, Darwin Correspondence Project. Hooker went on to say to Darwin, "Your affection for your children has been a great example to me, & there is no other living soul with whom I can talk of the subject.—it would make my wife ill if I went on so to her."

16. A. N. Wilson, *Charles Darwin: Victorian Mythmaker* (New York: HarperCollins, 2017). Wilson goes on to quote Darwin writing, in turn, to Asa Grey, an important American botanist—and supporter—that "children are one's greatest happiness, but often & often a still greater misery."

17. Peter Revers, "'. . . The Heart-Wrenching Sound of Farewell': Mahler, Rückert, and the Kindertotenlieder," in *Mahler and His World,* ed. Karen Painter (Princeton: Princeton University Press,

2002), 174. Luise, his youngest, died at the age of three on December 31, 1833, and Ernst, age five, on the following January 16. The poems were written in a burst of activity over the first six months of 1834, but Rückert kept them private, and they were published only posthumously in 1872. Musicologist Peter Revers quotes Rückert's wife's account of Ernst's death: "Suddenly he became so weak that we—especially his father—thought he would pass away instantly. Once more I had to hear the sound, the heart-wrenching sound of farewell to this world. . . . But not yet. The suffering would continue for eight more days." Revers goes on to say, "Her account and especially Rückert's 428 poems on the death of children became singular, almost manic documents of the psychological endeavor to cope with such loss . . . a private, almost obsessive testimony to the experience of pain" (174).

18. Henry-Louis de La Grange, *Gustav Mahler: Vienna: The Years of Challenge (1897–1904)* (Oxford: Oxford University Press, 1995), 368.

19. Friedrich Rückert and Gustav Mahler, "Kindertotenlieder," LiederNet Archive, www.lieder.net.

20. Egon Gartenberg, *Mahler: The Man and His Music* (New York: G. Schirmer Books, 1978), 288.

21. La Grange, *Gustav Mahler: Vienna: The Years of Challenge,* 713.

22. Henry-Louis de La Grange, *Gustav Mahler: Vienna: Triumph and Disillusion (1904–1907)* (Oxford: Oxford University Press, 1999), 691.

23. La Grange, *Gustav Mahler: Vienna: Triumph and Disillusion,* 690.

24. La Grange, *Gustav Mahler: Vienna: The Years of Challenge,* 711.

25. La Grange, *Gustav Mahler: Vienna: Triumph and Disillusion,* 697.

26. Henry-Louis de La Grange, *Gustav Mahler: A New Life Cut Short (1907–1911)* (Oxford: Oxford University Press, 2008), 90.

27. Edward Kravitt, "Mahler's Dirges for His Death," *Musical Quarterly* 64, no. 3 (July 1978): 335.

28. Joseph Ferretti and Werner Köhler, "History of Streptococcal Research," in *Streptococcus pyogenes: Basic Biology to Clinical Manifestations,* ed. Joseph J. Ferretti, Dennis L. Stevens, and Vincent A. Fischetti (Oklahoma City: University of Oklahoma Health Sciences Center, 2016). Pasteur made this statement in Paris more than a decade after the Hungarian physician Ignaz Semmelweis had shown at the Vienna Lying-In Hospital that the mortality rates of women giving birth in the ward

attended by the doctors and medical students were much higher than in the ward attended by midwives—and put that bowl of chloride of lime (the same disinfectant used by Darwin to clean his daughter) in front of the obstetric ward and made the medical men wash their hands. The infection rate and the mortality came down, but his findings were not taken seriously by his colleagues, and practices did not change.

29. Edith was quite a character, and she attracted a good deal of attention. She and her husband had four other children, a son and three daughters; she built a lavish Italian villa, Villa Turicum, in Lake Forest, Illinois, and her splendid jewel collection included emeralds that had belonged to Catherine the Great. In 1913, she went to Zurich to be treated for depression by Carl Jung; she spent eight years in Europe and ended up training as a lay analyst herself and serving as a patron to both Jung and James Joyce, who was writing *Ulysses*. The relationship ended when she pushed him to go into analysis with Jung. Edith returned to divorce her husband so he could marry a famous Polish opera singer, and in 1923, after the discovery of the tomb of Tutankhamun, she claimed to be the reincarnation of his first wife.

30. Margery Williams, *The Velveteen Rabbit* (New York: Open Road Media, 2014).

31. See Peter G. English, *Rheumatic Fever in America and Britain: A Biological, Epidemiological, and Medical History* (Rutgers: Rutgers University Press, 1999).

32. Certain strains of strep have a particular propensity for causing kidney damage, in a process called acute post-streptococcal glomerulonephritis; it's an autoimmune disease in which the body produces antibodies that attack its own glomeruli, the little clusters of blood vessels where fluid is filtered out of the blood and into urine. One theory about the death of Mozart, whose body became suddenly swollen before his tragically early demise, is that the swelling represented the edema and fluid retention of acute kidney disease; there was a major increase in edema as a cause of death in Vienna at the time, and it has been speculated that this represented an epidemic of streptococcal disease, perhaps starting in the military hospital. (Richard H. C. Zegers, Andreas Weigl, and Andrew Steptoe, "The Death of Wolfgang Amadeus Mozart: An Epidemiologic Perspective," *Annals of Internal Medicine* 151, no. 4 (September 2009): 274–78, W96.

33. Alcott, *Little Women*, 396.

34. Robert E. Gilbert, *The Tormented President: Calvin Coolidge, Death, and Clinical Depression* (Westport, CT: Greenwood, 2003), 153.

35. Calvin Coolidge, *Autobiography of Calvin Coolidge* (New York: Cosmopolitan Book Corporation, 1929): 190. Coolidge also suggested that he felt responsible: "We do not know what might have happened to him under other circumstances, but if I had not been President he would not have raised a blister on his toe, which resulted in blood poisoning. . . . In his suffering he was asking me to make him well. I could not" (190).

36. Dr. Ehrlich used the German term *Zauberkugel*, drawn from a nineteenth-century German opera, *Der Freischütz*, by Carl Maria von Weber, which revolves around a marksmanship contest in which magic bullets that will kill whatever the marksman wishes play an important role. The phase was recognizable enough to be used in a 1940 film, *Dr. Ehrlich's Magic Bullet*. Edward G. Robinson played the scientist—though the standards of Hollywood censorship that prevailed at the time made it difficult to mention syphilis.

37. William Rosen, *Miracle Cure: The Creation of Antibiotics and the Birth of Modern Medicine* (New York: Viking, 2017), 58. See also Allan M. Brandt, *No Magic Bullet: A Social History of Venereal Disease in the United States Since 1880* (1985; rev. ed., Oxford: Oxford University Press, 1987).

38. Rosen, *Miracle Cure*, 65–68.

39. "Gerhard Domagk Biographical," on nobelprize.org, https://www.nobelprize.org/prizes/medicine/1939/domagk/biographical/.

40. "YOUNG ROOSEVELT SAVED BY NEW DRUG; Doctor Used Prontylin in Fight on Streptococcus Infection of the Throat. CONDITION ONCE SERIOUS: But Youth, in Boston Hospital, Gains Steadily—Fiancee, Reassured, Leaves Bedside," *New York Times*, December 17, 1936.

41. There was also a World War II story that Winston Churchill's life (and thereby the whole war effort) had been saved by penicillin when he came down with pneumonia. It grew into a widely circulated urban legend that Churchill had been saved from drowning as a boy by Alexander Fleming's father, and the grateful Churchill family had paid to send the rescuer's son through school; the boy then grew up to discover penicillin and save Churchill's life all over again. This was a beautiful story and completely fictitious, right down to the antibiotic; Churchill was actually treated with Prontosil for his pneumonia, and recovered.

42. A British sulfa formulation, May & Baker, or M&B, was used to treat Winston Churchill's pneumonia in 1943, and in a radio speech, Churchill reached for a wartime metaphor: "This admirable M&B, from which I did not suffer any inconvenience, was used at the earliest moment; and after a week's fever, the intruders were repulsed."

43. Sir Alexander Fleming, "Banquet Speech," NobelPrize.org, https://www.nobelprize.org/nobel_prizes/medicine/laureates/1945/fleming-speech.html.

44. As William Rosen reports in *Miracle Cure:* "Chain's ability to summon every pertinent reference in the scholarly literature of biology and chemistry without recourse to a library made him the 1930s equivalent of a laboratory connection to the Internet. A dozen different colleagues would later recall his ability not merely to quote page and volume from relevant journal articles, but to quote text verbatim, even citing where on the page the important passage would be found." Both Chain and Florey were highly ambitious and not necessarily easy to get along with, but Florey proved particularly brilliant at the ongoing tricky task of funding the research, using his contacts at Rockefeller. Salvarsan and then the sulfa drugs had been developed by large German pharmaceutical companies; this would be a story of academic and philanthropic funding, always a little tenuous, never quite enough. But Florey managed to keep the lights on, and Chain pushed for better equipment; his overspending by fifteen pounds on a lab refrigerator, he later wrote, "caused a terrific upheaval and Florey never forgot this incident and reminded me of it until I left the Institute" (Rosen, *Miracle Cure,* 105–8).

45. In pursuing this elusive compound, they were wildly underfunded, but they were able to take advantage of the mechanical abilities of another research scientist in their group, Norman Heatley, who had a great ability to cobble together lab equipment from spare parts. Heatley was also able to devise methods for growing penicillin in much greater quantities, and even stabilizing it, two problems that had baffled Fleming. (Heatley, by the way, was not on good terms with Chain because of an earlier dispute about credit on a scientific article; Chain, for his part, ended up deeply resentful of Florey. And they all minded Fleming getting so much credit.) It was Heatley who took the bedpans and who rigged up a homemade machine made from spare parts, to filter the drug.

46. Rosen, *Miracle Cure,* 127.

47. Charles Fletcher, "First Clinical Use of Penicillin," *British Medical Journal* 289 (December 22–29, 1984): 1721–23.

48. Rosen, *Miracle Cure,* 77.

49. Lawrence K. Altman, "Dr. R. C. Lancefield, Bacteriologist, Dies," *New York Times,* March 4, 1981.

50. Maclyn McCarty, "Rebecca Craighill Lancefield: January 5, 1895–March 3, 1981," in National Academy of Sciences, *Biographical Memoirs,* vol. 57 (Washington, DC: National Academy Press, 1987), 230, https://doi.org/10.17226/1000.

51. Rockefeller University, "Masterminding Bacterial Classification," http://centennial.rucares.org/index.php?page=Bacterial_Classification.

52. Rebecca Lancefield, "A Serological Differentiation of Human and Other Groups of Hemolytic Streptococci," *Journal of Experimental Medicine* 57, no. 4 (March 1933): 571–95, doi: 10.1084/jem.57.4.571.

53. Cone, *History of American Pediatrics,* 215.

54. Wallace E Herrell and Roger L. J. Kennedy, "Penicillin: Its Use in Pediatrics," *Journal of Pediatrics* 25, no. 6 (December 1944): 505–16, 505.

55. Herrell and Kennedy, "Penicillin," 508.

Chapter 7: "Strides of Modern Medical Science"

1. Stephen E. Mawdsley, "'Dancing on Eggs': Charles H. Bynum, Racial Politics, and the National Foundation for Infantile Paralysis, 1938–1954," *Bulletin of the History of Medicine* 84, no. 2 (2010): 217–47.

2. Tad's death, which was without question due to lung disease, is usually attributed to tuberculosis and its complications; some accounts give other possible diagnoses, such as pneumonia, and it may well have been due to both.

3. Gretchen Holbrook Gerzina, *Frances Hodgson Burnett* (London: Chatto and Windus, 2004), 146. Gerzina goes on to describe how Burnett "wandered Europe like a ghost, attired in black dress, crepe veil, and bonnet. She thought incessantly of Lionel's body lying in St. Germain Cemetery."

4. Thomas M. Daniel, "The History of Tuberculosis," *Respiratory Medicine* 100, no. 11 (2006): 1862–70.

5. John F. Murray, "A Century of Tuberculosis," *American Journal of Respiratory and Critical Care Medicine* 169, no. 11 (June 1, 2004): 1181–86, https://doi.org/10.1164/rccm.200402-140OE.

6. Samuel H. Preston and Michael R. Haines, *Fatal Years: Child Mortality in Late Nineteenth-Century America* (Princeton: Princeton University Press, 1991), 6.

7. Murray, "A Century of Tuberculosis."

8. Daniel, "The History of Tuberculosis."

9. Maud Hart Lovelace, *"Betsy Was a Junior" and "Betsy and Joe"* (New York: William Morrow Paperbacks, 2009), 71–72.

10. Helen Bynum, *Spitting Blood: The History of Tuberculosis* (Oxford: Oxford University Press, 2012), 150.

11. Jessie C. Sleet Scales, "A Successful Experiment," in *On Nursing: A Literary Celebration; An Anthology,* ed. Margretta M. Styles and Patricia Moccia (1901; repr., National League for Nursing, 1993), 168.

12. J. Margo Brooks Carthon, "Life and Death in Philadelphia's Black Belt: A Tale of an Urban Tuberculosis Campaign, 1900–1930," *Nursing History Review* 19 (2011): 29–52.

13. Edith M. Lincoln "Course and Prognosis of Tuberculosis in Children," *American Journal of Medicine* 9, no. 5 (November 1950): 623–32.

14. Peter F. Donald, "Edith Lincoln, an American Pioneer of Childhood Tuberculosis," *Pediatric Infectious Disease Journal* 32, no. 3 (March 2013): 241–45.

15. David Oshinsky, *Polio: An American Story* (New York: Oxford University Press, 2005), 18.

16. Oshinsky, *Polio: An American Story,* 22–23.

17. Anne K. Gross, *The Polio Journals: Lessons from My Mother* (Greenwood Village, CO: Diversity Matters Press, 2011), 27.

18. Gross, *The Polio Journals,* 27.

19. The controversy played out yet again when the FDR memorial was built in Washington, DC, with disability activists insisting that the wheelchair, which he so avoided displaying, should be enshrined in stone. If you visit the FDR National Historic Site at Hyde Park, New York, the docents will show you the various stratagems that were employed to allow FDR to get from room to room and present himself to visitors without making his dependence on the wheelchair obvious. Thus, again, the polio sequela that he

most wanted to hide has become front and center in the place that
marks his legacy.

20. Gross, *The Polio Journals,* 10.

21. Gross, *The Polio Journals,* 41.

22. Gross, *The Polio Journals,* 43.

23. Gross, *The Polio Journals,* 47.

24. Oshinsky *Polio: An American Story,* 101.

25. Marc Shell, *Polio and Its Aftermath: The Paralysis of Culture* (Cambridge, MA: Harvard University Press, 2005), 28.

26. Moses Grossman, MD, interview by Jean D. Lockhart, August 1, 1996, San Francisco, Oral History Project, Pediatric History Center, American Academy of Pediatrics, pp. 13–14.

27. Neither Salk nor Sabin won a Nobel Prize; the only Nobel given for polio research went to John Enders and his colleagues, for figuring out how to grow the virus in tissue cultures, which was seen as vitally important for the whole field of virology.

28. Lee Edson, "Out of Favor for 20 Years, the Salk Vaccine Makes a Comeback," *New York Times,* January 25, 1981.

29. Steve Sternberg, "Which Polio Vaccine Is Really Better?" *Washington Post,* July 25, 1995.

30. Sternberg, "Which Polio Vaccine." After the vaccine, he got a fever, then recovered, and then progressed to the kind of terrifying story that parents had, as a group, left far behind them: "Then David lost his ability to crawl. Soon, when his father would hoist him to his feet, the baby's knees would buckle and his legs fold under him."

31. Helen E. Jenkins et al., "Mortality in Children Diagnosed with Tuberculosis: A Systematic Review and Meta-analysis," *Lancet: Infectious Diseases* 17, no. 3 (2017): 285–95, doi.org/10.1016/S1473-3099(16)30474-1.

Chapter 8: The Incubator Show

1. Judith Walzer Leavitt, "Under the Shadow of Maternity: American Women's Responses to Death and Debility Fears in Nineteenth-Century Childbirth," *Feminist Studies* 12, no. 1 (Spring 1986): 129–54.

2. Judith Walzer Leavitt, *Brought to Bed: Childbearing in America, 1750–1950* (Oxford: Oxford University Press, 1986), 20–21.

3. Nina Martin, Emma Cillekens, and Alessandra Freitas, "Lost Mothers," ProPublica, July 17, 2017, https://www.propublica.org/article/lost-mothers-maternal-health-died-childbirth-pregnancy.

4. John Zahorsky, "The Worlds Fair: The Louisiana Purchase Exposition," in *From the Hills: An Autobiography of a Pediatrician* (St. Louis: Mosby, 1949). Excerpted in "Neonatology on the Web," http://www.neonatology.org/classics/zahorsky/zahorsky.bio.html.

5. Michael Obladen, "Social Birth: Rites of Passage for the Newborn," *Neonatology* 112, no. 4 (2017): 317–23.

6. Peter M. Dunn, "Aristotle (384–322 BC): Philosopher and Scientist of Ancient Greece," *Archives of Disease in Childhood: Fetal and Neonatal Edition*, 2006, vol. 91, F77. Later experts on delivery continued to expect high mortality in the newborn period, and sometimes beyond; Viner points out that in 1849, the eminent American physician Charles D. Meigs said in his treatise on obstetrics that "a child that is born does not surely belong to its parents until it has obtained its sixth year; it seems to me that such a child is but a loan." From Russell Viner, "Abraham Jacobi and the Origins of Scientific Pediatrics in America," in *Formative Years: Children's Health in the United States, 1880–2000,* ed. Alexandra Minna Stern and Howard Markel (Ann Arbor: University of Michigan Press, 2002), 29.

7. Jeffrey P. Baker, *The Machine in the Nursery: Incubator Technology and the Origins of Newborn Intensive Care* (Baltimore: Johns Hopkins University Press, 1996), 27.

8. Baker, *The Machine in the Nursery*, 30

9. Baker, *The Machine in the Nursery*, 324.

10. Baker, *The Machine in the Nursery*, 60.

11. Baker, *The Machine in the Nursery*, 72.

12. William A. Silverman, "Incubator-Baby Side Shows," *Pediatrics* 64 (1979): 127–41. In her 2018 book, *The Strange Case of Dr. Couney: How a Mysterious European Showman Saved Thousands of American Babies* (New York: Blue Rider Press, 2018), Dawn Raffel carefully reconstructs not only the world of the midway but also Dr. Silverman's quest to tease out the "strange case" of this remarkable character, and his career of sideshow exhibitions and neonatology. She concludes that "every estimate puts the number of children whose lives he saved at between 6,500 and 7,000" (223).

13. Claire Prentice, "The Man Who Ran a Carnival Attraction That Saved Thousands of Premature Babies Wasn't a Doctor at All," *Smithsonian*, August 19, 2016, https://www.smithsonianmag.com/history/man-who-pretended-be-doctor-ran-worlds-fair-attraction-saved-lives-thousands-premature-babies-180960200/.

14. Silverman, "Incubator-Baby Side Shows," 130.

15. Silverman, "Incubator-Baby Side Shows," 131.

16. Silverman, "Incubator-Baby Side Shows," 132.

17. John Zahorsky, "The Worlds Fair."

18. Silverman, "Incubator-Baby Side Shows," 136.

19. Silverman "Incubator-Baby Side Shows,"137.

20. William A. Silverman, MD, interview by Lawrence M. Gartner, June 10, 1997, Greenbrae, CA, Oral History Project, Pediatric History Center, American Academy of Pediatrics, p. 5.

21. William A. Silverman, "Overtreatment of Neonates: A Personal Retrospective," *Pediatrics* 90, no. 6 (1992): 971.

22. Silverman, "Overtreatment of Neonates," 971.

23. Silverman, "Overtreatment of Neonates," 972.

24. Michael Obladen, "History of Neonatal Resuscitation—Part 1: Artificial Ventilation," *Neonatology* 94 (2008): 144–49.

25. Selma H. Calmes, "Virginia Apgar, M.D.: At the Forefront of Obstetric Anesthesia," *American Society of Anesthesiologists Newsletter* 56, no. 10 (October 1992): 9–12, 11.

26. Virginia Apgar, "A Proposal for a New Method of Evaluation of the Newborn Infant," *Current Researches in Anesthesia and Analgesia* 32, no. 4 (July–August 1953): 260–67, 260.

27. L. S. James, "Fond Memories of Virginia Apgar," *Pediatrics* 55, no. 1 (January 1975): 1–4, 3.

28. Apgar, "A Proposal for a New Method," 262.

29. James, "Fond Memories," 2.

30. Betty Smith, *A Tree Grows in Brooklyn* (1943; repr., New York: Harper-Collins 2001), 439–40. Sissy goes on to ask the doctor if he's *sure* the baby will live, and the doctor says yes, "unless you let him fall out of a three-story window." At that point she covers the doctor's hands with kisses, "and Dr. Aaron Aaronstein was not embarrassed about her emotionalism the way a Gentile doctor would have been."

31. Michael Obladen, "History of Neonatal Resuscitation—Part 2: Oxygen and Other Drugs," *Neonatology* 95 (2009): 91–96.

32. William A. Silverman, "A Cautionary Tale About Supplemental Oxygen: The Albatross of Neonatal Medicine," *Pediatrics* 113 (February 2004): 394–96, 394.

33. Silverman, "A Cautionary Tale," 394.

34. Silverman, "A Cautionary Tale," 395.

35. Mildred T. Stahlman, "Newborn Intensive Care: Success or Failure?," *Journal of Pediatrics* 105, no. 1 (July 1984): 162–67, 163. https://doi.org/10.1016/S0022-3476(84)80386-8.

36. Brian A. Darlow and Shahid Husain, "Primary Prevention of ROP and the Oxygen Saturation Targeting Trials," *Seminars in Perinatology* 43, no. 6 (2019): 333–40.

37. John Lantos, "OHRP and Public Citizen Are Wrong About Neonatal Research on Oxygen Therapy," Bioethics Forum Essay, Hastings Center, 2013, https://www.thehastingscenter.org/ohrp-and-public-citizen-are-wrong-about-neonatal-research-on-oxygen-therapy/.

38. Lantos, "OHRP and Public Citizen Are Wrong."

39. Lantos, "OHRP and Public Citizen Are Wrong."

40. John Zahorsky, "The Worlds Fair."

41. Silverman, "Incubator-Baby Side Shows," 140.

42. Stahlman, "Newborn Intensive Care," 167.

43. Mary Ellen Avery, interview by Lawrence M. Gartner, April 4, 1998, Chicago, Oral History Project, Pediatric History Center, American Academy of Pediatrics, p. 91.

44. Emanuel Lewis, "Mourning by the Family After a Stillbirth or Neonatal Death," *Archives of Disease in Childhood* 54 (1979): 303–6.

Chapter 9: *"Something Children Always Have"*

1. Jerome K. Jerome, *The Idle Thoughts of an Idle Fellow* (Philadelphia: Henry Altemus, 1912), 73. Jerome goes on to say of love, pursuing the infection metaphor: "Also like the measles, we take it only once. One never need be afraid of catching it a second time. The man who has had it can go into the most dangerous places, and play the most fool-hardy tricks with perfect safety. . . . He can keep his head through the whirl of the ravishing waltz, and rest afterwards in a dark conser-

vatory, catching nothing more lasting than a cold. . . . No, we never sicken with love twice" (73–74).

2. Eugene O'Neill, *Long Day's Journey into Night* (1956; repr., New Haven: Yale University Press, 1989), 90.

3. Frank B. Gilbreth Jr. and Ernestine Gilbreth Carey, *Cheaper by the Dozen* (New York: Thomas Y. Crowell, 1948), 99.

4. Frank B. Gilbreth Jr., *Time Out for Happiness* (New York: Thomas Y. Crowell, 1970), 111.

5. Cornelia Otis Skinner and Emily Kimbrough, *Our Hearts Were Young and Gay* (New York: Dodd, Mead, 1942), 78. Interestingly, neither of the young women, and neither of the two young doctors with whom they have been flirting on the boat, worry much about whether she might be exposing anyone to a dangerous disease; Cornelia's plan is that after she gets safely to England, where her parents are waiting, "Mother would in due course write the captain that what we'd thought was a cold had turned into measles, so they could fumigate the cabin and prevent any further spread of the disease,—as if, the preceding evening, I hadn't already spread it in a manner capable of starting an all-high European epidemic" (71–72).

6. Margaret Mitchell, *Gone with the Wind* (1936; repr., New York: Avon, 1973), 135. "The colonel would have wired earlier, but Charles, thinking his illness a trifling one, did not wish to have his family worried. The unfortunate boy had not only been cheated of the love he thought he had won but also of his high hopes of honor and glory on the battlefield."

7. Andrew Cliff, Peter Haggett, and Matthew Smallman-Raynor, *Measles: An Historical Geography of a Major Human Viral Disease from Global Expansion to Local Retreat, 1840–1990* (Oxford: Blackwell, 1993), 107.

8. Cliff, Haggett, and Smallman-Raynor, *Measles*, 81.

9. Thomas E. Cone, *History of American Pediatrics* (Boston: Little, Brown, 1979), 115.

10. Benjamin Spock, *The Pocket Book of Baby and Child Care* (New York: Pocket Books, 1946), 392. Dr. Spock promises parents that the complications of measles, unlike the measles itself, can be treated with "modern drugs," by which he probably means the use of sulfa drugs to treat pneumonia; he also recommends the use of measles antiserum if a child is exposed at a very young age, to ward off the disease or make it milder.

11. Francis Home, *Medical Facts and Experiments* (London: A. Millar, 1759), 266.

12. Home, *Medical Facts*, 283–84.

13. Samuel Lawrence Katz, MD, PhD, interview by Jeffrey P. Baker, March 7, 2002, and June 13, 2002, Durham, NC, Oral History Project, Pediatric History Center, American Academy of Pediatrics, p. 17.

14. Katz interview, 20.

15. Nothing is more indicative of his parsimoniousness—or, frankly, more difficult to believe as a lab legend—than that he apparently returned his unspent grant money to the NIH every year. See Jeffrey P. Baker, "The First Measles Vaccine," *Pediatrics* 128, no. 3 (2011): 435–37.

16. Katz interview, 23.

17. Katz interview, 71.

18. Baker, "The First Measles Vaccine," 436.

19. Katz interview, 71.

20. Katz interview, 33. Baker also describes the trial Dr. Saul Krugman from NYU carried out at the Willowbrook State School for the Retarded on Staten Island—an institution that would later become the subject of exposés for harsh mistreatment of the institutionalized patients, and also for dubious experimentation without consent, because of other trials in which Krugman deliberately exposed inmates to hepatitis B. Baker comments on the vulnerability of institutionalized children to measles, pointing out that "eight unvaccinated children at Willowbrook *died* of measles during the course of Krugman's study, an outcome that highlighted just how devastating the illness could be among profoundly handicapped children in an institutional setting." From Jeffrey P. Baker, "Immunization and the American Way," *American Journal of Public Health* 90, no. 2 (February 2000): 199–207, 205.

21. Samuel L. Katz, David C. Morley, and Saul Krugman, "Attenuated Measles Vaccine in Nigerian Children," *American Journal of Diseases of Children* 103, no. 3 (1962): 402–5. Katz recalled that when they did go to Nigeria, he saw how serious measles could be in children who were undernourished, children who "got terrible measles, who desquamated, who developed staphylococcal abscesses, who had terrible gastroenteritis" (Katz interview, 35).

22. Elena Conis, "Measles: How Vaccines Changed the Way We Think About Disease, *Sydney Morning Herald,* February 23, 2015.

23. Margaret Sidney, *Five Little Peppers and How They Grew* (Boston: Lothrop, 1881), 65.

24. Sidney, *Five Little Peppers,* 99.

25. "Vaccination Against Measles," editorial, *Journal of the American Medical Association* 194, no. 11 (December 13, 1965): 185.

26. Jonathan D. Moreno with Will Schupmann, "Will 'Measles Parties' Return?," *HuffPost,* January 30, 2018.

27. Ann Landers, "Child Needs Some Help," *Madera Tribune* 73, no. 233 (August 16, 1965), https://cdnc.ucr.edu/cgi-bin/cdnc?a=d&d=MT19650416.2.84.

28. Elena Conis, *Vaccine Nation: America's Changing Relationship with Immunization* (Chicago: University of Chicago Press, 2015).

29. *Measles Eradication 1967,* supplement to *Morbidity and Mortality Weekly Report* 16, no. 9 (March 4, 1967).

30. "Selected Endorsements," in *Measles Eradication 1967,* supplement to *Morbidity and Mortality Weekly Report* 16, no. 9 (March 4, 1967).

31. "Presidential Announcement on Measles Eradication," *Measles Eradication 1967,* supplement to *Morbidity and Mortality Weekly Report* 16, no. 15 (April 15, 1967).

32. Joy Miller, "Kim Is Example: Measles Can Cause Retardation," AP article, *Free Lance–Star* (Fredericksburg, VA), May 9, 1967, 5.

33. National Association for Retarded Children, *Closing the Gaps* (New York: National Association for Retarded Children, 1966), 5, https://mn.gov/mnddc/parallels2/pdf/60s/66/66-CTG-NARC.pdf.

34. National Association for Retarded Children, *Closing the Gaps*, 4.

35. *Measles Eradication 1967,* supplement to *Morbidity and Mortality Weekly Report* 16, no. 9 (March 4, 1967), third page.

36. James Colgrove, *State of Immunity: The Politics of Vaccination in Twentieth-Century America* (Berkeley: University of California Press, 2006), 149.

37. CDC, "Measles History," February 5, 2018, https://www.cdc.gov/measles/about/history.html.

38. Jennifer B. Rosen et al., "Public Health Consequences of a 2013 Measles Outbreak in New York City," *JAMA Pediatrics 172,* no. 9 (September 2018): 811–17, https://doi.org/10.1001/jamapediatrics.2018.1024.

39. Tyler Pager, "'Monkey, Rat and Pig DNA': How Misinformation Is Driving the Measles Outbreak Among Ultra-Orthodox Jews," *New York Times,* April 9, 2019.

40. Roald Dahl, "Measles: A Dangerous Illness," 1986, http://www
.roalddahl.com/roald-dahl/timeline/1960s/november-1962.

41. Ray Bradbury, *The Martian Chronicles* (1950; repr., New York: Simon
& Schuster, 2012), 66–67.

42. Moses Grossman, MD, interview by Jean D. Lockhart, August 1, 1996,
San Francisco, Oral History Project, Pediatric History Center, American Academy of Pediatrics, p. 23.

43. Meredith Wadman, *The Vaccine Race: Science, Politics, and the Human
Costs of Defeating Disease* (New York: Viking, 2017), 343.

44. Brian Wimer, Jacquelyn L. Emm, and Deren Bader, "Chickenpox Party: Developing Natural Varicella Immunity," *Mothering* 122
(January–February 2004). The publication's slogan is now "The home
for inclusive family living."

45. "Over the next few years, popularity of the parties swelled, achieving
a cult-like following and considerable press, particularly in upper-
middle-class enclaves from coast to coast," the historian Elena Conis
writes in her history of vaccination, arguing that parents spoke
almost religiously about their desire to help the body generate natural immunity and heal itself. This was, she argues, part of a more
general turning toward environmentalism, as well as a sense that
vaccines were polluting the body, rather than, in fact, activating
those same natural defenses. Conis, *Vaccine Nation: America's Changing Relationship with Immunization* (Chicago: University of Chicago
Press, 2015), 155.

Chapter 10: "Safe to Sleep"

1. Benjamin Spock, *The Pocket Book of Baby and Child Care* (New York:
Pocket Books, 1946), 3.

2. Julia Grant, in *Raising Baby by the Book: The Education of American Mothers* (New Haven: Yale University Press, 1998), emphasized Spock's
psychoanalytic orientation but described him as "child-centered"
rather than "permissive," writing, "Parents were urged to tailor their
child-rearing strategies to the nature and needs of their children.
Spock implied that if mothers were sufficiently in tune with these,
they would find ways to secure compliance through cooperation and
manipulation rather than traditional authoritarian discipline" (222).

3. Spock, *The Pocket Book of Baby and Child Care*, 399.

4. Spock, *The Pocket Book of Baby and Child Care*, 346.

5. Spock, *The Pocket Book of Baby and Child Care*, 403.

6. Sydney A. Halpern, "Medicalization as Professional Process: Postwar Trends in Pediatrics," *Journal of Health and Social Behavior* 31 (March 1990): 28–42, 28.

7. I feel compelled to add—it's almost a reflex—that nowadays the pediatric recommendation is to avoid bed-sharing (or co-sleeping) with infants; there is good evidence that it increases the risk of sudden infant death syndrome (SIDS) or sudden unexplained infant death (SUID). The current AAP recommendations for safe sleep, which include a firm sleeping surface with no crib bumpers, pillows, blankets, or stuffed animals, do also specify that the baby should sleep in the parents' room—though in a separate crib or bassinet—for the first six months of life and, if possible, for the first year—see the discussion later in this chapter. So we continue to be afraid of taking the infant into the parents' bed, though for different reasons.

8. T. Berry Brazelton, MD, interview by Steven Maron, February 19, 1997, Cambridge, MA, Oral History Project, Pediatric History Center, American Academy of Pediatrics, p. 22.

9. Ann Hulbert, *Raising America: Experts, Parents, and a Century of Advice About Children* (New York: Alfred A. Knopf, 2003), 226.

10. Spock, *The Pocket Book of Baby and Child Care*, 31.

11. Institute of Medicine Committee on Nutritional Status on Pregnancy and Lactation, *Nutrition During Lactation* (Washington, DC: National Academies Press, 1991), https://www.ncbi.nlm.nih.gov/books/NBK235588/.

12. Mary McCarthy, *The Group* (1963; repr., New York: Avon Books, 1980), 261.

13. McCarthy, *The Group*, 237.

14. Jacqueline H. Wolf, *Don't Kill Your Baby: Public Health and the Decline of Breastfeeding in the Nineteenth and Twentieth Centuries* (Columbus: Ohio State University Press, 2001), 197.

15. Lee Vinsel, "Doctors Inventing Auto Safety," Lemelson Center for the Study of Invention and Innovation, Smithsonian National Museum of American History, August 2, 2013, http://invention.si.edu/doctors-inventing-auto-safety.

16. Bridgespan Group, "Car Seats and Child Passenger Safety," case study accompanying "Audacious Philanthropy: Lessons from 15 World-Changing Initiatives," *Harvard Business Review,* September–October 2017, https://www.bridgespan.org/bridgespan/Images/articles/15 -success-stories-of-audacious-philanthropy/audacious-philanthropy -car-seats-and-child-passenger-safety.pdf.

17. Robert S. Sanders and Bruce B. Dan, "Bless the Seats and the Children: The Physician and the Legislative Process," *JAMA* 252 (1984): 2613–14.

18. Nick Charles, "Anton's Law," *People,* August 20, 2001.

19. Charles, "Anton's Law."

20. Much of this chronology is drawn from the "Key Moments in Safe to Sleep History" web page on the National Institute of Child Health and Human Development website, https://www1.nichd.nih.gov/sts/ campaign/moments/Pages/1994-2003.aspx.

21. CDC, "Data and Statistics," Sudden Unexpected Infant Death and Sudden Infant Death Syndrome, accessed June 28, 2018, https://www .cdc.gov/sids/data.htm. It's important to understand that the terminology changes over time and that each of these deaths has to be investigated to determine whether there is a cause; a baby who dies of SIDS by definition has not died of any other cause that can be determined—thus, in 2016, about 3,600 babies died in the United States from all forms of what is now called "sudden unexpected infant death." Some 1,500 of those deaths were classified as SIDS; the others were classified either as unknown cause (1,200) or as accidental suffocation or strangulation in bed (900). The combined SUID rate fell from 1990 to 1999, because of the safe sleep campaign, but the "unknown cause" deaths have actually been increasing since 1998, as have rates for accidental strangulation and suffocation in bed—the total rate for all SUIDs was 154.6 deaths per 100,000 live births in 1990 and 91.4 in 2016.

22. Geoff Watts, "Robert Johns Haggerty," *Lancet* 391, no. 10133 (May 2018): 1892, https://doi.org/10.1016/S0140-6736(18)31006-7.

23. Committee on Psychosocial Aspects of Child and Family Health, "Pediatrics and the Psychosocial Aspects of Child and Family Health," *Pediatrics* 79 (1982): 12–27.

24. Committee on Psychosocial Aspects of Child and Family Health, "The

New Morbidity Revisited: A Renewed Commitment to the Psychosocial Aspects of Pediatric Care," *Pediatrics* 108 (2001): 1227–30.

25. Halpern, "Medicalization as Professional Process," 36.

26. Brazelton interview, 8.

27. Spock, *The Pocket Book of Baby and Child Care*, 2.

Conclusion: The Promise of Safety

1. Bridget Onders et al., "Pediatric Injuries Related to Window Blinds, Shades, and Cords," *Pediatrics* 141, no. 1 (January 2018): e20172359, https://doi.org/10.1542/peds.2017-2359.

2. Examples of these stories can be found on the websites of the U.S. Consumer Product Safety Division and Kids in Danger: https://www.cpsc.gov/Business--Manufacturing/Business-Education/Business-Guidance/Drawstrings-in-Childrens-Upper-Outerwear and https://kidsindanger.org/family-voices/savannah/.

3. Rachel Rabkin Peachman, "You May Be Using Your Child's Car Seat Incorrectly," *New York Times*, March 20, 2018.

4. Mary Putnam Jacobi, *Life and Letters of Mary Putnam Jacobi* (New York: G. P. Putnam's Sons, 1925), 45.

5. Jacobi, *Life and Letters of Mary Putnam Jacobi*, 338–40.

Further Reading

Although I mention maternal mortality, the book does not go into the history of childbirth in great detail; this is well explored in Judith Walzer Leavitt's *Brought to Bed: Childbearing in America, 1750–1950*. The sad story of puerperal fever, and the reluctance of doctors to understand their own role in transmitting it, is told in *The Tragedy of Childbed Fever*, by Irvine Loudon. The history of modern neonatology in all its technological and moral complexity is covered in Jeffrey P. Baker's *The Machine in the Nursery: Incubator Technology and the Origins of Newborn Intensive Care*, and Dawn Raffel goes over the peculiar history of the "incubator baby shows" and the man who made them happen in *The Strange Case of Dr. Couney: How a Mysterious European Showman Saved Thousands of American Babies*.

Going back into more distant history, Hannah Newton's *The Sick Child in Early Modern England, 1580–1720* offers a fascinating perspective on childhood illness and on parental emotions.

Laurence Lerner's *Angels and Absences: Child Deaths in the Nineteenth Century* is full of insight about the ways children's deaths figured in life and in art during that era, and offers much wisdom about the connections between medical reality and cultural representations. *Pricing the Priceless Child: The Changing Social Value of Children*, by Viviana A. Zelizer, is an essential work of sociology for thinking about modern childhood.

The experience of enslaved children in the United States is carefully documented in Marie Jenkins Schwartz's *Born in Bondage: Growing Up Enslaved in the Antebellum South*, and there is also a tremendous wealth of relevant information in Daina Ramey Berry's *The Price for Their Pound of Flesh: The Value of the Enslaved, from Womb to Grave, in the Building of a Nation*.

Richard A. Meckel's *Save the Babies: American Public Health Reform and the Prevention of Infant Mortality, 1850–1929* is the definitive book on recognizing and attempting to come to grips with the problem of babies dying in the United States, in full historical context. *When Germs Travel: Six Major Epidemics That Have Invaded America Since 1900 and the Fears They Have Unleashed*, by Howard Markel, analyzes the ways that infectious diseases—and fears about infectious diseases—intersected with the history of immigration in twentieth-century America.

Evelynn Maxine Hammonds's *Childhood's Deadly Scourge: The Campaign to Control Diphtheria in New York City, 1880–1930* covers the remarkable history of battling back this terrible disease, now almost forgotten. David M. Oshinsky's *Polio: An American Story* brilliantly recounts a more recent story of vaccination and victory. *The Vaccine Race: Science, Politics, and the Human Costs of Defeating Disease*, by Meredith Wadman, tells the larger story of vaccine development.

For those who'd like more detail on two of the doctors who play large roles in this book, I would suggest reading Josephine Baker's remarkable autobiography, *Fighting for Life*, and Carla Bittel's excellent book *Mary Putnam Jacobi and the Politics of Medicine in Nineteenth-Century America*, which provides excellent perspective on women in medicine.

Molly Ladd-Taylor's *Raising a Baby the Government Way: Mothers' Letters to the Children's Bureau, 1915–1932* allows us to hear the questions and concerns of mothers desperate to do things right. *The End of American Childhood: A History of Parenting from Life on the Frontier to the Managed Child*, by Paula S. Fass, looks with lucidity and perspective across two centuries of parents and children and how they interact. In *Perfect Motherhood: Science and Childrearing in America*, Rima D. Apple traces the intersection of scientific expertise and maternal practice with sense and sympathy. *Raising America: Experts, Parents, and a Century of Advice About Children*, by Ann Hulbert, offers another valuable perspective on childhood, on parents, and on the people who told parents how to keep children safe and healthy.

Apple, Rima D. *Perfect Motherhood: Science and Childrearing in America*. New Brunswick: Rutgers University Press, 2006.

Baker, Jeffrey P. *The Machine in the Nursery: Incubator Technology and the Origins of Newborn Intensive Care*. Baltimore: Johns Hopkins University Press, 1996.

Baker, Josephine. *Fighting for Life*. 1939. Reprint, New York: NYRB Classics, 2013.

Berry, Daina Ramey. *The Price for Their Pound of Flesh: The Value of the*

Enslaved, from Womb to Grave, in the Building of a Nation. Boston: Beacon, 2017.

Bittel, Carla. *Mary Putnam Jacobi and the Politics of Medicine in Nineteenth-Century America.* Chapel Hill: University of North Carolina Press, 2009.

Fass, Paula S. *The End of American Childhood: A History of Parenting from Life on the Frontier to the Managed Child.* Princeton: Princeton University Press, 2016.

Hammonds, Evelynn Maxine. *Childhood's Deadly Scourge: The Campaign to Control Diphtheria in New York City, 1880–1930.* Baltimore: Johns Hopkins University Press, 1999.

Hulbert, Ann. *Raising America: Experts, Parents, and a Century of Advice About Children.* New York: Vintage, 2004.

Ladd-Taylor, Molly. *Raising a Baby the Government Way: Mothers' Letters to the Children's Bureau, 1915–1932.* New Brunswick, NJ: Rutgers University Press, 1986.

Leavitt, Judith Walzer. *Brought to Bed: Childbearing in America, 1750–1950.* Oxford: Oxford University Press, 1986.

Lerner, Laurence. *Angels and Absences: Child Deaths in the Nineteenth Century.* Nashville: Vanderbilt University Press, 1997.

Loudon, Irvine. *The Tragedy of Childbed Fever.* Oxford: Oxford University Press, 2000.

Markel, Howard. *When Germs Travel: Six Major Epidemics That Have Invaded America Since 1900 and the Fears They Have Unleashed.* New York: Pantheon, 2004.

Meckel, Richard A. *Save the Babies: American Public Health Reform and the Prevention of Infant Mortality, 1850–1929.* 1990. Reprint, Rochester, NY: University of Rochester Press, 2015.

Newton, Hannah. *The Sick Child in Early Modern England, 1580–1720.* Oxford: Oxford University Press, 2012.

Oshinsky, David M. *Polio: An American Story.* New York: Oxford University Press, 2005.

Raffel, Dawn. *The Strange Case of Dr. Couney: How a Mysterious European Showman Saved Thousands of American Babies.* New York: Blue Rider, 2018.

Schwartz, Marie Jenkins. *Born in Bondage: Growing Up Enslaved in the Antebellum South*. Cambridge, MA: Harvard University Press, 2009.

Wadman, Meredith. *The Vaccine Race: Science, Politics, and the Human Costs of Defeating Disease*. New York: Viking, 2017.

Zelizer, Viviana A. *Pricing the Priceless Child: The Changing Social Value of Children*. New York: Basic Books, 1985.

Index

Pages in *italics* refer to figures. Pages followed by *n* refer to notes.